Cancer Vaccines

From Research to Clinical Practice

Cancer Vaccines

From Research to Clinical Practice

Edited by

Adrian Bot, MD, PhD
Chief Scientific Officer, Kite Pharma, Inc.,
Los Angeles, California, USA

Mihail Obrocea, MD
Head, Clinical Development–Oncology,
Abbott Biotherapeutics Corporation, Redwood City, California, USA

and

Francesco Marincola, MD
Chief, Infectious Disease and Immunogenetics Section,
Department of Transfusion Medicine, Clinical Center; Associate Director,
Trans-NIH Center for Human Immunology, National Institutes of Health;
Director, CC/CHI FOCIS Center of Excellence; President Elect,
Society for the Immunotherapy of Cancer; President Elect,
International Society for Translational Medicine, Bethesda, Maryland, USA

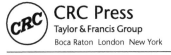

CRC Press
Taylor & Francis Group
Boca Raton London New York

CRC Press is an imprint of the
Taylor & Francis Group, an **informa** business

CRC Press
Taylor & Francis Group
6000 Broken Sound Parkway NW, Suite 300
Boca Raton, FL 33487-2742

First issued in paperback 2017

© 2011 by Taylor & Francis Group, LLC
CRC Press is an imprint of Taylor & Francis Group, an Informa business

No claim to original U.S. Government works

ISBN 13: 978-1-138-11260-5 (pbk)
ISBN 13: 978-1-84184-829-7 (hbk)

Visit the Taylor & Francis Web site at
http://www.taylorandfrancis.com

and the CRC Press Web site at
http://www.crcpress.com

A CIP record for this book is available from the British Library.

Library of Congress Cataloging-in-Publication Data

Cancer vaccines : from research to clinical practice / edited by Adrian Bot,
Mihail Obrocea, Francesco Marincola.
    p. ; cm.
  Includes bibliographical references and index.
    ISBN 978-1-84184-829-7 (hardback : alk. paper) 1. Cancer vaccines. I. Bot,
Adrian. II. Obrocea, Mihail. III. Marincola, Francesco M.
  [DNLM: 1. Cancer Vaccines--therapeutic use. QZ 266]
  RC271.I45C42 2011
  616.99'4061--dc23

                                                                    2011017121

For corporate sales please contact: CorporateBooksIHC@informa.com
For foreign rights please contact: RightsIHC@informa.com
For reprint permissions please contact: PermissionsIHC@informa.com

Typeset by Exeter Premedia Services Private Ltd., Chennai, India
Printed and bound in the United Kingdom.

The editors dedicate this book to all translational researchers, drug developers, clinicians, and entrepreneurs, who never gave up on the concept of active immunotherapy for cancer as a viable and promising option for oncology patients, for the present and future.

Contents

Contributors

Neeraj Agarwal Assistant Professor of Medicine, University of Utah, Huntsman Cancer Institute, Salt Lake City, UT, USA

Patrick A. Baeuerle Senior Vice President, Chief Scientific Officer, Micromet AG, Munich, Germany

Philip J. Bergman Chief Medical Officer, BrightHeart Veterinary Centers, Armonk, NY, USA; Adjunct Associate, Memorial Sloan-Kettering Cancer Center, New York, NY, USA

David Boczkowski Department of Surgery, Duke University Medical Center, Durham, NC, USA

Adrian Bot Chief Scientific Officer, Kite Pharma, Inc., Los Angeles, CA, USA

Vincent Brichard Vice President, Cancer Immunotherapeutics, GlaxoSmithKline Biologicals, Rixensart, Belgium

Cedrik M. Britten Johannes Gutenberg–University Mainz, Department of Internal Medicine III, Division of Experimental Oncology, and Ribological GmbH, Mainz, Germany

Mark Cameron Vaccine and Gene Therapy Institute, Port Saint Lucie, FL, USA

Glenda Canderan Vaccine and Gene Therapy Institute, Port Saint Lucie, FL, USA

Martin Cannon Department of Microbiology and Immunology, University of Arkansas for Medical Sciences, Little Rock, AR, USA

Denise L. Cecil Senior Fellow, Department of Medicine, University of Washington, Seattle, WA, USA

Maurizio Chiriva-Internati Director of Basic Research, Director of Translational Research, Division of Hematology/Oncology, Texas Tech University Health Sciences Center and Southwest Cancer Treatment and Research Center, Lubbock, TX, USA

Sarah Church Laboratory of Molecular and Tumor Immunology, Providence Cancer Center, Portland, OR, USA

Everardo Cobos Division of Hematology/Oncology, Texas Tech University Health Sciences Center and Southwest Cancer Treatment and Research Center, Lubbock, TX, USA

Brendan D. Curti Clinical Research, Robert W. Franz Cancer Research Center, Earle A. Chiles Research Institute, Providence Cancer Center, Providence Portland Medical Center, Portland, OR, USA

Pedro Miguel de Sousa Alves Senior Scientist, Cancer Immunotherapeutics, GlaxoSmithKline Biologicals, Rixensart, Belgium

David C. Diamond MannKind Corporation, Valencia, CA, USA

Mary L. Disis Professor, Division of Oncology, University of Washington; Seattle Cancer Care Alliance, Fred Hutchinson Cancer Research Center, Seattle, WA, USA

Benedetto Farsaci Laboratory of Tumor Immunology and Biology, Center for Cancer Research, National Cancer Institute, National Institutes of Health, Bethesda, MD, USA

Bernard A. Fox Chief, Laboratory of Molecular and Tumor Immunology, Earle A. Chiles Research Institute; Associate Professor, MMI and ENV and Biomolecular Systems; and Leader, Tumor Immunology Focus Group, Oregon Health & Science University Cancer Institute, Portland, OR, USA

Mark W. Frohlich EVP of Research & Development and Chief Medical Officer, Dendreon Corporation, Seattle, WA, USA

Cecile Gouttefangeas Institute for Cell Biology, Department of Immunology, University of Tübingen, Tübingen, Germany

Daniel R. Herendeen Senior Research Scientist, Department of Medicine, University of Washington, Seattle, WA, USA

William H. Hildebrand Department of Microbiology and Immunology, University of Oklahoma Health Sciences Center, Oklahoma City, OK, USA

James W. Hodge Laboratory of Tumor Immunology and Biology, Center for Cancer Research, National Cancer Institute, National Institutes of Health, Bethesda, MD, USA

Gregory E. Holt Assistant Professor, Department of Medicine, University of Miami, Miami, FL, USA

Axel Hoos Group Director, Immuno-oncology, Bristol-Myers Squibb, Wallingford, CT, USA

Hong-Ming Hu Cancer, Immunobiology, and Clinical Research, Robert W. Franz Cancer Research Center, Earle A. Chiles Research Institute, Providence Cancer Center, Providence Portland Medical Center, Portland, OR, USA

Leah Isakov Senior Director, Biostatistics, Data Management and Special Projects, Agenus, Inc., New York, NY, USA

Sylvia Janetzki ZellNet Consulting, Inc., Fort Lee, NJ, USA

Marjorie Jenkins Department of Internal Medicine, Department of Obstetrics and Gynecology, Division of Women's Health and Gender-Based Medicine, Laura W. Bush Institute for Women's Health, Amarillo, TX, USA

Shawn M. Jensen Laboratory of Molecular and Tumor Immunology, Providence Cancer Center, Portland, OR, USA

Bo Jin Professor of Medicine, Department of Gastroenterology, Naval General Hospital, Beijing, People's Republic of China

Michael Kalos Translational and Correlative Studies Laboratory, University of Pennsylvania School of Medicine, Philadelphia, PA, USA

W. Martin Kast Departments of Molecular Microbiology & Immunology, Obstetrics & Gynecology and Urology, Norris Comprehensive Cancer Center, University of Southern California, Los Angeles, CA, USA; and Cancer Center of Hawaii, University of Hawaii at Manao, Honolulu, HI, USA

Forrest Kievit Department of Materials Science and Engineering, University of Washington, Seattle, WA, USA

Anna Kwilas Laboratory of Tumor Immunology and Biology, Center for Cancer Research, National Cancer Institute, National Institutes of Health, Bethesda, MD, USA

Thomas M. Kundig Department of Dermatology, University Hospital Zurich, Zurich, Switzerland

Vy Phan-Lai Senior Fellow, Department of Medicine, University of Washington, Seattle, WA, USA

Jang-Won Lee Cedars-Sinai Medical Center, Maxine Dunitz Neurosurgical Institute, Los Angeles, CA, USA

Zhenhua Li Department of Neurosurgery, Cedars-Sinai Medical Center, Los Angeles, CA, USA

Francesco Marincola Chief, Infectious Disease and Immunogenetics Section (IDIS), Department of Transfusion Medicine, Clinical Center; Associate Director, Trans-NIH Center for Human Immunology, National Institutes of Health; Director, CC/CHI FOCIS Center of Excellence; President Elect, Society for the Immunotherapy of Cancer; President Elect, International Society for Translational Medicine, Bethesda, MD, USA

Sabrina Miles MannKind Corporation, Valencia, CA, USA

Leonardo Mirandola Department of Internal Medicine & Divisions of Hematology/Oncology, Texas Tech University Health Sciences Center and Southwest Cancer Treatment and Research Center, Lubbock, TX, USA

Debraj Mukherjee Cedars-Sinai Medical Center, Maxine Dunitz Neurosurgical Institute, Los Angeles, CA, USA

William J. Murphy Professor, Department of Dermatology, University of California, Davis, CA, USA

Cristina Musselli Senior Director, Preclinical Development and Translation Medicine, Agenus, Inc., New York, NY, USA

Smita Nair Associate Professor, Department of Surgery, Duke University Medical Center, Durham, NC, USA

Mihail Obrocea Head, Clinical Development–Oncology, Abbott Biotherapeutics Corporation, Redwood City, CA, USA

Christian Ottensmeier Department of Medical Oncology, Southampton University Hospitals, Southampton, UK

Christopher Paustian Division of Cellular and Gene Therapies, Center for Biologics Evaluation and Research, U.S. Food and Drug Administration, Bethesda, MD, USA; and Laboratory of Molecular and Tumor Immunology, Portland, OR, USA

Scott Pruitt Department of Surgery, Duke University Medical Center, Durham, NC, USA

Raj Puri   Division of Cellular and Gene Therapies, Office of Cellular, Tissue, and Gene Therapies, Center for Biologics Evaluation and Research, U.S. Food and Drug Administration, Bethesda, MD, USA

Sachin Puri   Laboratory of Molecular and Tumor Immunology, Providence Cancer Center, Portland, OR, USA

Zhiyong Qiu   Associate Director, Scientific Management and Project Lead, Oncology, MannKind Corporation, Valencia, CA, USA

Benno Rattel   Micromet, Inc., Bethesda, MD, USA, and Munich, Germany

Antoni Ribas   Professor of Medicine, Hematology-Oncology; Professor of Surgery, Surgical Oncology; Professor of Molecular and Medical Pharmacology; Director, Tumor Immunology Program, Jonsson Comprehensive Cancer Center (JCCC), University of California Los Angeles (UCLA), Los Angeles, CA, USA

Dar Rosario   MannKind Corporation, Valencia, CA, USA

Gail Sckisel   Department of Dermatology, UC Davis School of Medicine, Davis, CA, USA

John Schatzle   Vaccine and Gene Therapy Institute, Port Saint Lucie, FL, USA

Rafick-Pierre Sékaly   Professor and Associate Scientific Director (Basic Sciences and Strategy), CHUM, Université de Montréal; Scientific Director, National Immune-Monitoring Laboratory, Montreal, QC, Canada; and Co-Director and Scientific Director, Vaccine and Gene Therapy Institute, Port Saint Lucie, FL, USA

Kent A. Smith   Dockside Consultants and Properties, Ventura, CA, USA

Julia Tietze   Department of Dermatology, UC Davis School of Medicine, Davis, CA, USA

Chris Twitty   Laboratory of Molecular and Tumor Immunology, Providence Cancer Center, Portland, OR, USA

Walter J. Urba   Clinical Research, Robert W. Franz Cancer Research Center, Earle A. Chiles Research Institute, Providence Cancer Center, Providence Portland Medical Center, Portland, OR, USA

Johannes Urban   Department of Surgery, Duke University Medical Center, Durham, NC, USA

David Urdal   EVP and Chief Scientific Officer, Dendreon Corporation, Seattle, WA, USA

Sjoerd H. van der Burg   Department of Clinical Oncology, Leiden University Medical Center, Leiden, The Netherlands

Nicholas J. Vogelzang   Chair and Medical Director, Developmental Therapeutics and Member, GU Committee, U.S. Oncology Research, Las Vegas, NV, USA

Jon A. Weidanz   Center for Immunotherapeutic Research and Department of Biomedical Sciences, School of Pharmacy, Texas Tech University Health Sciences Center, Lubbock, and Receptor Logic, Inc., Abilene, TX, USA

Marij J. P. Welters Department of Clinical Oncology, Leiden University Medical Center, Leiden, The Netherlands

Kerry Wentworth VP Regulatory/Clinical/Quality, Agenus, Inc., New York, NY, USA

Peter Wilkinson Vaccine and Gene Therapy Institute, Port Saint Lucie, FL, USA

Jedd D. Wolchok Director, Immunotherapy Clinical Trials, Department of Medicine; Associate Director, Ludwig Center for Cancer Immunotherapy and Associate Attending Physician, Melanoma-Sarcoma Service, Memorial Sloan-Kettering Cancer Center, New York, NY, USA

Anthony E. T. Yeo Ingham Institute for Applied Medical Research, Liverpool, NSW, Australia

John S. Yu Director, Brain Tumor Center; Director, Surgical Neuro-Oncology, Department of Neurosurgery, Cedars-Sinai Medical Center, Los Angeles, CA, USA

Miqin Zhang Professor, Department of Materials Science and Engineering, University of Washington, Seattle, WA, USA

Foreword

The last few years witnessed considerable progress in the area of cancer vaccines, with the first active immunotherapies approved for oncologic indications in man and for veterinary use.

To herald the inception of a new era in cancer immunotherapy, Drs. Adrian Bot, Mihail Obrocea, and Francesco Marincola have edited this novel book entitled *Cancer Vaccines: From Research to Clinical Practice*. This book encompasses contributions by internationally recognized authorities from academia, industry, and regulatory agencies.

In addition to highlighting the path to approval of first licensed cancer vaccines, this book showcases some of the most important cancer vaccine programs currently in clinical development, discusses novel paradigms in support of development optimization, and presents new concepts that could lead to next generation immune interventions.

A wide range of readership will find this book informative, including opinion leaders, scientists and clinicians with interest in cancer immunotherapy, and more generally, immunotherapy and vaccination, drug developers, regulatory scientists, entrepreneurs in the life sciences arena, and oncology practitioners.

Samir N. Khleif, M.D.
Head, Cancer Vaccine Section
National Cancer Institute
National Institutes of Health
Bethesda, MD
USA

Preface

A perfection of means, and confusion of aims, seems to be our main problem.

Albert Einstein

The Editors and the Publisher are pleased to bring out a new edition entitled *Cancer Vaccines: From Research to Clinical Practice*, as we step into a new era in which active cancer immunotherapy ("cancer vaccines") is finally recognized as an integral component of the therapeutic arsenal against cancer. As these exciting and high-impact developments have opened the gates to new investigational vaccines and catalyzed interest more broadly in immunotherapy, this book emphasizes the promising technologies and strategies that are more likely to fulfill the aim of "cancer vaccines." Simply put, this is because they are increasingly based on lessons learned from the direct study of humans. We designed this book targeting a broad audience spanning academia, biotech and pharmaceutical researchers, and others who are interested in cancer immunotherapy for personal, not-for-profit, regulatory, or advocacy reasons.

As summarized by Albert Einstein's quote, the overarching message of the book is an invitation to all involved in this dynamic field of research to take a step back and "look at the forest," acknowledging the long-term goal of our efforts: effective control of cancer with cure still representing the ultimate aim. Perfecting the experimental aspects of the induction, control, and measurement of immunity should be ancillary to its clinical relevance linked to the impact on tumor progression, parameters that could be accurately assessed only by studying human reality. These two aspects—immunity and clinical impact—are complementary, feeding each other through a critical sequence of events to effectively unleash the potential of "cancer vaccines" and other immune interventions for cancer as shown below:

1. Define and focus on a limited number of immune interventions that yield measurable, consistent clinical responses.
2. Evaluate in depth the biological mechanisms that lead to objective responses in a clearly defined patient population.
3. Utilize this information to optimize and expedite development of current-generation vaccines, while designing superior strategies.

This means, effectively, transitioning from the current semi-empiric state of affairs in vaccine design and development to a systematic, rational process. As easy as it is to state, this goal may be difficult to achieve due to the limited frequency of objective clinical responses to cancer vaccines that reduce our opportunity to study them in clinical settings.

Why has progress been so slow? Perhaps it is time to question several paradigms (Box 1) that may need to be discarded, changed, or replaced by new ones. Perhaps, there is light at the end of the tunnel as several immune interventions are showing signs of statistically significant clinical benefit. This would offer a proof of concept and a fresh starting point for the sequence described above, breaking the cycle of "vaccine optimization" solely based on an immune response that we may only partially understand.

In addition to recently approved cancer vaccines—a landmark for modern medicine—and platform technologies in development, we take a look at several lessons learned from the past that uncovered hurdles, limitations, or opportunities for the development of current and future cancer vaccines and immune interventions in general.

We hope that this book provides more than a glance in this highly dynamic area of cancer research and conveys the overarching image that immune interventions carry the promise of viable and real long-term therapeutic benefit for the cancer patients. In addition, we hope to leave readers with several key questions (Box 2) that, along with others mentioned throughout the book, need to be kept in mind and eventually addressed, should we wish to fully realize the potential of cancer vaccines.

Box 1

Paradigms that need revisiting

Cancer vaccines are intrinsically applicable to minimal residual disease and would be largely ineffective in advanced, metastatic, measurable disease.

- *A range of immune interventions showed applicability to advanced cancers. What are the optimizations necessary to enable "vaccines" in such settings?*

Therapeutic vaccination is generally incompatible with chemotherapy or small-molecule targeted therapy.

- *With the advent of more selective targeted therapies, is there an opportunity for complementarity and even synergy between cancer vaccines and targeted therapies?*

Optimization of cancer vaccines is essentially guided by a quantitative enhancement of anti-vaccine immunity and supported through a narrow range of monitoring assays.

- *Standardization and harmonization of immune monitoring assays need to be preceded by critical review, selection, and optimization of immune assays based on joint mechanism-of-action and clinical response evaluation.*

Paradigm that needs wider acceptance

The timing and nature of clinical benefit afforded by immune interventions such as cancer vaccines are essentially different from that of other anti-cancer agents. RECIST criteria cannot be applied as such to guide treatment or quantify clinical responses.

- *Vaccine developers need to acknowledge that and optimize clinical trial designs accordingly. Regulatory agencies should negotiate new acceptable designs and surrogate endpoints with sponsors.*

Box 2

How do we amplify the clinical potency of cancer vaccines?

Could cancer vaccines, with cytostatic effects at best, be converted to cytoreductive treatments?

Is the concept of therapeutic vaccination applicable and clinically useful in advanced cancer?

How do we enhance the clinical predictability of cancer vaccines?

What are more reliable immune correlates of clinical response?

What are categories of targeted therapies that could facilitate or synergize with cancer vaccines or immune interventions in general?

Do cancer vaccines offer a means to control disease over long intervals?

What are the next generation target antigens that would facilitate the above?

What are the clinical settings with the best chance of technical success for cancer vaccines?

What are the clinical settings that, while offering a reasonable likelihood of technical success, would support an expedited development of cancer vaccines?

In light of this progress, opportunities, and challenges and rejoicing in the approval of the first therapeutic vaccines for cancer, Winston Churchill's famous quote comes naturally to mind: "Now this is not the end. It is not even the beginning of the end. But it is, perhaps, the end of the beginning."

Adrian Bot
Mihail Obrocea
Francesco Marincola

1 | Introduction: Cancer vaccines—mechanisms and a clinical overview

Antoni Ribas and Adrian Bot

INTRODUCTION

This book focuses on different avenues that have a common goal of fighting against cancer, resulting in safe and effective active immunotherapies (therapeutic "vaccines") against the disease, as described by recognized leaders in the field. Harnessing a cytotoxic T lymphocyte (CTL) response, or in general, an optimal immune response to cancer, can be achieved by several means that are not mutually exclusive: turning on immunity against specific tumor antigens using new generations of cancer vaccines, by nonspecifically inducing antitumor immune responses with the administration of immune stimulating cytokines or immune modulating antibodies, by manipulating the tumor microenviroment to enhance immune cell infiltration and function, or by creating large armies of tumor-specific T cells for adoptive cell transfer (ACT). Key to these efforts are first, to understand the roadblocks that are set against the generation of robust immune responses, operational within the tumor environment, and second, studying how the immune system is manipulated by the therapeutic interventions with the application of modern, informative, and relevant immune monitoring assays. The book aims to cover all these aspects from three points of view: (*i*) lessons learned from nearly two decades of efforts in developing various platform technologies culminating with the approval of first therapeutic vaccines for cancer; (*ii*) a perspective on several investigational agents in late- or early-stage development with companion immune monitoring and biomarker analysis technologies; (*iii*) a roadmap to future platform technologies that aim to integrate key advantages of diverse classes of immune intervention.

While the book is by no means a complete compendium of all cancer vaccine technologies studied or in development, it strives to cover the major platforms from a scientific and translational/developmental point of view. Since the realm of "cancer vaccines"—defined as approaches to generate in vivo safe and effective immune responses—is a subset of immune interventions, adoptive T-cell therapies, passive immunotherapy, and non-antigen-targeted immune interventions are outside the scope of the book. Nevertheless, lessons learned from such technologies in development have been extremely valuable for target antigen selection, design, and optimization of cancer vaccines as mono or combination therapies, hence will be referred to throughout the book.

The book has several sections: an introductory/scientific overview section, followed by a number of chapters dedicated to vaccines approved or in development for genitourinary (GU) tract cancers and non-GU cancers respectively, a section dedicated to innovative trial design and immune monitoring, one focused on emerging targets and platform technologies for active immunotherapy, and a last one dedicated to up and coming immune interventions that "borrow" features from vaccines along with other platform technologies. We are briefly setting up the stage for the rest of the book by discussing the major aspects of immune interventions in general—as they offer proof of principle that immunity could be harnessed against cancer—and of specific classes of vaccines, respectively.

NON-VACCINE IMMUNE INTERVENTIONS
Immune Stimulating Cytokines and Immunocytokines

Interleukin-2 (IL-2) and interferon alpha 2b (IFN- α2b) have been approved for the treatment of advanced melanoma and renal cell carcinoma, in the United States. They provide a low but reproducible clinical benefit that is hampered by the toxicities derived from high-dose systemic exposure (1,2). Other cytokines in clinical development for cancer treatment include IL-7, IL-12, IL-18, and IL-21, all of which have the recognized ability to activate cytotoxic

T cells (3). In an attempt to deliver the cytokines to the tumor sites and avoid systemic toxicities, immunocytokines have been developed (4). These are antibodies targeted to surface markers and are chemically or genetically linked to immune stimulating cytokines for intratumoral delivery (5).

Immune Modulating Antibodies

Co-stimulatory and co-inhibitory molecules are key players in the activation of a cellular immune response. They regulate the ability of antigen-specific T cells to expand, gain, and maintain effector functions. CTLA-4 plays a pivotal role in this interaction, dampening immune responses to self-antigens. A pioneering work by James Allison and colleagues provides evidence that murine tumors can respond to CTLA-4 blockade through monoclonal antibodies (6,7). In humans, the testing of the immunoglobulin G1 (IgG1), anti-CTLA-4 antibody ipilimumab (previously MDX-010), and the IgG2 antibody tremelimumab (previously CP-675,206) resulted in low (5–15%) objective tumor responses, but most are durable in terms of years (8). These benefits are achieved at the cost of clinically significant inflammatory and autoimmune toxicities (grade 3 or higher) in approximately 20% of patients. In a phase III clinical trial, ipilimumab was more effective than a peptide vaccine (9) and improved the overall survival of patients with previously treated metastatic melanoma, leading to the landmark approval of Yervoy® (Bristol-Myers-Squibb, New York, NY, USA) for the treatment of metastatic melanoma on March 25, 2011 (10).

The programmed-death 1 (PD-1) receptor is another negative immune-regulatory receptor expressed by activated lymphocytes. PD-1 blocking antibodies like MDX-1106/ONO-4538, and PD-1 ligand blocking antibodies like MDX-1105, are in clinical development with encouraging early evidence of anti-tumor activity (11). CD40 is a key molecule required for the generation of fully functional CD8+ CTL because it bypasses the need for CD4+ T helper cells (12). An activating antibody to CD40 (CP-870,893) is also in clinical development and has shown a single-agent activity in patients with metastatic melanoma in phase I trials (13). Also, it showed very encouraging results in a phase I trial, with objective responses in pancreatic carcinoma as adjunctive therapy to gemcitabine (14). This key study showed that an effective immune intervention does not necessarily need to act through antigen-specific T cells or even T cells in general, as long as it modifies the tumor environment, thereby enabling the activity of other immune effectors such as macrophages. This and other similar findings bring support to the paradigm proposed by Drs. Sckisel, Tietze, and Murphy in their chapter, emphasizing the pivotal importance of non-vaccine-specific immune effectors, generated independently or as a consequence of vaccination, for effectively harnessing cancer.

The tumor-necrosis factor (TNF) superfamily receptor CD137 (4-1BB) provides co-stimulatory signals to T cells. Activating antibodies to CD137 cause a regression of tumors in animal models (15). An activating antibody to CD137, BMS-663513, is under clinical development (16). OX40 is another member of the TNFR family (TNFR-4), which is expressed on activated, but not on resting, CD4 cells. Its primary role is to act as a late co-stimulatory receptor for CD4+ T cells (17). A fully murine antibody that activates OX40 has been tested with limited activity, and the humanized and fully human antibodies are advancing to the clinic. Altogether, these immune modulating antibodies have reproducible activity in a small subset of patients with metastatic melanoma (16).

Creating Large Quantities of Cancer-Fighting Cells: Adoptive Cell Transfer Immunotherapy

ACT approaches have the common goal of increasing the number of anti-tumor killer lymphocytes to overcome the lack of a natural or induced immune response against the cancer. Tumor-infiltrating lymphocytes (TILs) can be harvested from tumor biopsies, minced, and placed in ex vivo cell cultures with cytokines that allow the expansion of lymphocytes from them (18). TILs are expanded ex vivo to large numbers and are then infused back into the patients from whom the tumors were harvested. Depleting endogenous lymphocytes, using chemotherapy or radiotherapy conditioning therapy, before infusing the ex vivo expanded

TILs back into the patient, provide an advantage for the adoptively transferred lymphocytes to repopulate the host. Response rates of 50–70% have been achieved with this approach in arguably highly selected groups of patients (18). In addition, expansion of rare, blood-circulating T cells, specific for melanoma can be achieved by repetitive ex vivo stimulations of peripheral blood mononuclear cells with peptide antigens. This requires a prolonged process of weak antigen stimulation and cellular expansion of tumor antigen-reactive cells, eventually providing large quantities of antigen-specific lymphocytes for ACT. Through this approach, occasional patients with metastatic melanoma have had objective tumor responses against melanosomal and cancer testis antigens (19,20).

The fine antigen specificity of the tumor-specific lymphocytes used for ACT is provided by just two genes, the alpha and beta chains of their T-cell receptor (TCR). These two genes can be taken from the lymphocytes that have induced a specific anti-melanoma response in one patient and transferred to lymphocytes of another patient, using genetic engineering techniques. With this approach, the recipient lymphocytes are endowed with the tumor antigen and human leukocyte antigen (HLA) specificity of the donor lymphocytes (21). The pioneering work by investigators at the Surgery Branch, National Institute of Cancer, provided the first evidence that the ACT of TCR-engineered lymphocytes in humans is feasible and leads to objective tumor responses in patients with metastatic melanoma (22,23). In addition to gene modification with naturally occurring TCRs, lymphocytes can be genetically redirected with the use of chimeric antigen receptors (CARs). CARs are made up of an antibody-binding extracellular domain fused with intracellular signaling domains of co-stimulatory molecules. This approach provides very powerful means to redirect the specificity of T cells to specific surface proteins, merging the benefits of antibody targeting with the cytotoxic function of T cells (24). This concept could be translated to cell-free, recombinant molecules currently in various stages of development, such as T-cell engaging bispecific antibodies discussed in this book by Drs. Baeuerle and Rattel, or antibodies to major histocompatibility–peptide complexes by Drs. Weidanz and Hildebrand.

The merits and impacts of adoptive T-cell therapy findings to the field of cancer vaccines aiming to advance widely applicable therapies, is considerable and at multiple levels: (*i*) it showed that disease control, including tumor regression, could be achieved by antigen-specific immune intervention; (*ii*) it led to antigen target validation for a range of tumors, and (*iii*) it showed the importance of overcoming immune suppressive mechanisms as patient conditioning is key to the success of this approach.

CANCER VACCINES

The main body of the book is focused on active immunotherapies (therapeutic vaccines). The subsequent text gives a brief outline of several major platform technologies or cancer vaccine categories.

Polypeptide and Protein Vaccines

Vaccination with peptide epitopes recognized by T cells as antigenic in cancer cells has been broadly tested in the clinic for over 15 years (25). These peptides are usually administered together with immunological adjuvants as vaccines, and this requires the HLA matching between the peptide vaccine and the patient. Most studies have demonstrated that it requires a prolonged period of repeated immunizations to first detect peptide-specific T cells (26), which is a limitation in patients with progressive cancer. A phase II randomized trial tested the benefit of adding gp100 melanosomal antigen-derived peptides in an immunological adjuvant (Montanide-ISA, Seppic Inc., Fairfield, NJ) to the standard high-dose IL-2 regimen for patients with metastatic melanoma. This clinical trial demonstrated a statistically significant improvement in the response rate and progression-free survival of the combination compared with the response rate from IL-2 alone, with a nonstatistically significant trend toward a similar improvement in overall survival (27). Despite these data, the immunological potency of immunization with the minimal peptide epitopes of tumor antigens to induce T-cell responses is low (25,28), but it may be improved with the use of longer peptides (29). In this book, Drs. Lai, Cecil, Holt, Herenden, Kievit, Zhang, and Disis discuss the design, applicability, optimization, and testing of epitope-based vaccines for solid tumors such as breast carcinoma. In addition, in a distinct chapter, Drs. Alves and Brichard describe the development of a platform technology based on recombinant proteins and a range of adjuvants and aimed at overcoming HLA restriction. This program is accompanied by a biomarker analysis for predictive purposes. This platform technology (ASCI: Antigen Specific Cancer Immunotherapeutics) with its most advanced representative (MAGE-A3) has reached late development stages in lung cancer and melanoma.

Dendritic Cell Vaccines

Over 100 clinical trials of dendritic cell (DC) based immunotherapy have been conducted for cancer in the last 15 years. Overall, occasional tumor responses have been achieved in small subsets of patients, and the immunological responses have been much lower than it would have been predicted by preclinical models. A survival advantage has been demonstrated in two randomized clinical trials of one type of antigen-presenting cell (APC), not a fully developed DC, which was pulsed with a fusion protein containing a putative prostate cancer antigen (30). This led to a landmark approval of the first therapeutic cancer vaccine, namely sipuleucel-T (Provenge® Dendreon, Seattle, WA) for the treatment of metastatic prostate cancer—a milestone that had substantial positive impact in this field (31). In their chapter, Drs. Urdal and Frohlich outline the pivotal pathway to the approval of sipuleucel-T. In a distinct chapter, setting the stage, Drs. Agarwal and Vogelzang take a comprehensive look at all major classes of vaccines in development for treating GU cancers, leading in with DC-based vaccination. Last but not least, Drs. Chiriva-Internati, Cobos, Kast, Cannon, Mirandola, and Jenkins discuss several approaches for vaccination against hematological malignancies, with emphasis on DC vaccination and in general, cell-based therapies.

While DC vaccines were promising in the treatment prostate cancer, in a phase III randomized clinical trial, tumor antigen-loaded matured DC vaccines were inferior to dacarbazine in the treatment of metastatic melanoma (32). This, along with other efforts, outlines the need for further research and optimization of this promising class of vaccines.

Plasmid DNA, Recombinant Viral Vector, and Prime-Boost Immunizations

Tumor antigen genes have been administered as tumor vaccines. Initial efforts using tumor antigens expressed by a plasmid DNA or a viral vector administered intradermally, subcutaneously, or intramuscularly demonstrated low immunogenicity in humans. Interestingly, the first major breakthrough in this field was represented by a veterinarian vaccine based on DNA against canine melanoma. This was the very first approved therapeutic vaccine and its remarkable journey to market is outlined by Drs. Bergman and Wolchok in their chapter. The immunological potency of this genetic immunization strategy can be potentially applied to man and improved by using heterologous prime-boost approaches (33) and the intranodal immunization route (34), outlined in a separate chapter by Drs. Qiu, Diamond, Smith, Rosario, Miles, Obrocea, Kundig, and Bot.

With the advent of the first vaccine against prostate carcinoma, the interest and emphasis on "off-the-shelf" vaccines increased only as an alternative to personalized approaches. Drs. Farsaci, Kwilas, and Hodge discuss in detail the poxvirus-based vaccine technology with several exciting investigational agents in various stages of development, applicable to GU cancers and beyond.

NOVEL CONCEPTS AND VACCINE PLATFORM TECHNOLOGIES

Novel scientific information are being rapidly integrated in novel approaches. The realization that immune interventions could be utilized to target residual disease and possibly dormant "cancer stem cells", thus affording a more durable response compared with small molecule-targeted therapies, resulted in a significant interest in this area. Drs. Li, Mukherjee, Lee, and Yu introduce this concept in their chapter and discuss some of the efforts to target this category of cells, in general.

Another dimension of considerable interest to the whole field is positioning cancer vaccines vis-à-vis other therapies (approved or emerging), as combination approaches, to maximize the impact on disease. This idea, with a significant emphasis on T_{REG} cells as major roadblock to effective immunization against cancer, is discussed by Drs. Paustian, Jensen, Church, S. Puri, Twitty, Hu, Curti, Urba, R. Puri, and Fox in their chapter.

Yet, other areas of investigation consist of novel adjuvants and vectors that carry the promise of being superior relative to current or previously tested ones. As an example, Drs. Nair, Boczkowski, Pruitt, and Urban discuss the growing interest and novel developments in regards to RNA vaccines as a potential platform technology as compared with DNA or other categories of vaccines. In addition, in their chapter, Drs. Jin and Yeo present the realm of nucleic acid–based adjuvants that carry the promise of advancing safe and potent biological response modifiers which accompany the antigen-targeted vaccines or immune interventions in general.

IMMUNE MONITORING, BIOMARKERS, AND DEVELOPMENT STRATEGIES

Efficient means to quantitate and track T-cell responses to cancer is a key component of the development of effective immunotherapies in the clinic, to assist with the decisional process, especially in the absence of clinical response evaluation, help optimize a vaccine platform technology, or develop novel ones fitting the desired mechanisms of action. Established assays and new-generation immune monitoring assays, as well as whole-body molecular imaging, are being used for a thorough understanding of how the immune system can be harnessed to fight cancer. Current gold standard assays in immune monitoring include the enzyme-linked immunospot (35,36), the major histocompatibility complex tetramer binding assay, (37,38) and the intracellular cytokine flow cytometry assay (39,40). Their main advantage is allowing the enumeration of antigen-specific T lymphocytes at a single-cell level (41,42). Key to their adequate implementation is to prospectively define what change in assay results should be considered reflective of immune activation (41,43). New assays based on technical advances that allow a more comprehensive study of anti-tumor immune responses are being developed and provide additional required information to better understand the complex interplay between the immune system and cancer. These include polychromatic flow cytometry to define functional phenotypes of T cells (44,45) and the analysis of intracellular phosphorylated signaling proteins in permeabilized cells to study signaling networks through multiparameter flow cytometry (46). Even newer nanotechnology-based platforms have the promise of allowing a comprehensive study of limiting numbers of immune cells collected from tumor samples (47–49). In addition, modern metabolic imaging techniques, based on small molecule positron emission tomography (PET) tracers or reporter genes for PET imaging, can be used in humans and have the potential to allow longitudinal studies of the immune system interacting with cancer without disrupting the in vivo system (50,51). The incorporation of these types of assays to study how the immune system is modulated by immunotherapy is key to advance its use to treat cancer.

In their chapter, Drs. Britten, Janetzki, Hoos, Kalos, van der Burg, Gouttenfangeas, and Welters provide a concise and informative perspective of the evolving field of immune monitoring as a critical companion to developing cancer vaccines. In addition, Dr. Sekaly and collaborators discuss the need to implement a comprehensive systems biology approach involving transcriptome, immune gene signature analysis, proteomics, and other means to formulate more accurate models of how the immune system intervenes with disease; all with the aim of creating highly informative assays that could be more reliably utilized as prognostic, predictive, and response assessment tools.

Last but not the least, Drs. Musselli, Isakov, and Wentworth discuss novel concepts for clinical trial design and in general, for developing cancer vaccines, anchored in past lessons learned. As this class of investigational agents is very different—at multiple levels—from more conventional anti-cancer drugs, it is reasonable to consider a need to reevaluate efficacy end-points, clinical trial design principles, and success criteria. This could offer a veritable template for successful development and decision making in the cancer vaccine (active immunotherapy) field, barring regulatory and other considerations that need to be addressed.

CONCLUSIONS

New generations of immune stimulating strategies are being developed. The new experiences are built upon the well-documented anecdotes of patients with metastatic cancer who had spontaneous remissions or low frequency but durable remissions induced by a variety of immunotherapy approaches tested over many years. We have entered a new era, with two approved therapeutic cancer vaccines, one for veterinarian and the other for human use. The molecular understanding of how antigens can be presented to the immune system, the recognition of the relevance of modulating co-stimulatory and co-inhibitory molecules in an immunological synapse, of immune evasion mechanisms within the tumor environment, and the development of approaches to generate large cultures of tumor antigen–specific lymphocytes for ACT, are leading to significant advances in the use of immunotherapy for cancer. The development of efficient means to quantitate and track T-cell responses to cancer and more generally, of multiparametric biomarkers, is a key component to the development of effective immunotherapies in the clinic.

ACKNOWLEDGMENTS

A.R. is supported by The Fred L. Hartley Family Foundation, the Jonsson Cancer Center Foundation and the Caltech-UCLA Joint Center for Translational Medicine.

REFERENCES

1. Atkins MB, Kunkel L, Sznol M, Rosenberg SA. High-dose recombinant interleukin-2 therapy in patients with metastatic melanoma: long-term survival update. Cancer Journal from Scientific American 2000; 6(Suppl 1): S11–4.
2. Kirkwood JM, Manola J, Ibrahim J, et al. A pooled analysis of eastern cooperative oncology group and intergroup trials of adjuvant high-dose interferon for melanoma. Clin Cancer Res 2004; 10: 1670–7.
3. Ribas A, Butterfield LH, Glaspy JA, Economou JS. Current developments in cancer vaccines and cellular immunotherapy. J Clin Oncol 2003; 21: 2415–32.
4. Lode HN, Reisfeld RA. Targeted cytokines for cancer immunotherapy. Immunol Res 2000; 21: 279–88.
5. Ribas A, Kirkwood JM, Atkins MB, et al. Phase I/II open-label study of the biologic effects of the interleukin-2 immunocytokine EMD 273063 (hu14.18-IL2) in patients with metastatic malignant melanoma. J Transl Med 2009; 7: 68.
6. Leach DR, Krummel MF, Allison JP. Enhancement of antitumor immunity by CTLA-4 blockade. Science 1996; 271: 1734–6.
7. Chambers CA, Kuhns MS, Egen JG, Allison JP. CTLA-4-mediated inhibition in regulation of T cell responses: mechanisms and manipulation in tumor immunotherapy. Annu Rev Immunol 2001; 19: 565–94.
8. Agarwala SS, Ribas A. Current experience with CTLA4-blocking monoclonal antibodies for the treatment of solid tumors. J Immunother 2010; 33: 557–69.
9. Hodi FS, O'Day SJ, McDermott DF, Weber RW, Sosman JA, Haanen JB, et al. Improved survival with ipilimumab in patients with metastatic melanoma. N Engl J Med 2010.
10. FDA approves new treatment for a type of late-stage skin cancer. [Available from: http://www.fda.gov/newsevents/newsroom/pressannouncements/ucm1193237.htm].
11. Sznol M, Powderly JD, Smith DC, et al. Safety and antitumor activity of biweekly MDX-1106 (Anti-PD-1, BMS-936558/ONO-4538) in patients with advanced refractory malignancies. J Clin Oncol 2010; 28(suppl; abstract 2506): 15s.
12. Schoenberger SP, Toes RE, van der Voort EI, Offringa R, Melief CJ. T-cell help for cytotoxic T lymphocytes is mediated by CD40-CD40L interactions [see comments]. Nature 1998; 393: 480–3.

13. Vonderheide RH, Flaherty KT, Khalil M, et al. Clinical activity and immune modulation in cancer patients treated with CP-870,893, a novel CD40 agonist monoclonal antibody. J Clin Oncol 2007; 25: 876–83.
14. Beatty GL, Chiorean EG, Fishman MP, et al. CD40 agonists alter tumor stroma and show efficacy against pancreatic carcinoma in mice and humans. Science 2011; 331: 1612-6.
15. Melero I, Shuford WW, Newby SA, et al. Monoclonal antibodies against the 4-1BB T-cell activation molecule eradicate established tumors. Nat Med 1997; 3: 682–5.
16. Melero I, Hervas-Stubbs S, Glennie M, Pardoll DM, Chen L. Immunostimulatory monoclonal antibodies for cancer therapy. Nat Rev Cancer 2007; 7: 95–106.
17. Sugamura K, Ishii N, Weinberg AD. Therapeutic targeting of the effector T-cell co-stimulatory molecule OX40. Nat Rev Immunol 2004; 4: 420–31.
18. Rosenberg SA, Restifo NP, Yang JC, Morgan RA, Dudley ME. Adoptive cell transfer: a clinical path to effective cancer immunotherapy. Nat Rev Cancer 2008; 8: 299–308.
19. Yee C, Thompson JA, Byrd D, et al. Adoptive T cell therapy using antigen-specific CD8+ T cell clones for the treatment of patients with metastatic melanoma: in vivo persistence, migration, and antitumor effect of transferred T cells. Proc Natl Acad Sci USA 2002; 99: 16168–73.
20. Hunder NN, Wallen H, Cao J, et al. Treatment of metastatic melanoma with autologous CD4+ T cells against NY-ESO-1. N Engl J Med 2008; 358: 2698–703.
21. Schumacher TN. T-cell-receptor gene therapy. Nat Rev Immunol 2002; 2: 512–9.
22. Morgan RA, Dudley ME, Wunderlich JR, et al. Cancer regression in patients after transfer of genetically engineered lymphocytes. Science 2006; 314: 126–9.
23. Johnson LA, Morgan RA, Dudley ME, et al. Gene therapy with human and mouse T-cell receptors mediates cancer regression and targets normal tissues expressing cognate antigen. Blood 2009; 114: 535–46.
24. Sadelain M, Brentjens R, Riviere I. The promise and potential pitfalls of chimeric antigen receptors. Curr Opin Immunol 2009; 21: 215–23.
25. Rosenberg SA, Yang JC, Restifo NP. Cancer immunotherapy: moving beyond current vaccines. Nat Med 2004; 10: 909–15.
26. Slingluff CL Jr, Speiser DE. Progress and controversies in developing cancer vaccines. J Transl Med 2005; 3: 18.
27. Schwartzentruber DJ, Lawson D, Richards J, et al. A phase III multi-institutional randomized study of immunization with the gp100: 209-217(210M) peptide followed by high dose IL-2 compared with high dose IL-2 alone in patients with metastatic melanoma. J Clin Oncol 2009; 27(suppl; abstract CRA9011): 18s.
28. Sosman JA, Carrillo C, Urba WJ, et al. Three phase II cytokine working group trials of gp100 (210M) peptide plus high-dose interleukin-2 in patients with HLA-A2-positive advanced melanoma. J Clin Oncol 2008; 26: 2292–8.
29. Kenter GG, Welters MJ, Valentijn AR, et al. Phase I immunotherapeutic trial with long peptides spanning the E6 and E7 sequences of high-risk human papillomavirus 16 in end-stage cervical cancer patients shows low toxicity and robust immunogenicity. Clin Cancer Res 2008; 14: 169–77.
30. Kantoff PW, Higano CS, Shore ND, et al. Sipuleucel-T immunotherapy for castration-resistant prostate cancer. N Engl J Med 2010; 363: 411–22.
31. FDA Approves a Cellular Immunotherapy for Men with Advanced Prostate Cancer. [Available from: http://www.fda.gov/NewsEvents/Newsroom/PressAnnouncements/ucm210174.htm].
32. Schadendorf D, Ugurel S, Schuler-Thurner B, et al. Dacarbazine (DTIC) versus vaccination with autologous peptide-pulsed dendritic cells (DC) in first-line treatment of patients with metastatic melanoma: a randomized phase III trial of the DC study group of the DeCOG. Ann Oncol 2006; 17: 563–70.
33. Ramshaw IA, Ramsay AJ. The prime-boost strategy: exciting prospects for improved vaccination. Immunol Today 2000; 21: 163–5.
34. Ribas A, Weber JS, Chmielowski B, et al. Intra-lymph node prime-boost vaccination against melan A and tyrosinase for the treatment of metastatic melanoma: results of a phase 1 clinical trial. Clin Cancer Res. 2011. [Epub ahead of print].
35. Czerkinsky C, Andersson G, Ekre HP, et al. Reverse ELISPOT assay for clonal analysis of cytokine production. I. Enumeration of gamma-interferon-secreting cells. J Immunol Methods 1988; 110: 29–36.
36. Tanguay S, Killion JJ. Direct comparison of ELISPOT and ELISA-based assays for detection of individual cytokine-secreting cells. Lymphokine Cytokine Res 1994; 13: 259–63.
37. Altman JD, Moss PAH, Goulder PJR, et al. Phenotypic analysis of antigen-specific T lymphocytes. Science 1996; 274: 94–6.

38. Murali-Krishna K, Altman JD, Suresh M, et al. Counting antigen-specific CD8 T cells: a reevaluation of bystander activation during viral infection. Immunity 1998; 8: 177–87.
39. Labalette-Houache M, Torpier G, Capron A, Dessaint JP. Improved permeabilization procedure for flow cytometric detection of internal antigens. Analysis of interleukin-2 production. J Immunol Methods 1991; 138: 143–53.
40. Chikanza IC, Corrigal V, Kingsley G, Panayi GS. Enumeration of interleukin-1 alpha and beta producing cells by flow cytometry. J Immunol Methods 1992; 154: 173–8.
41. Keilholz U, Weber J, Finke JH, Gabrilovich D, Kast WM, Disis ML, et al. Immunologic monitoring of cancer vaccine therapy: Results of a workshop sponsored by the Society for Biological Therapy. J Immunother 2002; 25: 97–138.
42. Whiteside TL. Monitoring of antigen-specific cytolytic T lymphocytes in cancer patients receiving immunotherapy. Clin Diagn Lab Immunol 2000; 7: 327–32.
43. Comin-Anduix B, Gualberto A, Glaspy JA, et al. Definition of an immunologic response using the major histocompatibility complex tetramer and enzyme-linked immunospot assays. Clin Cancer Res 2006; 12: 107–16.
44. Perfetto SP, Chattopadhyay PK, Roederer M. Seventeen-colour flow cytometry: unravelling the immune system. Nat Rev Immunol 2004; 4: 648–55.
45. Seder RA, Darrah PA, Roederer M. T-cell quality in memory and protection: implications for vaccine design. Nat Rev Immunol 2008; 8: 247–58.
46. Perez OD, Nolan GP. Phospho-proteomic immune analysis by flow cytometry: from mechanism to translational medicine at the single-cell level. Immunol Rev 2006; 210: 208–28.
47. Soen Y, Chen DS, Kraft DL, Davis MM, Brown PO. Detection and characterization of cellular immune responses using peptide-MHC microarrays. PLoS Biol 2003; 1: E65.
48. Bailey RC, Kwong GA, Radu CG, Witte ON, Heath JR. DNA-encoded antibody libraries: a unified platform for multiplexed cell sorting and detection of genes and proteins. J Am Chem Soc 2007; 129: 1959–67.
49. Kwong GA, Radu CG, Hwang K, et al. Modular nucleic acid assembled p/MHC microarrays for multiplexed sorting of antigen-specific T cells. J Am Chem Soc 2009; 131: 9695–703.
50. Tumeh PC, Radu CG, Ribas A. PET imaging of cancer immunotherapy. J Nucl Med 2008; 49: 865–8.
51. Singh AS, Radu CG, Ribas A. PET imaging of the immune system: immune monitoring at the whole body level. Q J Nucl Med Mol Imaging 2010; 54: 281–90.

2 | Revisiting the paradigm on the putative need for antigen-specific responses in cancer

Gail D. Sckisel, Julia K. Tietze, and William J. Murphy

INTRODUCTION

Extensive efforts have been made in the development of antigen-specific immune therapies for cancer in hopes of developing targeted and sustained treatments to eliminate metastatic disease without "collateral" damage to normal tissues. This chapter will examine some of the biological aspects behind the interplay between the immune system and the tumor during tumorigenesis and tumor progression, to shed light on some of the potential reasons because of which antigen-specific therapies haven't necessarily translated clinically into the "magic bullet" that many thought they would be. We will also discuss the potential advantages of antigen-nonspecific therapies and how a rational combination of the two, based on their biology, may lead to the improvement of clinical immunotherapeutic responses.

PITFALLS OF ANTIGEN-SPECIFIC CANCER THERAPIES
Modest Efficacy of Antigen-Specific Cancer Therapies in Humans

A variety of approaches for vaccination against tumor-associated antigens (TAAs) have been attempted, including cell lysates, peptides, pulsed dendritic cells (DCs), recombinant viral vectors, whole-cell tumor preparations, nucleic acids, and others (1–3). From clinical trials involving these agents, it is evident that many of these cancer vaccines are able to induce functional TAA-specific immune responses. Unfortunately, large-scale clinical trials tend not to result in any significant differences in survival rates. One such example is the pancreatic cancer vaccine PANVAC™ (Therion Biologics Corporation, Cambridge, MA) trial in which ~70% of the patients surveyed tested positive for responses to carcinoembryonic antigen (an antigen immunized against in the study), yet a phase III trial showed no survival benefits relative to standard of care (4). In melanoma as well, immunization frequently elicits antigen-specific T-cell responses in most of the patients in the absence of tumor regression (5). In some cases, vaccination has even led to decreases in survival rates. A phase III trial in melanoma using the whole-cell vaccine Canvaxin™ (Rockville, MD) was terminated early due to decreased survival rates compared with placebo (6). In a retrospective study overlooking the 440 cancer vaccine trials conducted at the National Institutes of Health, Rosenberg and colleagues reported an overall response rate of only 2.6% (7). Another meta-analysis of 40 clinical studies involving 756 patients revealed a 4% response rate (8). Even in vaccine trials where survival is significant, only modest increases are noted. Provenge® (sipuleucel-T; Dendreon, Seattle, WA), a Food and Drug Administration–approved, novel treatment therapy for castration-resistant prostate cancer, yields a median increase of only 4.1 months in the overall survival time and yet no difference in the time to clinical disease progression (9).

These findings raise the question as to why antigen-specific responses are generated, yet do not translate into widespread anti-tumor immunity in a larger proportion of patients resulting in durable responses. We will next discuss hurdles to antigen-specific responses that likely contribute to the disappointing response rates of antigen-specific cancer therapies.

Mechanisms Contributing to Modest Cancer Vaccine Results
Weakly Immunogenic/Intracellular Antigens

In order for immune therapies to succeed, whether be it against cancer or a microorganism, an antigen is required for the immune system to target. With cancer this poses a problem as the cancer has arisen from "self" and to become tolerant to this, the immune system has gone through several rounds of selection. Therefore, one of the major challenges faced by antigen-specific therapies is the lack of a strong antigen to (*i*) distinguish the cancer from self and (*ii*) break the tolerance of the immune system.

In general, cancer antigens fall into five categories: (*i*) inappropriately expressed, tissue-specific proteins, (i.e., Her2/neu, microarray and gene expression), melanoma antigen recognized by T cells ([MART], NY-ESO, etc.), (*ii*) post-translationally modified proteins (i.e., MUC1, etc.), (*iii*) fusion proteins (i.e., B-cell receptor [BCR]-Abl, Gag-Abl, etc.), (*iv*) viral oncogenes (i.e., polyoma middle T, v-*src*, etc.), and (*v*) idiotypic antigens (i.e., BCR, T-cell receptor [TCR], etc.). With the exception of fusion proteins, viral oncogenes, and idiotypic proteins, most cancer antigens can be expressed on nontransformed cells as well. During the development of cancer, the thymus expresses proteins from throughout the body, and T cells recognizing them too strongly are deleted in a process known as central tolerance (10). For these reasons, the immune system remains ignorant to many cancer antigens, and the ones that it may recognize are also expressed on normal cells, making it difficult for malignant cells to distinguish on this basis.

In addition to being weakly immunogenic, many putative cancer antigens (oncogenes and tumor suppressor mutations) are expressed intracellularly. This poses a problem as T-cell recognition requires presentation of peptide fragments by major histocompatibility complex (MHC) molecules on antigen presenting cells (APCs). In order for an immune response to be generated, the antigens have to be released from the tumor cells and presented to T cells in the presence of the appropriate "danger" signals to elicit a cell-mediated response capable of eliminating and generating memory to transformed cells (11,12). This lack of "danger" signals during cancer progression, which can take place over many years, is thought to be a major impediment in allowing the induction of successful immune responses in cancer.

Immune Surveillance/Immune Editing

Despite the weakly immunogenic nature of most cancer antigens, there is a multitude of evidences which can vouch for the fact that the immune system is able to recognize and eliminate cells expressing them. Immune surveillance, a process in which the immune cells detect and eliminate tumor cells, was initially hypothesized by Burnet and Thomas in the 1950s, but was soon abandoned due to lack of experimental evidence. The theory was revived in the 1990s when a number of experiments were performed showing that the inability to produce interferon gamma (IFNγ) or perforin resulted in the increased incidence and shortened latency phase of chemically induced tumors (13). The most compelling evidence for this hypothesis came with the development of RAG2$^{-/-}$ mice that lacked T and B cells. These mice had significantly higher incidences of MCA-induced carcinomas as well as spontaneous epithelial cancers when bred in specific-pathogen-free environments compared to wild-type littermate controls (13,14). More recently, experiments have also been performed showing that deficiency in the natural killer (NK) cell-activating receptor, NKG2D, which can be used as a recognition mechanism by both NK cells and T cells, also leads to increased tumor incidence in a spontaneous prostate tumor model suggesting that this receptor pathway plays a role in tumor surveillance (15). In humans, immune surveillance is evident in immune suppressed individuals such as transplant recipients and AIDS patients, all of whom show greater susceptibility to virally and non–virally induced tumors (16). In addition to epidemiological data, there is a growing body of evidence correlating the presence of tumor infiltrating lymphocytes (TILs) with positive outcomes in patient survival (17–20). All of these data suggest that immune surveillance can indeed play a role in arresting cancer and thus can be exploited in cancer therapy.

More recently, Schreiber and colleagues have proposed the immunoediting hypothesis which acknowledges that while immune surveillance does occur (elimination), it exerts a selective pressure on the tumor to alter the immunogenicity (equilibrium) of the tumor itself eventually resulting in the development of a tumor that is able to grow with minimal immune intervention (escape) (21). This was evidenced by the observation that tumors grown in immunodeficient mice (RAG2$^{-/-}$, severe combined immunodeficiency disease [SCID]) were more frequently rejected when transplanted into immunocompetent mice. The same has been shown with tumors grown in perforin-deficient hosts. Further analysis of MCA-induced tumors grown in perforin-deficient mice has revealed an increased expression of the NKG2D ligand Rae-1γ indicating that the recognition by NKG2D (present on NK cells, T cells, and NK T cells) is one mechanism by which the immune system recognizes tumors (22). Clinically, melanoma patients have shown a progressive loss of the highly immunogenic MART-1/Melan-A tumor antigen expression in recurrent lesions and following adoptive transfer of MART-1 antigen-specific T cells (23,24). Analysis of patients with squamous cell carcinomas (SCC) and basal cell carcinomas (BCC) has shown decreases in TAAs along with increased MHC class I expression and CD8+ T-cell infiltration in SCC, whereas the opposite is true for BCC. This suggests that, in SCC, the expression of MHC class I has allowed for the recognition of TAA by CD8+ T cells ultimately driving immunoediting of SCCs to downregulate these antigens (25).

The aforementioned studies all provide evidence for the natural occurrence of immune editing. However, with increasing cancer vaccine experimentation over the past decade, there is enough evidence related to incidences of "accelerated" immune editing. In mice that have been engineered to inappropriately express the cancer antigen Her2/neu, vaccination against Her2/neu results in a delayed tumor onset with an eventual tumor growth correlating with mutations in Her2/neu epitopes targeted by the vaccine (26). In humans, specific targeting of Her2/neu and BCR-Abl, among other cancer antigens, with monoclonal antibodies results in dramatic clinical response rates (34% and 50% respectively); however, a significant proportion of patients eventually relapse presenting with malignancies deficient in the cancer antigens originally targeted (27,28). By these criteria, most cancers will have very low immunogenicity by the time they are discovered leaving little for an antigen-specific response to target. And if generated, an antigen-specific response will drive the eventual downregulation or loss of the targeted antigen rendering the antigen-specific cells useless, particularly in cases where the potential target antigen is not required for tumor survival.

Immune Evasion

The immune equilibrium and escape phases of the immunoediting process are in fact more complex than just downregulation of TAAs; instead they also involve active suppression of the immune system by the tumor itself. This can be achieved through a variety of mechanisms including downregulation of MHC class I, T-cell exhaustion and anergy, recruitment of inhibitory cells such as regulatory T cells (T$_{REGS}$), tumor-associated macrophages (TAMs), and myeloid-derived suppressor cells (MDSCs), and expression of suppressive molecules and death receptors (Fig. 2.1A–C).

Because expression of MHC is necessary for the presentation of tumor antigens, another mechanism by which the tumor can avoid antigen-specific recognition is to downregulate its expression of MHC class I or alter the expression of MHC class II on APCs. In numerous studies, the downregulation process of MHC class I is associated with abrogated immune responses and survival. Tumors achieve this through two main mechanisms: (*i*) mutations or altered expression of MHC class I structural components or (*ii*) altered expression of MHC class I loading machinery (29). Downregulation of MHC class I expression, however, leaves tumor cells vulnerable to NK-cell targeting through lack of triggering of inhibitory receptors expressed on NK cells toward "self" MHC (30). A clinical study looking at over 450 colorectal cancers showed that tumor cells expressing low, but not completely absent, MHC class I levels correlate with poor prognosis. The authors propose that tumor cells that are able to downregulate MHC to low-enough levels allowing them to avoid CD8 T-cell detection, yet maintain the NK-cell self-recognition status, incur a survival advantage (31). MHC class II expression is generally restricted to APCs; however, in certain cases it can be expressed on other cells including tumor cells. When expressed on tumor cells, CD4+ T cells have been shown to upregulate lytic molecules such as perforin and granzyme and death receptors resulting in tumor-cell destruction (32,33). Therefore, tumor cells expressing MHC class II have also been shown to downregulate expression of MHC class II and/or its loading machinery (34). In addition to altering MHC class II expression on themselves, tumor cells have also been shown to alter MHC class II expression on APCs through release of certain molecules. The TAA GA733-2 was recently shown to interfere with DC MHC class II antigen presentation thereby impairing CD4⁺ T-cell responses (35).

In addition to the need for antigenic stimulation, antigen-specific T cells are under strict regulatory control. In general, antigen-induced immune responses are meant to quickly control a challenge, contract, and retain a small number of antigen-specific cells for memory responses should the antigen be encountered again. During the contraction phase of the immune response,

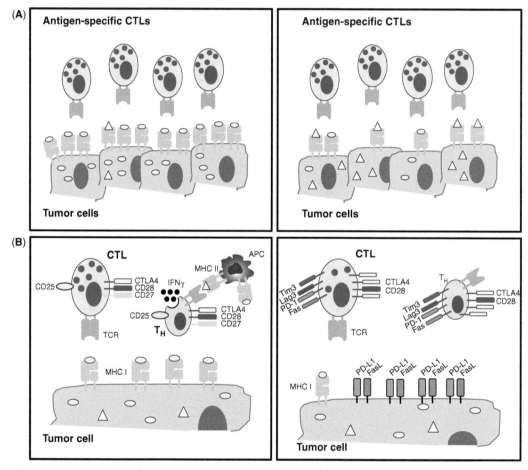

Figure 2.1 Tumor-cell mechanisms of escape from antigen-specific T-cell recognition. Panels on the left represent the interplay between the tumor and antigen-specific cells prior to immune editing and panels on the right represent the scenario afterward. (**A**) During the immune editing process, transformed cells that are not expressing an antigen that cytotoxic T-lymphocytes (CTLs) can recognize, or that are able to downregulate that particular antigen, incur a survival advantage over those that do not result in a tumor that is no longer able to be recognized by antigen-specific CTLs. Additionally, tumor cells that are able to downregulate major histocompatibility complex (MHC) presentation of the antigen incur a similar advantage. (**B**) As a result of the chronic immune stimulation that occurs during cancer, antigen-specific CTLs and TH cells that were once able to respond to transformed cells begin to upregulate inhibitory molecules and exhibit features of exhaustion including lack of interferon gamma (IFNγ) production, and expression of high levels of programmed death-1 (PD-1), CTLA-4, Lag3, Tim3, and Fas. In conjunction with this, tumor cells can upregulate ligands to some of these molecules, such as PD-L1 and FasL, resulting in an apoptosis of antigen-specific cells. (*Continued*)

(C)

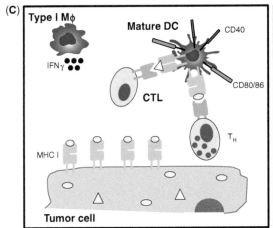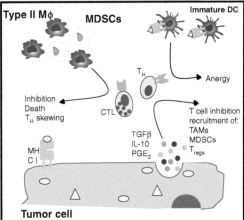

Figure 2.1 (*Continued*) (**C**) During the course of tumorigenesis, tumor cells secrete mediators that recruit immature myeloid cells including immature dendritic cells (iDCs) and myeloid-derived suppressor cells (MDSCs), as well as promote skewing of macrophage phenotypes from M1 to M2 and inhibit T-cell responses. iDCs work to anergize T cells because they lack the appropriate co-stimulation to correctly activate them. Tumor-associated macrophages (TAMs) and MDSCs work to dampen T-cell responses through a variety of mechanisms including nutrient sequestrations, reactive oxygen species generation, NO, as well as interference with trafficking into the tumor site. *Abbreviations*: APC, antigen presenting cell; IL, interleukin; PGE, prostaglandin E; TGF, transforming growth factor.

a number of molecules are expressed which aid in the elimination of cell types such as cytotoxic T-lymphocyte antigen-4 (CTLA-4), programmed death-1 (PD-1), Fas, lymphocyte activation gene-3 (LAG-3), etc. (36). During chronic infections, antigen-specific T cells never efficiently control the challenge and begin to overexpress many of these molecules, ultimately culminating in exhaustion (a state of terminal differentiation where cells are unable to proliferate or produce effector molecules such as IFNγ in response to stimulation). T-cell exhaustion can occur in tumors as well (37). In melanoma patients, TAA-specific CD4$^+$ and CD8$^+$ T cells (specific for MART-1 and NY-ESO) were shown to have elevated PD-1 expression (38,39). Furthermore, MART-1-specific CD4$^+$ and CD8$^+$ T cells were shown to express high levels of CTLA-4 and lack expression of CD25 and interleukin (IL) 7Rα, and MART-1-specific CD8$^+$ T cells failed to produce IFNγ upon stimulation (38). In Hodgkin's lymphoma, LAG-3 expression accompanies diminished IFNγ production on tumor-specific CD8$^+$ T cells (40). The use of "check-point" blockade in which PD-1 and CTLA-4 are targeted is being assessed clinically with favorable results being reported. However, toxicities due to autoreactivity are pressing issues and whether antigen-specific responses are generated and maintained and contribute to the anti-tumor effects remains to be delineated. Many tumors take advantage of the T-cell expression of some of the markers associated with exhaustion by upregulating the expression of ligands for these molecules resulting either in inhibition or death or both of activated immune cells. Fas ligand (FasL) expression is seen in many different tumor types, and increases in the FasL/Fas ratio within tumors have been associated with poor prognosis (41). PD-L1 expression has also been observed in a wide variety of tumors (42). In addition to exhaustion, tumor-specific T cells may become anergic or hyporesponsive. This is due to the lack of co-stimulation as well as presence of various inhibitory cell types at the tumor site (43).

Finally, tumors have been shown to secrete factors that attract suppressive cells and/or actively suppress effector cells at the tumor site. This results in a highly immunosuppressive tumor microenvironment making it extremely difficult for antigen-specific cells to become activated. Tumoral expression of numerous suppressive cytokines including transforming growth factor-beta (TGF-β), IL-10, and prostaglandin E2 (PGE2) is well documented. These molecules suppress adaptive immune responses through induction of T_{REGS}, T_H skewing, recruitment of suppressive cell types, etc. (44). In addition to secreted factors, tumor-associated leukocytosis has been observed; it is a negative prognostic factor for many types of human cancer including lung, colorectal, and skin (melanoma) and a variety of hematological malignancies, to name a few (45). Increased myelopoiesis is often the root of the leukocytosis resulting in increases in immature myeloid cells such as MDSCs and immature DCs (iDCs), and also the recruitment and accumulation of tumor-associated macrophages (TAMs). MDSCs and TAMs act to negatively regulate T cells through a variety of mechanisms including nutrient metabolism/sequestration, reactive oxygen species, NO, induction of T_{REGS}, and interference of trafficking mechanisms (46). iDCs induce T-cell anergy as they fail to upregulate co-stimulatory molecules during antigen presentation, thereby rendering the T cells specific to antigens from the tumor site hyporesponsive (47).

ANTIGEN-NONSPECIFIC/IMMUNOMODULATORY THERAPIES

In the prior section, we reviewed some of the mechanisms which tumors can employ to actively suppress and evade antigen-specific immune responses. In this section, we discuss antigen-nonspecific (immunomodulatory) therapies that aim to induce both innate and adaptive immune responses and highlight some of the advantages they allow for in contrast to antigen-specific therapies. In general, immunomodulatory therapies induce widespread immune activation leading to changes in the immunosuppressive environment of tumors toward one that favors immune activation. Additionally, through the production of effector molecules such as IFNγ, they can cause increases in the overall immunogenicity of tumor cells. Finally, immunomodulatory therapies induce the activation of multiple cell types including APCs, NK cells, and non–classically activated T cells such as "bystander" CD8 T cells which are different both functionally and regulation-wise than traditionally activated T cells and therefore may represent an advantage over antigen-specific T cells in the case of cancer.

An Overview of Immunomodulatory Therapies

Antigen-nonspecific therapies generally include cytokine-based and monoclonal antibody treatments. Cytokine-based therapies involve the use of proinflammatory cytokines to systemically, or locally, induce immune responses. Cytokine therapies that have been experimented with clinically include IL-2, IL-12, IL-21, tumor necrosis factor alpha (TNFα), type I IFNs, and granulocyte-macrophage colony stimulating factor (GM-CSF) (48,49). In addition to cytokine-based therapies, monoclonal antibodies can also be used to elicit immune activation. Monoclonal antibodies used in cancer can be agonistic to stimulatory receptors or can block membrane-bound inhibitory receptors against immune cells. Examples of these include agonistic CD40 antibodies, anti-CTLA-4 and anti-PD-1, which block the generation of suppressive signals by these molecules. Other stimulatory regimens include the use of various toll-like receptor (TLR) agonists such as CpGs and imiquimod.

Despite impressive preclinical data and clear advantages over antigen-specific therapies which will be discussed subsequently, clinical outcomes associated with immunomodulatory therapies have been modest as well. To date, IL-2 and IFNα are the only immunomodulatory therapies that are FDA approved for the treatment of metastatic melanoma. A recent meta-analysis of 35 independent immunotherapy trials including 765 patients demonstrated an overall response rate of 3.3%. Response rates and overall survival vary with individual therapies depending on the type of cancer and regimen of administration. However, in general, response rates rarely exceed 15% (48,49). Because of their high dose and systemic nature, many of these therapies tend to induce a range of toxicities and/or immune-related adverse events when used clinically (50-54). Consequently, significantly lower doses are given during clinical trials and may contribute to the discrepancies in responses between preclinical and clinical studies.

Advantages of Antigen-Nonspecific Attack over Antigen-Specific Therapies

When immunomodulatory therapies are given systemically or locally, they have been shown to enhance the immune response through a variety of mechanisms. The mechanisms depend highly upon the therapy but in general fall into two categories. The first is the alteration of the immunosuppressive environment either directly through monoclonal antibody-based targeting or indirectly through inflammatory cytokine production. The second involves the activation of cytotoxic lymphocytes.

Reversal of the Immunosuppressive Tumor Microenvironment

Numerous monoclonal antibodies have been developed to target and activate myeloid antigen-presenting cells for use as cancer immunotherapeutics. These therapies have been generated with a rationale of altering the immunosuppressive environment as well as improving antigen presentation/activation of T cells. Examples of targets for these monoclonal antibodies include CD40, FLT3, and OX40. In preclinical studies, agonistic anti-CD40, when used in combination with IL-2 or IL-15, has been shown to alter the expression of various chemokines within the tumor microenvironment resulting in a greater infiltration of effector cells with a concomitant reduction in T_{REG} infiltration (55). Certain cytokines such as GM-CSF are also capable of improving anti-tumor responses, presumably through improvement of antigen presentation. Many tumor vaccines consisting of tumor cells, which are genetically engineered to express GM-CSF, have been generated. These agents have shown tremendous success in preclinical models, especially when combined with inhibitory blockades such as aCTLA-4 and have since spawned clinical trials in humans (56,57). TLR agonists have also been promising in this area. Among other functions, CpGs have been shown to inhibit the regulatory function of MDSCs and promote their maturation and differentiation (58). Lastly, cytokine activation of NK and gd T cells results in the expression of various chemokines that recruit T cells, including MIP1α, MIP1β, IL-8, MDC, and RANTES (59).

Inflammatory cytokines, especially IFNγ, are shown to be expressed after various immunotherapies and, in many cases, instrumental in observed anti-tumor effects (60,61). IFNγ, in particular, is responsible for numerous changes within the tumor itself as well as to the immune system that result in enhanced immune responsiveness (62). The cytostatic properties of IFNγ have been described well. IFNγ has been shown to arrest the growth of tumor cells in the S phase of the cell cycle (63). In addition to growth arrest, it causes upregulation of MHC class I antigen presentation which leads to improved recognition by antigen-specific cytotoxic T cells (64). IFNγ also polarizes the immune system toward a type I response, thereby inhibiting Th2 skewing that some tumors use to overcome immunity (65). With type I skewing comes the activation and repolarization of TAMs, MDSCs, and iDCs present at the tumor site resulting in greater phagocytosis and antigen presentation of tumor cells and their antigens. Lastly, IFNγ activates cytotoxic cells such as CD8$^+$ T cells and NK cells resulting in greater recognition and elimination of transformed cells (66). Conversely, we have shown that IFNγ can also inhibit immune responses, particularly CD4$^+$ T cells (67). Thus, the same molecules that the immune system uses to mediate anti-tumor effects can also be inhibitory toward allowing sustained responses.

Lymphocyte Activation

In addition to altering the tumor microenvironment, strong immunostimulatory therapies often result in the massive expansion and activation of lymphocytes. This population consists of innate NK cells as well as T cells including NKT, $\gamma\delta$ T, $\alpha\beta$ T, and both antigen specific and nonspecific. Since this chapter is geared more toward antigen-specific versus antigen-nonspecific $\alpha\beta$ T-cell activation, we will mainly focus on these cell types.

The $\alpha\beta$ T cells that become activated and expand during immune stimulation are probably a combination of antigen-specific and antigen-nonspecific effectors. When agonistic αCD40 is combined with IL-2, it results in tumor elimination in a metastatic model of renal carcinoma, even bypassing the need for CD4+ T-cell help (60). Upon rechallenge, mice were able to specifically reject the tumor they were initially inoculated with, but not a chemically mutated form of it, suggesting the formation of antigen-specific memory. Another example is the administration of tumor vaccines expressing GM-CSF in combination with aCTLA-4 in mouse models of various cancers, including melanoma and prostate cancer. In these models, a complete regression of established tumors is observed in addition to organ-specific autoimmunity in the same tissue from which the tumor had arisen (56,57).

Because immunomodulatory therapies can lead to massive activation and proliferation of lymphocytes in the absence of vaccination, it suggests that most of the activated cells present are not specific to any TAA, yet play a critical role in mediating anti-tumor effects. While the expansion of antigen-nonspecific $\alpha\beta$ T cells following immunotherapy is marked, the role for these cells has not been clearly delineated. Several studies have documented the induction of TCR-independent anti-tumor effects following cytokine-based immunotherapies. In vitro culture of lymphocytes in the presence of high-dose IL-2 leads to the conversion of NK and T cells into lymphokine-activated killer (LAK) cells which are able to kill through an antigen-independent mechanism (68). In vitro studies show that IL-2 stimulation leads to the proliferation and activation of a subset of CD44^{high} CD8+ T cells that expresses high levels of various NK receptors including NKG2D and that these cells preferentially lyse syngeneic targets expressing NKG2D ligands (69). Similarly, we have shown that in vivo administration of IL-2 with αCD40 or IL-2 with IL-12 leads to the proliferation of similar subset of CD25$^-$CD44^{high} CD8+ T cells that highly upregulate NKG2D. These cells are highly activated and capable of killing through an NKG2D-dependent mechanism (manuscript submitted). In other monotherapy models involving IL-12 or IL-21, cytokine-induced rejection of tumors occurs partly through an NKG2D-dependent mechanism that likely includes NK cells and T cells (70–72). T cells expressing NK receptors have also been described in human melanoma patients and expression of these receptors is thought to play a role in their cytotoxicity (68,73). Thus, it appears that both antigen-specific and antigen-nonspecific immune pathways work together to produce the greatest anti-tumor effects.

Antigen-Nonspecific $\alpha\beta$ T Cells

The activation and expansion of antigen-nonspecific (bystander) cells during viral and bacterial infections have been extensively described (74). During these infections, memory phenotype (CD44^{high}) CD8+ T cells of multiple specificities are expanded both in the secondary lymphoid organs as well as in the periphery. Whether these cells play a crucial role in pathogenic clearance is debatable, as conflicting reports have been generated (75-77). For this review we will focus on bystander $\alpha\beta$ CD8+ T cells; however, $\alpha\beta$ CD4+ T cells are capable of bystander activation as well (78). Bystander cells are generally induced in high-cytokine environments (79–81) such as those present during the acute phase of an immune response or during high-dose cytokine-based immunotherapies and thus are highly dependent on cytokine stimulation for survival and function. Due to their TCR–MHC independent nature and the widespread abundance of cells capable of being activated in this fashion, activation of bystander T cells presents an attractive option for cancer immunotherapies. Additionally, because they do not become activated through TCR engagement, bystander cells differentially express regulatory molecules associated with contraction making them an attractive target for overcoming some of the regulatory mechanisms induced within the tumor microenvironment. The potential advantages of antigen-nonspecific T cells in cancer immunotherapy are depicted in Figure 2.2.

Since bystander cells do not recognize target cells through TCR–MHC interactions, they need another mechanism in place to determine which cells need to be eliminated. NK cell–activating receptors are known to be expressed on T cells (69,73,82) and may be instrumental in this process. These receptors recognize stress ligands that are expressed on virally infected and transformed cells (83). Data from our lab suggest that in influenza infection, CD25$^-$CD44^{high}NKG2D+ CD8 T cells are capable of lysing NKG2DL+ targets suggesting that they may

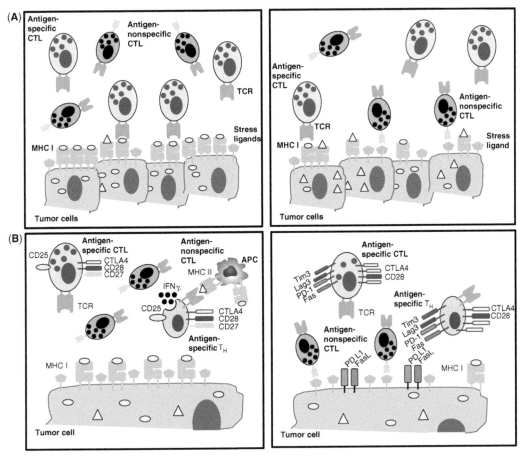

Figure 2.2 Antigen-nonspecific T cells are not evaded by the same mechanisms as antigen-specific T cells. Panels of left represent interplay between the tumor and antigen-specific cells prior to immune editing and panels on the right represent the scenario afterward. (**A**) During the immune editing process, transformed cells are able to downregulate antigen or antigen presenting machinery to avoid detection by antigen-specific T cells. Since antigen-nonspecific cells recognize other molecules present on transformed cells such as stress ligands or damage associated molecular patterns (DAMPs), they are still able to detect and lyse tumor cells. (**B**) During the chronic immune stimulation that occurs in cancer, antigen-specific T cells downregulate CD25 and upregulate molecule-associated, activation-induced cell death and exhaustion such as programmed death-1 (PD-1), cytotoxic T-lymphocyte antigen-4 (CTLA-4), Fas, Tim3, and Lag3. This can be accompanied by tumor associated upregulation of PD-L1 and FasL resulting in inhibition and/or apoptosis of antigen-specific T cells. Since antigen-nonspecific T cells are not activated through TCR engagement, they are differentially regulated and do not respond to these molecules in the same fashion as antigen-specific cells. *Abbreviations*: APC, antigen presenting cell; IFNγ, interferon gamma; IL, interleukin; MHC 1 major histocompatibility complex 1; MDSCs, myeloid-derived suppressor cells; PGE, prostaglandin E; TAMs, tumor-associated macrophages; TGF, transforming growth factor.

play a role in the clearance of virally infected cells expressing stress ligands (manuscript in preparation). In addition to models of pathogen exposure, NKG2D⁺ T cells have also been shown to play a role in autoimmunity and the immunosurveillance of tumor cells. In celiac disease, it has been shown that induction of IL-15 in the gut leads to conversion of CTLs to LAK cells (84). Tumors generated from mice deficient in the effector molecules IFNγ or TNF-related apoptosis inducing ligand (TRAIL) express high levels of Rae1γ. Tumors generated from mice deficient in either NK or T cells exhibit little to no Rae1γ expression suggesting that T cells and NK cells both use NKG2D-dependent mechanisms to surveil transformed tissues (22). Because bystander cells use TCR-independent mechanisms to recognize targets, they are resistant to some of the immune escape tactics that tumors use against traditional αβ T cells, such as antigen loss and MHC downregulation (Fig. 2.2A).

Cytokine-induced bystander proliferation generally occurs in CD44high (antigen experienced) populations of T cells which is likely due to the differential expression of cytokine receptors. For instance, CD122, the low affinity IL-2/IL-15 receptor has five to six-fold higher expression in CD44high (memory) cells than CD44low (naïve) cells (85,86). This is important and advantageous for two reasons. First, CD44high populations are present in secondary lymphoid organs as well as within tissues as tissue resident effector memory T cells. This means that bystander memory T cells can be activated and expanded directly at the tumor site from effector memory T cells already present in surrounding tissues making them faster to respond than T cells activated during primary antigen exposure which can take up to two weeks to become generated. Furthermore, since they are already memory cells, it is assumed that they have been vetted through multiple rounds of immune selection in order to ensure that they will not cause undesirable autoimmunity after nonspecific activation (Fig. 2.2B).

Since bystander memory T cells are directly induced by cytokine activation and have not been activated through TCR engagement, their regulation occurs through different mechanisms as well. Bystander activation is dependent on continuous exposure to cytokines. This can be evidenced by the fact that discontinuance of cytokine administration results in their rapid contraction. Furthermore, in the case of IL-2 activation, since antigen-nonspecific cells have not been activated through TCR engagement, they do not express CD25 and therefore rely on high doses of IL-2 in order to remain activated. Other markers upregulated upon TCR engagement and during contraction, including PD-1 and CTLA-4, seem to be differentially regulated in antigen-nonspecific T cells as well. PD-1 is not upregulated at all and CTLA-4 is not upregulated to the same extent (manuscript in preparation). This makes antigen-nonspecific cells more attractive effector cells at the tumor site because they are less susceptible to tumor-induced immunosuppression through mechanisms related to these markers.

COMBINATION OF ANTIGEN-SPECIFIC AND ANTIGEN-NONSPECIFIC THERAPIES

In the previous sections, we have addressed the reasons why antigen-specific therapies have not been as successful as hypothesized, as well as some of the ways that antigen-nonspecific therapies can compensate for these shortcomings. Next we will discuss the potential mechanisms of how antigen-specific and antigen-nonspecific T-cell responses may work together to maximize the benefits of each other. Since the interplay of antigen-specific and bystander cells under physiological conditions is not well understood, we will also consider how the timing of induction of different types of T cells can complement each other and analyze situations in which each would be beneficial. By understanding the advantages of alternatively timing antigen-specific and antigen-nonspecific activation, it may be possible to rationally design regimens of therapies combining vaccination with immunomodulation.

Antigen-Specific Followed by Nonspecific T-Cell Responses

Generation of antigen-specific cells prior to the induction of antigen-nonspecific cells as a way to supplement antigen-specific responses would be most advantageous in tumors that are highly immunogenic to ensure that antigen-specific cells are capable of being generated (Fig. 2.3A). In this scenario, antigen-specific T cells generated through vaccination traffic to the tumor site. At the tumor site, antigen-specific cells may induce a proinflammatory environment capable of causing bystander activation and recruitment of nearby tissue resident and circulating memory T cells. Administration of cytokines or other immunomodulators at this point may improve the activation and proliferation of nonspecific cells. IFNγ, produced as a result of immune stimulation, induces tumor growth arrest and increased MHC expression. This may allow for the better targeting of transformed cells by expanded antigen-specific CD8 T cells.

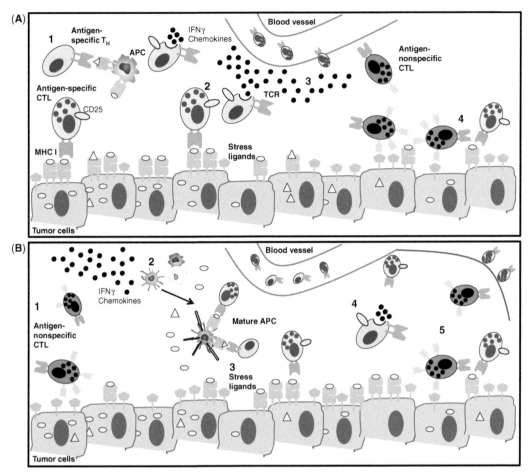

Figure 2.3 Coordination of antigen-specific and antigen-nonspecific T-cell responses. (**A**) Antigen-specific cells may recruit antigen-nonspecific cells to the tumor site in more immunogenic tumors. (1) Circulating tumor-specific T cells, presumably generated from vaccination, traffic to the tumor site and begin to perform effector functions. (2) Th cells secrete cytokines and chemokines thereby attracting the circulating and tissue resident CD44^{high} CD8$^+$ T cells to the site. (3) These memory cells then become bystander activated due to the cytokine rich environment, and begin expressing activating NK receptors such as NKG2D. (4) Both antigen-specific and nonspecific CD8 T cells lyse tumor cells through complementary mechanisms. Antigen-specific cells maintain antigen-nonspecific activation through cytokine production. (**B**) Antigen-nonspecific cells may debulk less immunogenic tumors thereby releasing antigen and initiating antigen-specific activation. (1) Antigen-nonspecific cells, generated through immunomodulation, traffic to the tumor site and lyse tumor cells via NK receptor–stress ligand recognition leading to antigen release. (2) Immunomodulation also conditions antigen presenting cells (APCs) and myeloid cells at the tumor site toward a proinflammatory phenotype. (3) Antigen release and APC maturation lead to migration and activation of antigen-specific T cells to the tumor site. (4) Antigen-specific cells complement antigen-nonspecific T cells in tumor destruction. (5) Cytokines and chemokines generated by antigen-specific cells maintain and recruit additional antigen-nonspecific cells at the tumor site. *Abbreviations*: CTL, cytotoxic T-lymphocytes; IFnγ, interferon gamma.

Tumor cells not expressing CD8 epitopes, recognized by antigen-specific cells are targeted by nonspecific CD8 T cells via the NK receptor–stress ligand pathways. Generally, once immune stimulation is halted, the expansion of antigen-nonspecific cells is reversed. However, cytokines produced by the antigen-specific cells may be sufficient for the expansion to continue locally within the tumor allowing for more efficient tumor clearance.

A recent paper suggests that the situation described above may be more indicative of what occurs within the tumor under normal physiological conditions. The presence of antigen-nonspecific cells within tumors has been observed. Ghani and colleagues describe antigen-specific cells as "pioneers" that facilitate the recruitment of other effector/memory T cells to the site regardless of their antigen specificity. They went on to show that IFNγ and TNFα are necessary for recruitment into the tumor (87).

Antigen-Nonspecific Followed by Specific T-Cell Responses

When induced initially, antigen-nonspecific T-cell responses may mediate tumor debulking and antigen release to enhance subsequent antigen-specific responses. Induction of nonspecific T-cell responses generally requires a proinflammatory, cytokine-rich environment (Fig. 2.3B). The proinflammatory environment may reverse some of the immune suppression created by the tumor as well as promote activation and maturation of APCs. Antigen-nonspecific CD8 T cells express high amounts of IFNγ, leading to tumor growth arrest and upregulation of MHC. Furthermore, nonspecific CD8 T cells express the effector molecules perforin, granzyme, and FasL as well as NKG2D, which can be used to recognize tumor cells that express stress-related NKG2D ligands. Tumor killing releases an antigen which, in coordination with the proinflammatory environment, fosters the development of antigen-specific responses. The newly generated, multivalent adaptive response would then be responsible for perpetuating the immune response against residual disease.

This situation would likely involve some sort of immune activation to initially induce the activation of antigen-nonspecific cells. It may also be advantageous to boost the induction of antigen-specific responses with vaccination. Again, the optimal dosage and timing of when to administer a vaccination would be highly important so as to achieve the maximum utilization of the proinflammatory, high antigen environment, yet avoid crippling of antigen-specific CD4 responses that may occur as a result of high-dose immunomodulation. One example of this type of treatment schema is the oncolytic virus OncoVEX[GM-CSF]. OncoVEX is a herpes virus that has been attenuated to selectively reproduce in tumor cells. Furthermore, a virulence gene-limiting antigen presentation was deleted and replaced by GM-CSF to enhance the visibility of and response to cancer antigens released upon viral lysis of tumor cells (88). OncoVEX[GM-CSF] leads to selective lysis of tumor cells releasing tumor antigens in the presence of virally induced danger signals and GM-CSF, which increases DC maturation and antigen presentation, leading to sustainable antigen-specific responses. Intratumoral treatment with OncoVEX[GMCSF] leads to both local and systemic anti-tumor effects. In preclinical studies using athymic nude mice, it has been shown that while the local effects were due to oncolytic properties of the virus, systemic effects were mediated through an adaptive immune response (89). Clinical data thus far have remained promising. In a phase II study in stage III/IV squamous cell cancer of the head and neck, 13/17 patients achieved objective responses by CT (90). In another phase II study, in stage III/IV unresectable metastatic melanoma, the overall response rate was 28%, with the overall survival being 58% at one year and 52% at two years (91); a dramatic improvement from the estimated survival rate of 25.5% at one year of current treatments (92). Currently, OncoVEX is being tested in phase III trials for both cancer types.

CONCLUSIONS

While neither vaccination nor immune modulation has been widely successful as monotherapies, they each provide advantages where the other fails. Combination of different aspects of the two types of responses may result in superior anti-tumor effects. Order and timing of induction of antigen-specific and nonspecific T-cell responses will be crucial for success and may need to be different depending on the tumor itself. Clearly, inducing antigen-nonspecific responses prior to antigen-specific vaccination may be more advantageous for poorly immunogenic tumors, whereas providing immune stimulation after vaccination may be sufficient for highly immunogenic tumors. In either case, the induction of adverse immune events and other side effects will need to be carefully monitored.

REFERENCES

1. Brinckerhoff LH, Thompson LW, Slingluff CL Jr. Melanoma vaccines. Curr Opin Oncol 2000; 12: 163–73.
2. Bystryn JC. Vaccines for melanoma. Design strategies and clinical results. Dermatol Clin 1998; 16: 269–75.
3. Bystryn JC, Shapiro RL, Harris M, Roses DF, Oratz R. Use of vaccines in treatment of malignant melanoma. Clin Dermatol 1996; 14: 337–41.
4. Madan RA, Arlen PM, Gulley JL. PANVAC-VF: poxviral-based vaccine therapy targeting CEA and MUC1 in carcinoma. Expert Opin Biol Ther 2007; 7: 543–54.
5. Meijer SL, Dols A, Jensen SM, et al. Induction of circulating tumor-reactive CD8+ T cells after vaccination of melanoma patients with the gp100 209-2M peptide. J Immunother 2007; 30: 533–43.
6. Morton DL. Immune response to postsurgical adjuvant active immunotherapy with Canvaxin polyvalent cancer vaccine: correlations with clinical course of patients with metastatic melanoma. Dev Biol (Basel) 2004; 116: 209–17; discussion 229–36.
7. Rosenberg SA, Yang JC, Restifo NP. Cancer immunotherapy: moving beyond current vaccines. Nat Med 2004; 10: 909–15.
8. Eggermont AM. Therapeutic vaccines in solid tumours: can they be harmful? Eur J Cancer 2009; 45: 2087–90.
9. Nabhan C. Sipuleucel-T immunotherapy for castration-resistant prostate cancer. N Engl J Med 2010; 363: 1966–67; author reply 1968.
10. Hogquist KA, Baldwin TA, Jameson SC. Central tolerance: learning self-control in the thymus. Nat Rev Immunol 2005; 5: 772–82.
11. Fuchs EJ, Matzinger P. Is cancer dangerous to the immune system? Semin Immunol 1996; 8: 271–80.
12. Matzinger P. Tolerance, danger, and the extended family. Annu Rev Immunol 1994; 12: 991–1045.
13. Dunn GP, Bruce AT, Ikeda H, Old LJ, Schreiber RD. Cancer immunoediting: from immunosurveillance to tumor escape. Nat Immunol 2002; 3: 991–8.
14. Shinkai Y, Rathbun G, Lam KP, et al. RAG-2-deficient mice lack mature lymphocytes owing to inability to initiate V(D)J rearrangement. Cell 1992; 68: 855–67.
15. Guerra N, Tan YX, Joncker NT, et al. NKG2D-deficient mice are defective in tumor surveillance in models of spontaneous malignancy. Immunity 2008; 28: 571–80.
16. de Visser KE, Coussens LM. The inflammatory tumor microenvironment and its impact on cancer development. Contrib Microbiol 2006; 13: 118–37.
17. Liakou CI, Narayanan S, Ng Tang D, Logothetis CJ, Sharma P. Focus on TILs: Prognostic significance of tumor infiltrating lymphocytes in human bladder cancer. Cancer Immun 2007; 7: 10.
18. Oble DA, Loewe R, Yu P, Mihm MC Jr. Focus on TILs: prognostic significance of tumor infiltrating lymphocytes in human melanoma. Cancer Immun 2009; 9: 3.
19. Uppaluri R, Dunn GP, Lewis JS Jr. Focus on TILs: prognostic significance of tumor infiltrating lymphocytes in head and neck cancers. Cancer Immun 2008; 8: 16.
20. Yamada N, Oizumi S, Kikuchi E, et al. CD8+ tumor-infiltrating lymphocytes predict favorable prognosis in malignant pleural mesothelioma after resection. Cancer Immunol Immunother 2010; 59: 1543–9.
21. Dunn GP, Old LJ, Schreiber RD. The three Es of cancer immunoediting. Annu Rev Immunol 2004; 22: 329–60.
22. Smyth MJ, Swann J, Cretney E, et al. NKG2D function protects the host from tumor initiation. J Exp Med 2005; 202: 583–8.
23. Maeurer MJ, Gollin SM, Martin D, et al. Tumor escape from immune recognition: lethal recurrent melanoma in a patient associated with downregulation of the peptide transporter protein TAP-1 and loss of expression of the immunodominant MART-1/Melan-A antigen. J Clin Invest 1996; 98: 1633–41.
24. Yee C, Thompson JA, Byrd D, et al. Adoptive T cell therapy using antigen-specific CD8+ T cell clones for the treatment of patients with metastatic melanoma: in vivo persistence, migration, and antitumor effect of transferred T cells. Proc Natl Acad Sci USA 2002; 99: 16168–73.
25. Walter A, Barysch MJ, Behnke S, et al. Cancer-testis antigens and immunosurveillance in human cutaneous squamous cell and basal cell carcinomas. Clin Cancer Res 2010; 16: 3562–70.
26. Singh R, Paterson Y. Immunoediting sculpts tumor epitopes during immunotherapy. Cancer Res 2007; 67: 1887–92.
27. Nahta R, Esteva FJ. HER-2-targeted therapy: lessons learned and future directions. Clin Cancer Res 2003; 9: 5078–84.

28. Scott SD. Rituximab: a new therapeutic monoclonal antibody for non-Hodgkin's lymphoma. Cancer Practice 1998; 6: 195–7.
29. Kasajima A, Sers C, Susano H, et al. Down-regulation of the antigen processing machinery is linked to a loss of inflammatory response in colorectal cancer. Hum Pathol 2010; 41: 1758–69.
30. Lanier LL. NK cell recognition. Annu Rev Immunol 2005; 23: 225–74.
31. Watson NF, Ramage JM, Madid Z, et al. Immunosurveillance is active in colorectal cancer as downregulation but not complete loss of MHC class I expression correlates with a poor prognosis. Int J Cancer 2006; 118: 6–10.
32. Quezada SA, Simpson TR, Peggs KS, et al. Tumor-reactive CD4(+) T cells develop cytotoxic activity and eradicate large established melanoma after transfer into lymphopenic hosts. J Exp Med 2010; 207: 637–50.
33. Zennadi R, Abdel-Wahab Z, Seigler HF, Darrow TL. Generation of melanoma-specific, cytotoxic CD4(+) T helper 2 cells: requirement of both HLA-DR15 and Fas antigens on melanomas for their lysis by Th2 cells. Cell Immunol 2001; 210: 96–105.
34. Satoh A, Toyota M, Ikeda H, et al. Epigenetic inactivation of class II transactivator (CIITA) is associated with the absence of interferon-gamma-induced HLA-DR expression in colorectal and gastric cancer cells. Oncogene 2004; 23: 8876–86.
35. Gutzmer R, Li W, Sutterwala S, et al. A tumor-associated glycoprotein that blocks MHC class II-dependent antigen presentation by dendritic cells. J Immunol 2004; 173: 1023–32.
36. Prlic M, Bevan MJ. Exploring regulatory mechanisms of CD8+ T cell contraction. Proc Natl Acad Sci USA 2008; 105: 16689–94.
37. Kim PS, Ahmed R. Features of responding T cells in cancer and chronic infection. Curr Opin Immunol 2010; 22: 223–30.
38. Ahmadzadeh M, Johnson LA, Heemskerk B, et al. Tumor antigen-specific CD8 T cells infiltrating the tumor express high levels of PD-1 and are functionally impaired. Blood 2009; 114: 1537–44.
39. Fourcade J, Kudela P, Sun Z, et al. PD-1 is a regulator of NY-ESO-1-specific CD8+ T cell expansion in melanoma patients. J Immunol 2009; 182: 5240–9.
40. Gandhi MK, Lambley E, Duraiswamy J, et al. Expression of LAG-3 by tumor-infiltrating lymphocytes is coincident with the suppression of latent membrane antigen-specific CD8+ T-cell function in Hodgkin lymphoma patients. Blood 2006; 108: 2280–9.
41. Rivoltini L, Carrabba M, Huber V, et al. Immunity to cancer: attack and escape in T lymphocyte-tumor cell interaction. Immunol Rev 2002; 188: 97–113.
42. Blank C, Gajewski TF, Mackensen A. Interaction of PD-L1 on tumor cells with PD-1 on tumor-specific T cells as a mechanism of immune evasion: implications for tumor immunotherapy. Cancer Immunol Immunother 2005; 54: 307–14.
43. Staveley-O'Carroll K, Sotomayor E, Montgomery J, et al. Induction of antigen-specific T cell anergy: An early event in the course of tumor progression. Proc Natl Acad Sci USA 1998; 95: 1178–83.
44. Wojtowicz-Praga S. Reversal of tumor-induced immunosuppression: a new approach to cancer therapy. J Immunother 1997; 20: 165–77.
45. Wilcox RA. Cancer-associated myeloproliferation: old association, new therapeutic target. Mayo Clin Proc 2010; 85: 656–63.
46. Ostrand-Rosenberg S. Myeloid-derived suppressor cells: more mechanisms for inhibiting antitumor immunity. Cancer Immunol Immunother 2010; 59: 1593–600.
47. Gabrilovich D. Mechanisms and functional significance of tumour-induced dendritic-cell defects. Nat Rev Immunol 2004; 4: 941–52.
48. Sivendran S, Glodny B, Pan M, Merad M, Saenger Y. Melanoma immunotherapy. Mt Sinai J Med 2010; 77: 620–42.
49. Donnelly RP, Young HA, Rosenberg AS. An overview of cytokines and cytokine antagonists as therapeutic agents. Ann NY Acad Sci 2009; 1182: 1–13.
50. Weber J. Ipilimumab: controversies in its development, utility and autoimmune adverse events. Cancer Immunol Immunother 2009; 58: 823–30.
51. Yang JC, Hughes M, Kammula U, et al. Ipilimumab (anti-CTLA4 antibody) causes regression of metastatic renal cell cancer associated with enteritis and hypophysitis. J Immunother 2007; 30: 825–30.
52. Weber J. Review: anti-CTLA-4 antibody ipilimumab: case studies of clinical response and immune-related adverse events. Oncologist 2007; 12: 864–72.
53. Lentsch AB, Miller FN, Edwards MJ. Mechanisms of leukocyte-mediated tissue injury induced by interleukin-2. Cancer Immunol Immunother 1999; 47: 243–8.
54. Genetics Institute suspends phase II study of rhiL-12. J Int Assoc Physicians AIDS Care 1995; 1: 34.

55. Weiss JM, Back TC, Scarzello AJ, et al. Successful immunotherapy with IL-2/anti-CD40 induces the chemokine-mediated mitigation of an immunosuppressive tumor microenvironment. Proc Natl Acad Sci USA 2009; 106: 19455–60.

56. Hurwitz AA, Foster BA, Kwon ED, et al. Combination immunotherapy of primary prostate cancer in a transgenic mouse model using CTLA-4 blockade. Cancer Res 2000; 60: 2444–8.

57. van Elsas A, Hurwitz AA, Allison JP. Combination immunotherapy of B16 melanoma using anti-cytotoxic T lymphocyte-associated antigen 4 (CTLA-4) and granulocyte/macrophage colony-stimulating factor (GM-CSF)-producing vaccines induces rejection of subcutaneous and metastatic tumors accompanied by autoimmune depigmentation. J Exp Med 1999; 190: 355–66.

58. Zoglmeier C, Bauer H, Nörenberg D, et al. CpG blocks immune suppression by myeloid-derived suppressor cells in tumor-bearing mice. Clin Cancer Res 2011; 17: 1765–75.

59. Subleski JJ, Wiltrout RH, Weiss JM. Application of tissue-specific NK and NKT cell activity for tumor immunotherapy. J Autoimmun 2009; 33: 275–81.

60. Murphy WJ, Welniak L, Back T, et al. Synergistic anti-tumor responses after administration of agonistic antibodies to CD40 and IL-2: coordination of dendritic and CD8+ cell responses. J Immunol 2003; 170: 2727–33.

61. Wigginton JM, Gruys E, Geiselhart L, et al. IFN-gamma and Fas/FasL are required for the antitumor and antiangiogenic effects of IL-12/pulse IL-2 therapy. J Clin Invest 2001; 108: 51–62.

62. Dunn GP, Koebel CM, Schreiber RD. Interferons, immunity and cancer immunoediting. Nat Rev Immunol 2006; 6: 836–48.

63. Gooch JL, Herrera RE, Yee D. The role of p21 in interferon gamma-mediated growth inhibition of human breast cancer cells. Cell Growth Differ 2000; 11: 335–42.

64. Yang Y, Xiang Z, Ertl HC, Wilson JM. Upregulation of class I major histocompatibility complex antigens by interferon gamma is necessary for T-cell-mediated elimination of recombinant adenovirus-infected hepatocytes in vivo. Proc Natl Acad Sci USA 1995; 92: 7257–61.

65. Murphy KM, Reiner SL. The lineage decisions of helper T cells. Nat Rev Immunol 2002; 2: 933–44.

66. Schroder K, Hertzog PJ, Ravasi T, Hume DA. Interferon-gamma: an overview of signals, mechanisms and functions. J Leukoc Biol 2004; 75: 163–89.

67. Berner V, Liu H, Zhou Q, et al. IFN-gamma mediates CD4+ T-cell loss and impairs secondary antitumor responses after successful initial immunotherapy. Nat Med 2007; 13: 354–60.

68. Kalland T, Belfrage H, Bhiladvala P, Hedlund G. Analysis of the murine lymphokine-activated killer (LAK) cell phenomenon: dissection of effectors and progenitors into NK- and T-like cells. J Immunol 1987; 138: 3640–5.

69. Dhanji S, Teh HS. IL-2-activated CD8+CD44high cells express both adaptive and innate immune system receptors and demonstrate specificity for syngeneic tumor cells. J Immunol 2003; 171: 3442–50.

70. Ma HL, Whitters MJ, Konz RF, et al. IL-21 activates both innate and adaptive immunity to generate potent antitumor responses that require perforin but are independent of IFN-gamma. J Immunol 2003; 171: 608–15.

71. Smyth MJ, Swann J, Kelly JM, et al. NKG2D recognition and perforin effector function mediate effective cytokine immunotherapy of cancer. J Exp Med 2004; 200: 1325–35.

72. Takaki R, Hayakawa Y, Nelson A, et al. IL-21 enhances tumor rejection through a NKG2D-dependent mechanism. J Immunol 2005; 175: 2167–73.

73. Tarazona R, Casado JG, Soto R, et al. Expression of NK-associated receptors on cytotoxic T cells from melanoma patients: a two-edged sword? Cancer Immunol Immunother 2004; 53: 911–24.

74. Tough DF, Borrow P, Sprent J. Induction of bystander T cell proliferation by viruses and type I interferon in vivo. Science 1996; 272: 1947–50.

75. Brice GT, Graber NL, Carucci DJ, Doolan DL. Optimal induction of antigen-specific CD8+ T cell responses requires bystander cell participation. J Leukoc Biol 2002; 72: 1164–71.

76. Lertmemongkolchai G, Cai G, Hunter CA, Bancroft GJ. Bystander activation of CD8+ T cells contributes to the rapid production of IFN-gamma in response to bacterial pathogens. J Immunol 2001; 166: 1097–105.

77. Zarozinski CC, Welsh RM. Minimal bystander activation of CD8 T cells during the virus-induced polyclonal T cell response. J Exp Med 1997; 185: 1629–39.

78. Di Genova G, Savelyeva N, Suchacki A, Thirdborough SM, Stevenson FK. Bystander stimulation of activated CD4+ T cells of unrelated specificity following a booster vaccination with tetanus toxoid. Eur J Immunol 2010; 40: 976–85.

79. Sun S, Zhang X, Tough DF, Sprent J. Type I interferon-mediated stimulation of T cells by CpG DNA. J Exp Med 1998; 188: 2335–42.

80. Zhang X., Sun S, Hwang I, Tough DF, Sprent J. Potent and selective stimulation of memory-phenotype CD8+ T cells in vivo by IL-15. Immunity 1998; 8: 591–9.

81. Ramanathan S, Gagnon J, Ilangumaran S. Antigen-nonspecific activation of CD8+ T lymphocytes by cytokines: relevance to immunity, autoimmunity, and cancer. Arch Immunol Ther Exp (Warsz) 2008; 56: 311–23.

82. Ogasawara K, Lanier LL. NKG2D in NK and T cell-mediated immunity. J Clin Immunol 2005; 25: 534–40.

83. Wu J, Lanier LL. Natural killer cells and cancer. Adv Cancer Res 2003; 90: 127–56.

84. Meresse B, Chen Z, Ciszewski C, et al. Coordinated induction by IL15 of a TCR-independent NKG2D signaling pathway converts CTL into lymphokine-activated killer cells in celiac disease. Immunity 2004; 21: 357–66.

85. Ku CC, Murakami M, Sakamoto A, Kappler J, Marrack P. Control of homeostasis of CD8+ memory T cells by opposing cytokines. Science 2000; 288: 675–8.

86. Cho BK, Wang C, Sugawa S, Eisen HN, Chen J. Functional differences between memory and naive CD8 T cells. Proc Natl Acad Sci USA 1999; 96: 2976–81.

87. Ghani S, Feuerer M, Doebis C, et al. T cells as pioneers: antigen-specific T cells condition inflamed sites for high-rate antigen-non-specific effector cell recruitment. Immunology 2009; 128: e870–80.

88. Liu BL, Robinson M, Han ZQ, et al. ICP34.5 deleted herpes simplex virus with enhanced oncolytic, immune stimulating, and anti-tumour properties. Gene Ther 2003; 10: 292–303.

89. Toda M, Rabkin SD, Kojima H, Martuza RL. Herpes simplex virus as an in situ cancer vaccine for the induction of specific anti-tumor immunity. Hum Gene Ther 1999; 10: 385–93.

90. Coffin RS, Hingorani M, McNeish I, et al. Phase I/II trial of OncoVEX[GM-CSF] combined with radical chemoradiation (CRT) in patients with newly diagnosed node-positive stage III/IV head and neck cancer (HNC). Journal of Clinical Oncology, ASCO Annual Meeting Proceedings Part I 2007; 25: 14095.

91. Senzer NN, Kaufman HL, Amatruda T, et al. Phase II clinical trial of a granulocyte-macrophage colony-stimulating factor-encoding, second-generation oncolytic herpesvirus in patients with unresectable metastatic melanoma. J Clin Oncol 2009; 27: 5763–71.

92. Korn EL, Liu PY, Lee SJ, et al. Meta-analysis of phase II cooperative group trials in metastatic stage IV melanoma to determine progression-free and overall survival benchmarks for future phase II trials. J Clin Oncol 2008; 26: 527–34.

3 | Development of novel immune interventions for genito-urinary cancers

Neeraj Agarwal and Nicholas J. Vogelzang

IMMUNE SYSTEM AND CANCER

From the perspective of immunotherapy, the adaptive immune response is of more interest, since it can be instructed and taught to act against foreign antigens versus self antigens. The adaptive immune system is comprised of the antigen-presenting cells (APCs, which include dendritic cells [DCs], the most effective APCs), and CD4$^+$ and CD8$^+$ T cells (1). CD4$^+$ T cells include both helper T cells (T$_{H17}$) and regulatory T cell (T$_{REG}$) populations. APCs, such as DCs and Langerhan cells, can activate T cells by efficiently processing exogenous, as well as endogenous antigens, and present them to T cells at the plasma membrane through the major histocompatibility complex (MHC) antigen processing machinery (Fig. 3.1).

Stimulation of T cells through T-cell receptors (TCR) *alone* often results in a nonresponsive state (anergy), which results in the failure of T cells to respond to antigens, as well as becoming refractory to re-stimulation (2). Co-stimulation of other cell surface receptors on T cells is required for the avoidance of anergy and optimal T-cell activation. Among these, CD28 is the most potent co-stimulatory molecule, and is expressed at constant levels on both resting and activated T cells, and promotes T-cell proliferation, cytokine production, cell survival, and cellular metabolism. In addition to CD28, multiple other T-cell surface receptors have co-stimulatory functions, including CD2, CD5, CD30, 4-1BB, OX40 (CD134), inducible co-stimulator (ICOS), and leukocyte function-associated antigen-1. The CD28 receptor on T cells interacts with the B7 receptors (B7.1/CD80 and B7.2/CD86) on APCs. Additionally, CD28 also enhances the expression of other co-stimulatory molecules (such as ICOS, OX40, and 4-1BB), which are important for the formation of memory T cells (3). Conversely, the timely activation of negative regulatory signals in T cells is required to prevent an unduly, inappropriate immune response. The inhibitors of TCR signaling include adaptor proteins (such as Dok-1 and Dok-2), Cbl proteins (c-Cbl, Cbl-b), kinases (Csk, HPK1), phosphatases (SHP1 and Sts-1), and feedback inhibitory receptors such as cytotoxic T-lymphocyte antigen-4 (CTLA-4) and programmed death-1 (PD-1). As a negative feedback, peak expression of inhibitor receptors occurs approximately 24–48 hours after stimulation of T cells and is essential for maintaining tolerance for self antigens (2).

MECHANISMS OF IMMUNE EVASION BY CANCER

These include defective antigen presentation by APCs, immunosuppressive microenvironment and cytokines, T-cell co-inhibition, T-cell receptor dysfunction, and upregulation of regulatory T cells (4–6).

Defective Antigen Presentation

Presentation of tumor-associated antigens (TAAs) with MHC class I antigen by APCs is a crucial step for the differentiation and expansion of CD8+ cytotoxic T lymphocytes (CTLs) against TAAs and the eventual destruction of tumor cells. However, tumor cells can downregulate the expression of MHC class I antigens which allows them to escape presentation and subsequent recognition by CTLs. The diminished expression of human leukocyte antigen (HLA) class I antigens has been reported in several prostate cancer lines, as well as in primary and metastatic prostate tumors and is associated with poor prognosis in clear cell metastatic renal cell carcinoma (mRCC) (4,7–9). Furthermore, in spite of normal HLA expression, defective antigen processing by DCs can occur due to diminished expression of transporter-associated antigen processing (4,10).

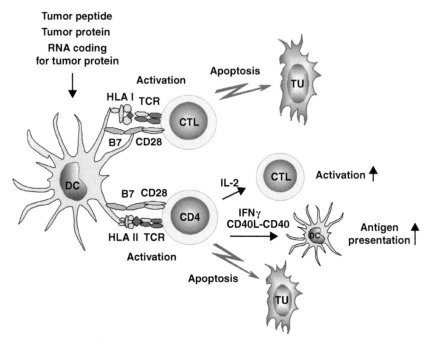

Figure 3.1 Dendritic cell (DC) based immunotherapeutic strategies for prostate cancer. DCs display a unique capacity to induce and maintain T-cell responses and have emerged as promising candidates for vaccination strategies in prostate cancer therapy. Thus, DCs are loaded with prostate cancer-associated antigen-derived peptides, protein, or RNA. Due to their high surface expression of HLA-peptide complexes and co-stimulatory molecules, DCs efficiently activate and expand CD8⁺ CTLs and CD4⁺ T cells. CD8⁺ CTLs possess a profound capability to recognize and destroy tumor cells. CD4⁺ T cells enhance the capacity of DCs to induce CTLs by the interaction between CD40 on DCs and CD40 ligand on activated CD4⁺ T cells. In addition, they provide help for the maintenance and expansion of CTLs by secreting cytokines and are able to eradicate tumor cells directly. *Abbreviations*: CTLs, cytotoxic T cells; DCs, dendritic cells; HLA, human leukocyte antigen; IL, interleukin; IFN, interferon; TCR, T cell receptor; TU, tumor cells. *Source*: Ref. 32.

Immunosuppressive Tumor Microenvironment and Cytokines

An imbalance in the production of proinflammatory (Th1) cytokines with respect to anti-inflammatory (Th2) cytokine with resulting skewing toward the Th2 response and upregulation of immunosuppressive cytokines, such as interleukin (IL)-4, IL-6, and IL-10 may promote cancer cell proliferation, as well as T-cell anergy. Higher levels of these Th2 cytokines have been reported in patients with prostate cancer, when compared with normal controls (4,11,12). Furthermore, the tumor microenvironment can promote upregulation of other immunosuppressive cytokines, such as tumor necrosis factor (TNF), transforming growth factor-beta (TGF-β), vascular endothelial growth factor (VEGF), and granulocyte monocyte colony stimulating factor (GM-CSF). These cytokines promote the accumulation of immunosuppressive, myeloid-derived suppressive cells (MDSCs), tumor-associated macrophages (TAMs), or tolerogenic DCs in the tumor microenvironment (5,13,14). Higher expression of immunosuppressive cytokines such as TGF β-1 correlates with a higher pathologic grade and stage in mRCC (15). MDSCs promote not only immunosuppression but also tumor growth by stimulating angiogenesis. Tivozanib (AV-951, AVEO Pharmaceuticals Inc., Cambridge, MA) is an orally active, ATP-competitive, small molecule that selectively inhibits VEGFR- 1, 2 and 3 tyrosine kinases. In a phase II trial of patients with advanced renal cell carcinoma (RCC) (n = 272), treatment with tivozanib was associated with an overall response rate of 25.4% and a median progression-free survival (PFS) of 11.8 months (16). However, there was a variation in sensitivity to tivozanib that impacts patient outcome. In mice, resistance to treatment with tivozanib is predicted by a 42-gene resistance signature defining a specific tumor infiltrating myeloid population. Analysis of 21 patient samples from the above-mentioned phase II trial demonstrated a significant correlation between the percent myeloid cell composition in the tumors and clinical anti-tumor activity of tivozanib (17). MDSCs also promote expansion of immunosuppressive T_{REGS} (described later). An important feature of MDSC is the overexpression of arginase 1 and eventual T-cell dysfunction. In addition, expression of arginase in MDSCs can be induced and upregulated by Th2 cytokines, such as IL-4 and IL-13. MDSCs also secrete NO, which can further promote tumor growth and induce T-cell dysfunction directly (5,18).

Upregulation of T-Cell Co-Inhibitory Signals

Optimal effector T-cell functioning requires a fine balance between T-cell co-stimulatory and T-cell co-inhibitory signals. However, in the tumor microenvironment, this balance is often skewed toward co-inhibition (19). Co-inhibitory signaling pathways such as PD-L1/PD-1 are upregulated in the prostate cancer microenvironment and are highly expressed in prostate cancer tumor infiltrating immune cells (6). More than 90% of CD8$^+$ cytotoxic T cells have been shown to express PD-1 in some patients (20). These CD8$^+$ T cells also displayed restricted T-cell receptor or TCRV-β gene uses, suggesting a limited tumor infiltration, or expansion of T-cell clones in prostate cancer, associated with upregulated PD-1 expression (6). Similarly, PD-L1 is expressed by RCC tumor cells and is associated with poor prognosis independent of other risk factors (21). Among other co-inhibitory molecules, the B7 family has been recognized to play an important role in downregulating immunity against prostate cancer. B7x, upon binding with receptors on activated T cells, downregulates T-cell proliferation and activation (6,19). Overexpression of B7x and related co-inhibitory ligand B7-H3 is also associated with a higher risk of invasive disease, metastases, and recurrence in prostate and renal cell carcinomas (22–24).

Upregulation of Regulatory T Cells

Normally, (T_{REGS}) comprise 5–10% of the peripheral CD4$^+$ T-cell population (25). The key role of T_{REGS} is to inhibit cytotoxic T-cell response against self antigens and maintain peripheral T-cell tolerance to self antigens (26). T_{REGS} constitutively express CD25 (IL-2 receptor α chain) on their cell surface and suppress CD4$^+$ and CD8$^+$ effector T cells through the release of immunosuppressive cytokines, consumption of IL-2, and direct cell-to cell contact. An increased number of T_{REGS} in peripheral blood as well as in the tumor infiltrate has been reported in various human cancers, including prostate cancer, and is associated with reduced survival. The blocking of the T_{REGS} (CD4$^+$, CD25$^+$ T cells) using an anti-CD25 monoclonal antibody is known to reduce prostate cancer growth in mice (4,5,25). Sunitinib decreases T_{REGS} and improves type-1 T-cell cytokine response in mRCC patients while reducing T_{REG} function which may be an additional mechanism of its anti-tumor effect in mRCC (27).

RATIONALE FOR IMMUNOTHERAPY IN GENITOURINARY CANCERS

Spontaneous remissions in mRCC occasionally occur after removal of primary RCC, particularly in the lungs (28,29). This provided the rationale for testing various immunotherapeutic strategies in mRCC. Among these, the immunomodulatory cytokines, IL-2, and interferon alpha (IFNα) were found to be associated with clinically relevant antitumor activities. This led to the establishment of high-dose IL-2 therapy as the standard of care for mRCC in patients with good organ function, in the 1990s.

On the other hand, immunotherapy with modified autologous DCs pulsed with tumor antigen has recently been approved for the treatment of prostate cancer, which provides an appropriate setting for vaccine-based therapies for many reasons (30). First, prostate cancer is a relatively slow growing cancer with a long natural history, which provides a period of opportunity for vaccine therapy to generate an optimal anti-tumor immune response. Second, prostate cancer expresses several tumor-associated antigens, such as prostate specific antigen (PSA), prostatic acid phosphatase (PAP), and prostate specific membrane antigen (PSMA), each of which has been used for the development of vaccines. Third, because of the expendable nature of the prostate as an organ and the immune response generated against prostate tissue, immunotherapy is not a significant health concern. Fourth, because of a reliable tumor marker such as PSA, metastatic prostate cancer is often diagnosed very early, thus providing the opportunity for employment of immunotherapy in the presence of minimal residual disease, when the immunosuppressive effects of the tumor are relatively milder.

IMMUNOTHERAPEUTIC APPROACHES IN GENITOURINARY CANCERS

Traditionally, cancer immunotherapy has been categorized into passive immunotherapy, when the immunotherapeutic agent has direct anti-tumor effects, and active immunotherapy, where the immunotherapeutic agent induces a host anti-tumor immune response. Both the active and passive immunotherapy can further be classified into a nonspecific therapy, where the immunotherapeutic agent induces a generalized upregulation of the host immune system, or a specific immunotherapy, where the immune activation is targeted toward a specific tumor-associated antigen (31). Several active immunotherapy-based approaches (both specific and nonspecific) have been tested in prostate and renal cell carcinomas, some of which have advanced to mature stages of clinical development and are reviewed in this chapter.

Dendritic Cell Vaccines

DCs are professional APCs and are critical for the induction of adoptive immune response against tumor antigens. In vivo activation and maturation of DCs is induced by several tumor-derived molecules such as heat shock proteins, high-mobility-group box 1 protein, and inflammatory cytokines derived from immune cells populating the tumor microenvironment (32). In vitro, mature DCs can be generated by exposing multipotent CD34+ hematopoietic progenitor cells, first to stem cell factor and Flt3 ligand (FL), and second to GM-CSF, IL-4, and TNF-α, or by exposing myeloid progenitor CD14+ cells to GM-CSF and IL-4, which can then be pulsed with the TAA (33) with an objective of enabling them to present both MHC-I- and MHC-II-derived TAA on their cell surface. During this process, DCs can be pulsed with tumor antigens which are then phagocytosed, processed, and presented by the DCs to the CTLs in the context of MHC machinery. Although a successful and widely utilized strategy is to use peptides or fusion protein to pulse DCs in vitro, clinical trials employing m-RNA encoding TAAs to transfect DCs or using tumor lysates to pulse DCs have been reported in prostate cancer (34) and RCC (35,36).

Dendritic Cell-Based Vaccine in Prostate Cancer and Sipuleucel-T

Significant advancements in the development of vaccines, based on DC modified to enhance the presentation of tumor antigens to CTLs, have been made in last two decades. This has culminated in the recent approval of sipuleucel-T (Provenge®, APC8015, Dendreon Corp., Seattle, WA) which consists of autologous APCs enriched for a CD54+ DC fraction harvested by leukapheresis and cultured with a fusion protein (PA2024) comprising of PAP and GM-CSF (8,37). In a phase III trial (IMmunotherapy Prostate AdenoCarcinoma Treatment trial) 512 men with asymptomatic chemo-naive metastatic castration refractory prostate cancer (CRPC) were randomized in a 2:1 ratio to sipuleucel-T or placebo (38). The primary and secondary end points of the IMPACT trial were overall survival and PFS, respectively. The median overall survival was significantly improved in the sipuleucel-T group, when compared with the placebo group (25.8 months vs. 21.7 months, hazard ratio, 0.77; p = 0.02), with a relative reduction of 22% in the risk of death in the

Table 3.1 Adjuvant Immunotherapy Trial in RCC

	Study	Treatment	Eligibility	Design	End Points	Results
1	Clark et al. (39) (n = 69)	One course of high-dose IL-2 or observation	Locally advanced (LA; T3b-4 or N1-3) or metastatic (M1) RCC, no prior systemic therapy, and excellent organ function	1:1 randomized, phase III	DFS	No difference in DFS
2	Messing et al. (40) (n = 283)	IFN α-NL (Wellferon, Burroughs-Wellcome, Durham, NC) given daily for 5 days every 3 wks for up to 12 cycles or observation	Pathologic stage T3-4a and/or node-positive disease after radical nephrectomy and lymphadenectomy	1:1 randomized, phase III	OS and DFS	No difference in OS or DFS
3	Pizzocaro et al. (41) (n = 247)	Recombinant IFN α-2b 6 million IU, IM 3 times per week for 6 mo	Pathologic stages II and III RCC (1987 tumor-node-metastasis categories T3aN0M0 and T3bN0M0 or T2/3N1-3M0)	1:1 randomized, phase III	OS and DFS	No difference
4	Jocham et al. (42) (n = 558)[a]	Autologous tumor vaccine, Reniale® (LipoNova, Hannover, Germany); 6 intradermal applications at 4-wk intervals postoperatively or observation	Pathologic stage T2-3b pN0-3 M0RCC	1:1 randomized, phase III	DFS	5-year PFS rate 77.4% vs. 67.8% in vaccine vs. control group respectively (p = 0.0204)[b]
5	Wood et al. (43) (n = 728)	Vitespen a heat-shock protein (glycoprotein 96)-peptide complex derived from autologous tumors; intradermally once a week for 4 wks, then every 2 wk until vaccine depletion	Clinical stage T1b-T4 N0 M0, or Tany N1-2 M0, prior to radical nephrectomy	1:1 randomized, phase III	DFS	No difference

[a]379 patients were assessable for the intention-to-treat analysis.
[b]In an updated analysis, patients with pT3 stage RCC revealed 5- and 10-year OS rates of 71.3 and 53.6% in the study group and 65.4 and 36.2% in the control group (p = 0.022) (44).
Abbreviations: DFS, disease-free survival; RCC, renal-cell carcinoma; OS, overall survival.

sipuleucel-T group (hazard ratio 0.78; p = 0.03). Notably, the time to objective disease progression was similar in both groups. Thus, overall survival was improved without any measurable anti-tumor effect. Antibody response against the immunizing antigen PA2024 was observed in 66% of patients in the sipuleucel-T group and 3% in the placebo group. It is interesting to note that while both T-cell and antibody responses to sipuleucel-T were observed, only antibody responses were associated with an extension of survival. Majority of adverse events were mild to moderate and included chills, fever, fatigue, nausea, and headache. Notably, the survival benefit of sipuleucel-T was observed consistently across the subgroup of patients, including those with adverse prognostic factors, such as increased levels of PSA, lactate dehydrogenase, and alkaline phosphatase, as well as increased number of bone metastases, increased Gleason score, decreased performance status, and the presence of pain. Subsequently, sipuleucel-T was approved by the Food and Drug Administration (FDA) on April 29, 2010 for the treatment of patients with symptomatic or minimally asymptomatic CRPC.

Strategies using treatment with DCs transfected with tumor RNA have also been shown to be safe and feasible in prostate cancer and are capable of stimulating the expansion of tumor-specific, polyclonal T cells in immunized patients (32). Multiple early phase studies have shown that vaccines, using RNA from autologous or allogeneic tumor cells to transfect autologous DCs, induced a cytotoxic T-cell response, and in many instances PSA responses (34,45,46).

Dendritic Cell–Based Vaccines in mRCC

In a nonrandomized study, 27 patients with progressive cytokine-refractory mRCC were treated with DCs pulsed with either a cocktail of survivin and telomerase peptides (in HLA-A2 positive) or tumor lysate (in HLA-A2 negative), along with concomitant low-dose IL-2. Although, there were no objective responses, almost half the patients (13/27) had stable disease for >8 weeks and of these, 30% had disease stability for >6 months. In patients who were HLA-A2 negative and who attained the stage of stable disease during treatment, a spontaneous predominance of Th1-secreting tumor lysate-specific T cells was observed prior to vaccination, whereas patients with continued progressive disease had a mixed Th1/Th2 response, suggesting pre-vaccination cytokine levels to be predictors of response to subsequent vaccinations (36,47).

In mRCC, treatment with DCs transfected with tumor RNA has also been shown to be safe and feasible, and stimulated expansion of tumor-specific, polyclonal T cells. In a phase I trial, 10 patients with metastatic RCC were treated with DCs transfected with their renal tumor RNA. No vaccine-related adverse effects, including autoimmunity, were seen. In six of the seven evaluable subjects, the expansion of tumor-specific T cells was detected after immunization. These T cells were reactive against a broad set of renal tumor-associated antigens, including telomerase reverse transcriptase, G250, and oncofetal antigens, but not against self antigens expressed by normal renal tissues. Although most patients underwent secondary therapies after vaccination, tumor-related mortality was unexpectedly low, with only 3 of 10 patients dying from disease after a mean followup of 19.8 months (35). In a subsequent phase I study by the same group, immuno-stimulatory efficacy of RNA-transfected DCs was further enhanced when patients underwent a prior depletion of T_{REGS} by treatment with the recombinant IL-2 diphtheria toxin conjugate DAB_{389} IL-2 (denileukin diftitox/ONTAK, Eisai Inc, Woodcliff Lake, NJ) (48). Denileukin diftitox is a fusion protein consisting of full length IL-2 fused to the enzymatically active and translocating domain of diphtheria toxin, which allows for the targeting of CD25 expressing cells. After internalization into the cytoplasm of the CD25 expressing cells, diphtheria toxin is released intracellularly leading to an inhibition of protein synthesis (5,48).

In vivo presentation of tumor antigens by autologous DCs can be further enhanced by the manipulation of CD40L/CD40 pathway or by the use of growth factors such as FL.

Enhancement of CD40L/CD40 Pathway

The CD40 receptor is a member of the TNF receptor superfamily and is expressed on a variety of normal cells, such as B cells; macrophages; DCs; epithelial, stromal, endothelial cells and platelets (49). The ligand for CD40 (CD40L) is expressed on activated CD4[+] helper T cells and platelets. The binding of the CD40L to the CD40 receptor on DCs promotes expression of MHC and co-stimulatory molecules and stimulates the production of proinflammatory cytokines, such as IL-2, and migration of DCs to regional lymph nodes, following antigen exposure and induction of T cell activation, all of which are essential to cell-mediated immune responses (49).

Mature DCs presenting TAAs can initiate productive anti-tumor T cell responses. However, in the tumor microenvironment, DCs often become tolerogenic after being exposed to tumor-derived immunosuppressive factors, such as VEGF, TGFb, IL-6, and IL-10 (50). These tolerogenic DCs tend to anergize T cells and prevent them from mounting an anti-tumor response. Interventions targeted toward ligand-dependent or ligand-independent activation of CD40 receptors have the potential to overcome the tolerogenicity of the DCs, and promote an effective cell-mediated response against TAAs.

The systemic administration of agonist anti-CD40 Abs in mice leads to the maturation of DCs, without binding with CD40L. In a phase I study, treatment with a CD40 agonist monoclonal Ab (CP-870,893) was well tolerated, biologically active, and was associated with anti-tumor activity. The most common adverse event was cytokine release syndrome (grade 1 to 2), which included chills, rigors, and fever (51). Other studies with recombinant soluble CD40L protein, and CD40L-expressing autologous tumor cells showed similar results (50). However, systemic activation of CD40 could potentially induce autoimmuity, as is evident from the increased CD40 signaling in several autoimmune diseases. This problem can be circumvented by CD40 ligation in the tumor microenvironment. A novel strategy to achieve this is to engineer tumor-reactive T cells, which deliver stimulatory signals to DCs in the tumor microenvironment (50). In a transgenic adenocarcinoma of mouse prostate (TRAMP) model, tumor-reactive CD8[+] T cells were used to deliver the CD40L signal to activate tolerogenic DCs. Most of the cytoplasmic domain of CD40L was deleted to increase the level and duration of CD40L expression on the surface of CD8[+] T cells. These tumor-reactive CD8[+] T cells expressed the truncated form of CD40L and stimulated the maturation of DCs in vitro and in vivo in prostate draining lymph nodes. The anti-tumor CD8[+] T cell response was further enhanced if TRAMP mice were also immunized with a tumor-specific antigen (50).

Drug-inducible CD40 (iCD40) is a ligand-independent approach to enhance CD40 signaling in DCs. In iCD40, CD40 is reengineered by fusing the cytoplasmic domain of CD40 to drug-binding domains, allowing it to respond to the lipid-permeable, high-affinity dimerizer drug, AP20187. Administration of AP20187, a chemical inducer of dimerization in mice, led to a prolonged ligand-independent induction of CD40-dependent signaling cascades, while circumventing ectodomain-dependent negative-feedback mechanisms. Furthermore, the iCD40-mediated DC activation exceeded that achieved by stimulating the full-length, endogenous CD40 receptor, both in vitro and in vivo. Because iCD40 is insulated from the extracellular environment and can be activated within the context of an immunological synapse, iCD40-expressing DCs have a prolonged lifespan and should lead to more potent vaccines, possibly even in immune compromised patients (52,53).

Treatment with Recombinant Human Flt3 Ligand

Flt3 ligand (FL) is a growth factor for early hematopoietic progenitor cells. Treatment with recombinant FL produces high concentrations of circulating, functionally competent, human DCs, both in healthy volunteers and in patients with metastatic colon cancer (54). In a phase I study, treatment of patients with castration refractory nonmetastatic prostate cancer with recombinant FL, was well tolerated and associated with a remarkable increase in the number of peripheral blood DCs. Although, overall PSA levels remained unchanged with FL treatment,

11 of 33 treated patients had a decrease or only a minor increase (<25%) in PSA. The median relative velocity was significantly less in patients after FL treatment (54).

Vaccines with Viral Vectors

The use of viruses as vehicles to deliver tumor antigens in to the APCs in vivo is a very promising strategy for many reasons. The inherent immunogenicity of the virus leads to a strong inflammatory response, directed against the viral protein. This inflammatory response in turn may lead to an improved immune response against the tumor antigens being expressed by the virus itself (55). This immune response is further enhanced by the high level of gene expression seen with viral vectors. Other factors in favor of a viral-based vaccine include the relative ease to engineer viral vectors and their ability to carry a large amount of genetic material. Poxviral vectors are utilized the most in the vaccines. The prototype is the vaccinia virus, which has been used worldwide in the eradication of smallpox (56,57). The poxvirus family is composed of double-stranded DNA viruses that do not integrate with the host cell genome, and instead replicate within the cytoplasm of infected cells. The host immune response to the vaccinia virus leads to strong neutralizing antibody titers, following which a proportion of these undergoes cell death. Cellular debris, including the encoded antigen (such as PSA) is then taken up by infiltrating APCs, which in turn present the antigens to helper and cytotoxic T cells in a proinflammatory atmosphere. Another way poxvirus vectors can induce an immune response is the direct infection of APCs, such as Langerhan cells, present in the skin. A major limitation of poxvirus-based vectors is the rapid appearance of strong neutralizing antibodies against the vaccinia vector. This renders a booster vaccination using the same virus (*homologous* prime/ boost vaccination) ineffective, as the antibody response to viral proteins dominates over the intended response to encoded antigens (such as PSA) (56,58). This can be circumvented by using avipox viral vectors encoding the same antigens as the booster vaccination (*heterologous* prime/boost vaccination). The avipox virus is a family of pox viruses that infects birds and does not replicate in mammalian cells. Since infections with avipox viruses do not produce new virions, the degree of neutralizing antibodies which are generated, following mammalian infection, is quite low. This allows avipox viral particles to persist for a longer period of time and to express foreign transgenes, resulting in a significantly enhanced T-cell immunity. Further studies in the animal models suggested that heterologous prime/boost vaccination schedules using two different poxvirus vectors (i.e., vaccinia vector followed by avipox vector), expressing tumor antigens and co-stimulatory factors induced stronger immune responses against foreign antigens compared with single-agent immunization protocols. An example of heterologous prime/boost vaccination strategy is Prostvac®-VF (Therion Biologics Corporation, Cambridge, MA), which comprises two recombinant viral vectors (vaccinia vector and fowlpox vector), each encoding transgenes for PSA and TRICOM. TRICOM consists of three co-stimulatory molecules, including ICAM (intercellular addition molecules)-1 (CD54), B7.1 (CD80), and leukocyte function-associated antigen-3 (CD58). Preclinical studies demonstrated TRICOM to be superior compared with a transgene containing only one or two of the co-stimulatory molecules (33).

In a recently reported double-blind randomized phase II trial of patients with chemonaïve, minimally symptomatic metastatic CRPC, 82 patients received Prostvac-VF and 40 received control vectors. PFS was similar in both groups (hazard ratio, 0.884; 95% CI, 0.568 to 01.375, p=0.56) and originally, the trial was reported as negative. However, at three years post study, patients treated with Prostvac-VF were found to have significantly improved overall survival (25.1 vs. 16.6 months, p=0.0061), a better 3-year survival (30% vs. 17%), and a 44% reduction in death rate. Based on these encouraging results, multiple clinical trials have been planned in various stages of prostate cancer including a large phase III registrational study (59).

In mRCC, the modified vaccinia Ankara (MVA) engineered to express the tumor antigen 5T4 (TroVax) showed encouraging results (60). In a phase II study, MVA-5T4 vaccine administered alone or in combination with IFNα-2b was safe and well tolerated. Of the 23 intent-to-treat patients tested for immune responses, 22 (96%) mounted 5T4-specific antibody and/or cellular responses, post vaccination. One patient treated with MVA-5T4, plus IFNα, had a partial response for >7 months, whereas an additional 14 patients (7 receiving MVA-5T4 plus IFN and 7 receiving MVA-5T4 alone) showed periods of disease stabilization, ranging from 1.73 to 9.60 months. Median PFS and overall survival were 3.8 months (range: 1–11.47 mo) and 12.1 months (range 1–27 months), respectively (60). Encouraging results were also seen in a phase II study using a pox viral vector expressing MUC1 antigen (TG4010 vaccine) in patients with breast, kidney, prostate, and lung cancers, warranting further investigation (61).

DNA-Based Vaccines

DNA-based vaccines provide an additional avenue for cancer immunotherapy and comprise naked DNA plasmids encoding specific tumor antigens. The primary advantage is the ease and preciseness with which DNA can be synthesized and target selected antigens (56). However, because of the absence of a concurrent inflammatory response seen with viral vaccines, DNA-based vaccines are poorly immunogenic. Another disadvantage is the low level of in vivo infection of APCs by these vaccines (30,56). Several approaches have been developed to circumvent the poor immunogenicity of DNA-based vaccines and include multiple immunizations, simultaneous administration of cytokines (GM-CSF or IL-2) (62), concomitant use of plasmids encoding non-self antigens (i.e. hepatitis B surface antigen) (63), modification of the plasmid-encoded antigens (64), and improved delivery system (gene gun, cationic liposomes) (55,65). Several phase I and II clinical trials using DNA-based vaccines targeting PSA and PAP have been reported in patients with prostate cancer (66,67). In a phase I trial, nine patients with CRPC were treated with a plasmid vector carrying a gene coding for the full-length human PSA protein (pVAX/PSA). The objectives were to assess the feasibility, safety, and immunogenicity of DNA vaccines at three different dose levels. Patients also received GM-CSF and IL-2 as vaccine adjuvants. Of the eight evaluated patients, a PSA-specific cellular immune response (measured by IFNγ production against recombinant PSA protein) and a rising anti-PSA IgG, were detected in two of three patients in the highest dose cohort (66). In another phase I/II trial, 22 patients with castration-sensitive prostate cancer with biochemical recurrence only were treated with plasmid DNA encoding PAP at three different dose levels, along with GM-CSF as a vaccine adjuvant (67). Patients received six immunizations delivered at 2-week intervals and were followed for one year; 3/22 patients (14%) developed PAP-specific IFNγ-secreting CD8+ T cells immediately after the treatment course, and 9/22 patients (41%) developed PAP-specific CD4+ and/or CD8+ T-cell proliferation. No antibody response to PAP was detected. The median serum PSA doubling time increased from 6.5 months in the pretreatment phase to 8.5 months during treatment (p = 0.033) and 9.3 months in the one year post-treatment followup (P = 0.054).

Messenger RNA–Based Vaccine

Messenger RNA (mRNA) has emerged as a promising alternative in the field of nonviral gene delivery (68). This strategy has several advantages over naked plasmid DNA and viral vector-based vaccines: (i) the nuclear membrane, which is a major obstacle for plasmid DNA, is avoided because mRNA exerts its function in the cytoplasm; (ii) there is no risk of insertional mutagenesis; (iii) there is no need for determination and use of an efficient promoter; (iv) it allows repeated application; (v) there is increased effectiveness of mRNA in nondividing cells, and (vi) it avoids vector-induced immunogenicity. Other advantages are the ease of producing mRNA in large amounts with very high purity and lack of induction of antibodies (69). In addition, the same mRNA molecule not only provides an antigen source for adaptive immunity but can simultaneously bind to pattern recognition receptors, thus stimulating innate immunity. Vaccination with mRNA can be achieved by several delivery methods: (i) the direct injection of naked mRNA, (ii) the injection of mRNA encapsulated in liposomes, (iii) the gene gun delivery of mRNA loaded on gold beads, or (*iv*) in vitro transfection of the mRNA in cells, followed by reinjection of cells (described in the section, "DC-Based Vaccines") (69).

CV9103 (CureVac GmbH, Tübingen, Germany) is an mRNA-based vaccine that encodes for four PSAs, three of which are membrane bound. The preliminary results of a phase I/II study were recently reported, in which 44 patients with metastatic CRPC were treated with CV9103. CV9103 was shown to be safe, well tolerated, and biologically active. Over 70% of the study patients responded to at least one out of the four CV9103 antigens (70).

Peptide-Based Vaccines

Advantages of peptide-based vaccines are (*i*) faster and more cost-effective production, storage, and distribution; (*ii*) the ability to select specific TAA as targets by the vaccine, and (*iii*) avoidance of self-antigens capable of generating autoimmune response (55). Disadvantages are (*i*) weak immunogenicity of a single protein or, especially, a single epitope; (*ii*) the possibility of tumor escape from immune recognition through antigen mutation or loss; (*iii*) restricted use of HLAs (mainly for epitope-based vaccines), (*iv*) limitation to a subset of patients (usually HLA-A2+), and (*v*) the poor ability to induce balanced activation of CD4 and CD8 subsets, which is believed to be essential for effective, long-lasting anti-tumor immunity (55). Heat shock protein (HSP gp96) and MUC1 glycoprotein are expressed differently in RCC and prostate cancer, respectively and are targets of peptide-based vaccine strategies.

Vitespen (HSPPC-96, Oncophage; Antigenics Inc., New York, NY) is a heat-shock protein (glycoprotein 96) peptide complex derived from autologous tumors (71). In mice, vitespen has shown a high degree of effectiveness for micrometastatic disease, and less so for progressively growing tumors (72). In phase I and II trials, treatment with vitespen has been shown to be safe and feasible in melanoma, colorectal cancer, RCC, and glioma; encouraging signals of clinical activity and tumor-specific immune response seen in a phase III melanoma trial (73). This led to a phase III randomized study to compare adjuvant therapy with vitespen to observation, in patients with RCC at a high risk of recurrence post nephrectomy (of 728 patients, 361 received vitespen). There was no difference in the recurrence-free survival (the primary endpoint) in the ITT population. However, in a predefined exploratory analysis of recurrence-free survival, by American Joint Committee on Cancer stage, fewer patients with early-stage (stage I or II) RCC who received vitespen recurred, compared with the observation group, although this difference was not statistically significant (hazard ratio 0·576, 95% CI 0·324–1·023; p = 0·056) (73) (Table 3.1).

MUC1 is a type 1 glycoprotein and is overexpressed on various tumors, including lung and prostate cancer, making it an excellent target for immunotherapy (55). Stimuvax (Oncothyreon Inc., Seattle, WA) consists of MUC1 lipopetide BLP25, an immunoadjuvant monophosphoryl lipid A, and three lipids (cholesterol, dimyristoyl phosphatidylglycerol, and dipalmitoyl phosphatidylcholine), forming a liposomal product. It is designed to induce a cellular immune response that may lead to immune rejection of tumor tissues that express MUC1 antigen (74). Early-phase trials in lung cancer have shown encouraging results and Stimuvax holds promise in the treatment of prostate cancer, as well (55).

Tumor Cell–Based Immunotherapy

Tumor cells themselves are poorly immunogenic and do not induce effective immune response. However, tumor cells can be engineered to express proinflammatory cytokines or administered with adjuvants to improve anti-tumor immune response (75). In theory, simultaneous administration of proinflammatory cytokines such as GM-CSF or adjuvants such as BCG, improves the presentation of tumor associated antigens though recruitment and maturation of DCs at the injection site. DCs then migrate to the lymph nodes and activate antigen-specific CD4+ T cells. Furthermore, using the whole cell instead of a specific antigen or peptide provides the advantage of presentation of a large number of tumor antigens simultaneously with the potential to induce a more generalized cytotoxic T-cell response against multiple antigens (56).

Although both autologous and allogeneic tumor cells have been used, the advantage of using allogeneic tumor cell lines is their easy availability, unlike autologous tumor cells which are difficult to obtain in large numbers.

This strategy is exemplified by prostate-GVAX (Cell Genesys, South San Francisco, CA), which consists of two irradiated allogeneic human prostate cancer cell lines, LNCaP and PC-3, genetically modified to secrete GM-CSF. This genetic modification is achieved by in vitro trans-duction of these tumor cells with an adeno-associated viral vector encoding the human GM-CSF gene (55). After encouraging clinical and immunological responses in five phase I and II trials with approximately 200 prostate cancer patients, two phase III trials of GVAX, VITAL-1, and VITAL-2 respectively were initiated (55). VITAL-1 trial randomized 626 CRPC patients without pain to either GVAX monotherapy for up to six months or standard docetaxel/predni-sone therapy and completed accrual in 2007. Primary end point was overall survival. VITAL-2 was designed to evaluate the efficacy of GVAX plus docetaxel in comparison with that of docetaxel/prednisone in metastatic CRPC patients with pain. In this case also, the primary endpoint was the overall survival. Disappointingly, after accrual of 408 patients, VITAL-2 trial was terminated prematurely after a safety review which revealed an imbalance in deaths, with 67 deaths in the GVAX/docetaxel arm and 47 deaths in the standard arm and a shorter median survival in the GVAX/docetaxel arm (12.2 vs. 14.1 months, $p = 0.0076$). Subsequently, an unplanned futility analysis of the VITAL-1 trial indicated <30% chance of meeting the primary endpoint, following which VITAL-1, despite having completed the accrual of 626 patients, was also terminated (33,55). Owing to these negative results, further development of GVAX in pros-tate cancer has become uncertain.

An example of an autologous tumor vaccine is Reniale (LipoNova, Hannover, Germany), which is prepared with the lysate of autologous renal tumor cells, preincubated with IFNγ and tocopherol acetate. The incubation of renal carcinoma cells with IFN leads to the increased expression of not only MHC class I and II but also of ICAM1 (intercellular adhesion molecule 1), transporter associated with antigen processing 1, and LMP2 (low molecular weight peptide), thus increasing the antigenicity of these cells. Tocopherol acetate, a lipid-soluble radical-scavenging agent, protects the inner and outer cell membranes during the incubation process with IFNγ (76). Between January 1997 and September 1998, 558 patients with a localized RCC who were scheduled for radical nephrectomy, were randomized to receive adjuvant therapy with Reniale or no adjuvant treatment (control group). The primary endpoint was PFS (77). Of the 379 patients assessable for the intent-to-treat analysis, the five-year PFS rate for patients of all tumor stages was 77·4% in the vaccine group and 67·8% in the control group ($p = 0·0204$). The vaccine was well tolerated, with only 12 treatment-associated adverse events reported.

Interestingly, in a subset analysis, there was an even more remarkable difference in the five-year PFS, favoring vaccine in the T3 group (67·5% vs. 49·7%). This suggests that there is a higher risk group, who could potentially derive a greater benefit from the adjuvant vaccine therapy (76,77). Methodological problems with this study were (*i*) a high number of patients lost after initial randomization (174/553, 32%), (*ii*) the imbalance of this loss (99 from the Reniale arm and 75 from the placebo arm), and (*iii*) the absence of tabulation of overall survival (77). Nonetheless, these data point toward beneficial effects of adjuvant vaccine therapy in patients with localized RCC of more than 2.5 cm in diameter.

Blockade of Immune Checkpoints

Multiple co-stimulatory and co-inhibitory pathways in T cells work in tandem to ensure optimal T-cell response against a foreign antigen, while simultaneously protecting self antigens from immune recognition. Many co-inhibitory pathways are known to be present and upregulated in the tumor microenvironment and are known to attenuate cytotoxic T-cell response against tumor antigens. These include pathways that are mediated through CTLA-4, PD-1, B7-H3, or B7x. In addition, blocking the CD25 receptor on T_{REGS} is another avenue, which can be exploited to downregulate T_{REG} cells (CD4+, CD25+), in order to optimize cytotoxic T-cell response.

Blockade of CTLA-4 Signaling

Cytotoxic T lymphocyte antigen 4 (CTLA-4) is a key negative regulator of T-cell responses, inhibits recognition of self antigens by T cells, and can downregulate the antitumor immune response. Ipilimumab (MDX-010, Bristol-Myers Squibb, New York, NY) and tremelimumab (CP-675206, Pfizer, New York, NY) are fully human, monoclonal antibodies against CTLA-4 and have reached advanced phases of clinical trials in cancer therapy (78). Ipilimumab was recently reported to significantly improve the overall survival rate in patients with metastatic melanoma in a phase III trial. Notably, in this group of heavily pretreated patients, ipilimumab, compared with the peptide vaccine, showed a near doubling of the rates of survival at 12 months (46% vs. 25%) and 24 months (24% vs. 14%) (79). This led to the FDA approval of the agent for metastatic melanoma in March 2011. Many phase I and phase II clinical trials have been conducted in patients with prostate cancer with ipilimumab with objective clinical responses and PSA responses being described (80,81) (Table 3.2). Based on these encouraging results, phase III clinical trials of ipilimumab versus placebo have been initiated in men with castration refractory metastatic prostate cancer, with or without prior exposure to chemotherapy with results expected in near future (87,88).

Blockade of PD-1/PD-L1 Pathway

Interaction between (PD-1) receptor and its ligand PD-L1 (also known as B7-H1) leads to the inhibition of T-cell function (56). Blockade of this pathway is associated with anti-tumor immune response being encouraged in animal models (89,90). Unlike early lethality in CTLA-4 knockout mice, PD-1-deficient animals demonstrate a mild form of late-onset strain-specific autoimmunity (20). B7-H1 has been shown to be upregulated in a variety of human tumors and is associated with poor clinical outcomes (91). The presence of PD-1 and PD-L1 in the prostate cancer microenvironment provides a rationale for the blockade of the PD-1 pathway in prostate cancer immunotherapy. Results of a phase I study of fully human monoclonal antibody targeting PD-1, MDX-1106 (Bristol-Myers Squibb-936558) was reported in 39 patients with advanced solid tumors (92). This included patients with colorectal cancer (N=14), melanoma (N=10), prostate cancer (N=8), non-small-cell lung cancer (N=6), and RCC (N=1). MDX-1106 binds PD-1 with high affinity, promotes tumor antigen-specific T-cell proliferation and secretion of cytokines in vitro. Patients received MD-1106 in four escalating dose cohorts of 0.3–10 mg/kg and an expansion cohort of 10 mg/kg. Median age was 62 years. MDX-1106 was remarkably well tolerated and the maximum tolerated dose was not defined in the study. One serious adverse event, inflammatory colitis, was observed in a patient with metastatic ocular melanoma, following five doses of MDX-1106 (1 mg/kg) administered over eight months, and responded to steroids and infliximab. One durable complete response (in colorectal cancer) and two partial responses (in melanoma and RCC, respectively) were seen. Although no objective responses were seen in any patients with prostate cancer, it is too early to rule out the role of PD-1 blockade in the treatment of prostate cancer. Especially, given its remarkable tolerability, blockade of the PD-1 pathway remains a very promising therapy in combination with other immunotherapeutic approaches. Several clinical trials using the blockade mechanism of PD-1 are ongoing with results expected in the near future.

Depletion of T-Regulatory Cells by Targeting CD25

The physiologic role of T_{REGS} (CD4+, CD25+) is to inhibit cytotoxic T cells from mounting an immune response against self antigens. Since tumor antigens largely comprise of self antigens, T_{REGS} may inhibit cytotoxic T cells from mounting an immune response against tumor-associated antigens. Depletion of T_{REGS}, using anti-CD25 antibodies in mice, improves anti-tumor immune response (48,93). Furthermore, anti-CD25 therapy improves the therapeutic efficacy of GM-CSF-secreting B16 tumor cells in animals (94). These data provide the rationale for using anti-CD25 therapy to deplete T_{REGS} prior to cancer vaccine therapy. Recently, depletion of T_{REGS} using denileukin diftitox was reported to be capable of enhancing a vaccine-induced T-cell response in patients with advanced RCC (see section "Dendritic

Table 3.2 Ipilimumab trials in prostate cancer

	Study	Treatment	Eligibility	Design	End points	Results
1	Fong et al. (82) (n = 24)	Ipilimumab with GM-CSF (day 1–14)	Metastatic, castration-resistant chemotherapy naïve prostate cancer	Phase I escalating doses of ipilimumab (0.5 mg/kg to 3 mg/kg) with a fixed dose of GM-CSF	Safety	3 of 6 patients in the highest dose cohort (3 mg/kg) experienced a PSA response (>50%)
2	Small et al. (83) (n = 14)	Ipilimumab	Metastatic CRPC (prior chemotherapy allowed)	Phase I: ipilimumab given at a fixed dose of 3 mg/kg	Safety	2 of 14 showed a PSA response (>50%)
3	Tollefson et al. (84) (n = 108)	AA or AA with Ipilimumab	Unresectable prostate cancer (castration sensitive)	1:1 randomized, phase II	Safety, PSA and clinical response	Patients treated with ipilimumab and AA were more likely to have an undetectable PSA by 3 mo (55% vs. 38%)
4	Slovin et al. (85) (n = 45)	Ipilimumab (IPI) 10 mg/kg q3 wks × 4 in 3 groups: (1) IPI alone n = 16, (2) IPI + XRT n = 15 chemotherapy naïve, and (3) IPI + XRT n = 14 chemotherapy experienced	Metastatic CRPC	Randomized phase III	Safety and efficacy	10 of 45 patients (22%) had a PSA response (≥50%)
5	Gerritsen et al. (86) (n = 28)	Ipilimumab (escalating doses of 0.3, 1, 3, or 5 mg/kg) with GVAX	Metastatic CRPC (chemonaive)	Phase I: dose escalation (n = 12), dose expansion (n = 16)	Safety	6 of 28 patients had a PSA response (>50%)

cell-based vaccines in mRCC") (48). In this study, denileukin diftitox treatment resulted in selective elimination of T_{REGS} from peripheral blood in a dose-dependent manner and without apparent bystander toxicity to other cellular subsets with intermediate or low expression of CD25. T_{REG} cell depletion resulted in enhanced stimulation of proliferative and cytotoxic T-cell responses in vitro, but only when denileukin diftitox was used prior to, and omitted during the T-cell priming phase. In these six patients with mRCC, depletion of T_{REG} cells, followed by vaccination with tumor RNA-transfected DCs, led to improved stimulation of tumor-specific T cells when compared with vaccination alone (48). In a pilot study, 18 patients with mRCC were treated with a combination therapy of high-dose IL-2 and denileukin diftitox (95). There was a significant improvement in the peak absolute lymphocyte count and a decrease in T_{REGS} compared to a historical control of 15 patients treated with high-dose IL-2 alone. An encouraging overall response rate of 33% was noted. These results support that denileukin diftitox has the potential for targeting CD25 and depleting $T_{REGs'}$ prior to the administration of cancer vaccines in combinatorial regimens.

Passive Immunotherapy

Monoclonal antibodies (MoAbs), targeting a specific protein expressed on the surface of tumor cells, exemplify passive immunotherapy and are commonly utilized in the treatment of several malignancies (56). Examples include antibodies targeting CD20 (rituximab) and human epidermal growth factor receptor 2 (transtuzumab). In their primary form, MoAbs can block receptors or activate immune response against the targeted protein. In addition, MoAbs can be modified as vehicles to deliver cytotoxic radionuclides, drugs, or toxins to the targeted cancer cell population (96). In urologic oncology, MoAbs targeting PSMA are in the most advanced phase of development. PSMA is a type II membrane glycoprotein which is universally expressed on the prostate epithelial cells and is markedly upregulated in prostate cancer. It is one of the folate-binding proteins, also expressed on neovasculature. These characteristics make PSMA an ideal target for therapy with MoAbs (96). Murine MoAb J591 (muJ591) has been chosen as the vehicle to deliver radioisotopes because of its high affinity (1 nm) for PSMA in animal models. To avoid human anti-mouse response seen with murine antibodies which precludes repetitive dosing, muJ591 has to be deimmunized. Deimmunization is done by identifying murine immunoglobulin sequence motifs recognizable by human B and/or T lymphocytes and their replacement by human homologous sequences (97). Among various radioisotopes used with muJ591, 90 Yttrium (90 Y-muJ591) and 177 Lutetium (177 Lu-muJ591) provide better dosimetry because of longer intracellular half-lives and can be delivered using fractionated dosing, thus providing higher cumulative doses. Early-phase trials have shown radio-labeled J591 to be safe and non-immunogenic and that it effectively targets metastatic prostate tumors with resulting PSA declines. Between 90 Y-muJ591 and 177 Lu-muJ591, the latter has been favored for further development as it can be administered in higher doses with comparatively less radiation to the marrow and because of its gamma emission, it enables imaging to be performed using the treatment doses (96).

CONCLUSIONS

The improvement in the overall survival with sipuleucel-T has led to its approval for the treatment of castration refractory metastatic prostate cancer. It is the first vaccine ever approved for the treatment of cancer. However, the survival benefit is modest and the need for more effective immune-based therapies is paramount. Encouraging results from early-phase immunotherapy-based clinical trials have led to multiple, ongoing phase III trials in genitourinary cancers. An example is ipilimumab, an immune checkpoint inhibitor, which is associated with improved survival in metastatic melanoma and is being tested in multiple clinical trials in prostate cancer. The poxvirus-based vaccine therapy is another promising strategy and was associated with an overall survival benefit (~8 months) in a randomized phase II trial in CRPC. The use of combinatorial regimens, which simultaneously target multiple steps in the immune system, is expected to optimize the overall efficacy, while minimizing component drug toxicities. Using a DC-based vaccine, along with inhibitors of T_{REGS} (such as denileukin diftitox or sunitinib) or agonist anti-CD40 Abs/drug-inducible CD40 or Flt3 ligand, exemplifies this approach. Combinatorial regimens may be applicable, especially for immunologically weaker vaccine approaches, such as DNA, messenger RNA, or peptide-based vaccines which otherwise provide several advantages, including faster and more cost-effective production, storage, and distribution as well as the ability to select specific TAA as targets. Androgen deprivation therapy has been evinced to reverse age-related thymic involution, improve T and B cell response, and has the potential to improve responses, when used in conjunction with immunotherapy. Additionally, a high tumor burden is immunosuppressive, and cytoreduction prior to immunotherapy is known to improve outcomes in the metastatic setting, providing the rationale for the use of chemotherapy prior to immunotherapy. Furthermore, chemotherapeutic drugs, such as cyclophosphamide may downregulate T_{REGS}, independent of their cytotoxic effect and improve the efficacy of subsequent immunotherapy. However, the failure of GVAX when used concurrently with docetaxel chemotherapy will likely remain an impediment to designing future immunotherapy-based trials, which include chemotherapy. Immunotherapy may particularly be more effective in the adjuvant setting, when there is a significantly lower tumor burden. Although the phase III trial that used vitespen for RCC in the adjuvant setting did not show an overall survival benefit, there was a trend toward an improved PFS in early-stage tumors. Despite these negative results, immunotherapy remains a promising strategy in adjuvant setting in genitourinary cancers.

REFERENCES

1. Iwasaki A, Medzhitov R. Regulation of adaptive immunity by the innate immune system. Science 2010; 327: 291–5.
2. Smith-Garvin JE, Koretzky GA, Jordan MS. T cell activation. Annu Rev Immunol 2009; 27: 591–619.
3. Watts TH. TNF/TNFR family members in costimulation of T cell responses. Annu Rev Immunol 2005; 23: 23–68.
4. Miller AM, Pisa P. Tumor escape mechanisms in prostate cancer. Cancer Immunol Immunother 2007; 56: 81–7.
5. Kusmartsev S, Vieweg J. Enhancing the efficacy of cancer vaccines in urologic oncology: new directions. Nat Rev Urol 2009; 6: 540–9.
6. Barach YS, Lee JS, Zang X. T cell coinhibition in prostate cancer: new immune evasion pathways and emerging therapeutics. Trends Mol Med 2010. [E pub ahead of print].
7. Blades RA, Keating PJ, McWilliam LJ, George NJ, Stern PL. Loss of HLA class I expression in prostate cancer: implications for immunotherapy. Urology 1995; 46: 681–6; discussion 686–7.
8. Zhang H, Melamed J, Wei P, et al. Concordant down-regulation of proto-oncogene PML and major histocompatibility antigen HLA class I expression in high-grade prostate cancer. Cancer Immun 2003; 3: 2.
9. Kitamura H, Honma I, Torigoe T, et al. Down-regulation of HLA class I antigen is an independent prognostic factor for clear cell renal cell carcinoma. J Urol 2007; 177: 1269–72; discussion 1272.
10. Sanda MG, Restifo NP, Walsh JC, et al. Molecular characterization of defective antigen processing in human prostate cancer. J Natl Cancer Inst 1995; 87: 280–5.
11. Filella X, Alcover J, Zarco MA, et al. Analysis of type T1 and T2 cytokines in patients with prostate cancer. Prostate 2000; 44: 271–4.
12. Elsasser-Beile U, Gierschner D, Jantscheff P, et al. Different basal expression of type T1 and T2 cytokines in peripheral lymphocytes of patients with adenocarcinomas and benign hyperplasia of the prostate. Anticancer Res 2003; 23: 4027–31.
13. Mantovani A, Allavena P, Sica A, Balkwill F. Cancer-related inflammation. Nature 2008; 454: 436–44.
14. Murdoch C, Muthana M, Coffelt SB, Lewis CE. The role of myeloid cells in the promotion of tumour angiogenesis. Nat Rev Cancer 2008; 8: 618–31.
15. Yang SD, Sun RC, Mu HJ, Xu ZQ, Zhou ZY. The expression and clinical significance of TGF-beta1 and MMP2 in human renal clear cell carcinoma. Int J Surg Pathol 2010; 18: 85–93.
16. De Luca A, Normanno N. Tivozanib, a pan-VEGFR tyrosine kinase inhibitor for the potential treatment of solid tumors. IDrugs 2010; 13: 636–45.

17. Robinson MO, Lin J, Feng B, et al. Correlation of a tivozanib response biomarker identified in a preclinical model with clinical activity in a phase II study in renal cell carcinoma (RCC). J Clin Oncol 2010; 28 (suppl; abstract e13564).
18. Ochoa AC, Zea AH, Hernandez C, Rodriguez PC. Arginase, prostaglandins, and myeloid-derived suppressor cells in renal cell carcinoma. Clin Cancer Res 2007; 13: 721s-6s.
19. Zang X, Allison JP. The B7 family and cancer therapy: costimulation and coinhibition. Clin Cancer Res 2007; 13: 5271–9.
20. Nishimura H, Okazaki T, Tanaka Y, et al. Autoimmune dilated cardiomyopathy in PD-1 receptor-deficient mice. Science 2001; 291: 319–22.
21. Thompson RH, Kuntz SM, Leibovich BC, et al. Tumor B7-H1 is associated with poor prognosis in renal cell carcinoma patients with long-term follow-up. Cancer Res 2006; 66: 3381–5.
22. Zang X, Thompson RH, Al-Ahmadie HA, et al. B7-H3 and B7x are highly expressed in human prostate cancer and associated with disease spread and poor outcome. Proc Natl Acad Sci USA 2007; 104: 19458–63.
23. Chavin G, Sheinin Y, Crispen PL, et al. Expression of immunosuppresive B7-H3 ligand by hormone-treated prostate cancer tumors and metastases. Clin Cancer Res 2009; 15: 2174–80.
24. Krambeck AE, Thompson RH, Dong H, et al. B7-H4 expression in renal cell carcinoma and tumor vasculature: associations with cancer progression and survival. Proc Natl Acad Sci USA 2006; 103: 10391–6.
25. Buonaguro L, Petrizzo A, Tornesello ML, Buonaguro FM. Translating tumor antigens into cancer vaccines. Clin Vaccine Immunol 2011; 18: 23–34.
26. Sakaguchi S. Naturally arising Foxp3-expressing CD25+CD4+ regulatory T cells in immunological tolerance to self and non-self. Nat Immunol 2005; 6: 345–52.
27. Finke JH, Rini B, Ireland J, et al. Sunitinib reverses type-1 immune suppression and decreases T-regulatory cells in renal cell carcinoma patients. Clin Cancer Res 2008; 14: 6674–82.
28. Vogelzang NJ, Priest ER, Borden L. Spontaneous regression of histologically proved pulmonary metastases from renal cell carcinoma: a case with 5-year followup. J Urol 1992; 148: 1247–8.
29. Gleave ME, Elhilali M, Fradet Y, et al. Interferon gamma-1b compared with placebo in metastatic renal-cell carcinoma. Canadian Urologic Oncology Group. N Engl J Med 1998; 338: 1265–71.
30. Becker JT, Olson BM, Johnson LE, et al. DNA vaccine encoding prostatic acid phosphatase (PAP) elicits long-term T-cell responses in patients with recurrent prostate cancer. J Immunother 2010; 33: 639–47.
31. Longo DL. New therapies for castration-resistant prostate cancer. N Engl J Med 2010; 363: 479–81.
32. Jahnisch H, Fussel S, Kiessling A, et al. Dendritic cell-based immunotherapy for prostate cancer. Clin Dev Immunol 2010; 2010: 517493.
33. Sonpavde G, Slawin KM, Spencer DM, Levitt JM. Emerging vaccine therapy approaches for prostate cancer. Rev Urol 2010; 12: 25–34.
34. Su Z, Dannull J, Yang BK, et al. Telomerase mRNA-transfected dendritic cells stimulate antigen-specific CD8+ and CD4+ T cell responses in patients with metastatic prostate cancer. J Immunol 2005; 174: 3798–807.
35. Su Z, Dannull J, Heiser A, et al. Immunological and clinical responses in metastatic renal cancer patients vaccinated with tumor RNA-transfected dendritic cells. Cancer Res 2003; 63: 2127–33.
36. Berntsen A, Trepiakas R, Wenandy L, et al. Therapeutic dendritic cell vaccination of patients with metastatic renal cell carcinoma: a clinical phase 1/2 trial. J Immunother 2008; 31: 771–80.
37. Small EJ, Fratesi P, Reese DM, et al. Immunotherapy of hormone-refractory prostate cancer with antigen-loaded dendritic cells. J Clin Oncol 2000; 18: 3894–903.
38. Kantoff PW, Higano CS, Shore ND, et al. Sipuleucel-T Immunotherapy for Castration-Resistant Prostate Cancer. N Engl J Med 2010; 363: 411–22.
39. Clark JI, Atkins MB, Urba WJ, et al. Adjuvant high-dose bolus interleukin-2 for patients with high-risk renal cell carcinoma: a cytokine working group randomized trial. J Clin Oncol 2003; 21: 3133–40.
40. Messing EM, Manola J, Wilding G, et al. Phase III study of interferon alfa-NL as adjuvant treatment for resectable renal cell carcinoma: an Eastern Cooperative Oncology Group/Intergroup trial. J Clin Oncol 2003; 21: 1214–22.
41. Pizzocaro G, Piva L, Colavita M, et al. Interferon adjuvant to radical nephrectomy in Robson stages II and III renal cell carcinoma: a multicentric randomized study. J Clin Oncol 2001; 19: 425–31.
42. Jocham D, Richter A, Hoffmann L, et al. Adjuvant autologous renal tumour cell vaccine and risk of tumour progression in patients with renal-cell carcinoma after radical nephrectomy: phase III, randomised controlled trial. Lancet 2004; 363: 594–9.

43. Wood C, Srivastava P, Bukowski R, et al. An adjuvant autologous therapeutic vaccine (HSPPC-96; vitespen) versus observation alone for patients at high risk of recurrence after nephrectomy for renal cell carcinoma: a multicentre, open-label, randomised phase III trial. Lancet 2008; 372: 145–54.

44. May M, Brookman-May S, Hoschke B, et al. Ten-year survival analysis for renal carcinoma patients treated with an autologous tumour lysate vaccine in an adjuvant setting. Cancer Immunol Immunother 2010; 59: 687–95.

45. Mu LJ, Kyte JA, Kvalheim G, et al. Immunotherapy with allotumour mRNA-transfected dendritic cells in androgen-resistant prostate cancer patients. Br J Cancer 2005; 93: 749–56.

46. Heiser A, Coleman D, Dannull J, et al. Autologous dendritic cells transfected with prostate-specific antigen RNA stimulate CTL responses against metastatic prostate tumors. J Clin Invest 2002; 109: 409–17.

47. Soleimani A, Berntsen A, Svane IM, Pedersen AE. Immune responses in patients with metastatic renal cell carcinoma treated with dendritic cells pulsed with tumor lysate. Scand J Immunol 2009; 70: 481–9.

48. Dannull J, Su Z, Rizzieri D, et al. Enhancement of vaccine-mediated antitumor immunity in cancer patients after depletion of regulatory T cells. J Clin Invest 2005; 115: 3623–33.

49. Khalil M, Vonderheide RH. Anti-CD40 agonist antibodies: preclinical and clinical experience. Update Cancer Ther 2007; 2: 61–5.

50. Higham EM, Wittrup KD, Chen J. Activation of tolerogenic dendritic cells in the tumor draining lymph nodes by CD8+ T cells engineered to express CD40 ligand. J Immunol 2010; 184: 3394–400.

51. Vonderheide RH, Flaherty KT, Khalil M, et al. Clinical activity and immune modulation in cancer patients treated with CP-870,893, a novel CD40 agonist monoclonal antibody. J Clin Oncol 2007; 25: 876–83.

52. Hanks BA, Jiang J, Singh RA, et al. Re-engineered CD40 receptor enables potent pharmacological activation of dendritic-cell cancer vaccines in vivo. Nat Med 2005; 11: 130–7.

53. Lapteva N, Seethammagari MR, Hanks BA, et al. Enhanced activation of human dendritic cells by inducible CD40 and Toll-like receptor-4 ligation. Cancer Res 2007; 67: 10528–37.

54. Higano CS, Vogelzang NJ, Sosman JA, et al. Safety and biological activity of repeated doses of recombinant human Flt3 ligand in patients with bone scan-negative hormone-refractory prostate cancer. Clin Cancer Res 2004; 10: 1219–25.

55. Vergati M, Intrivici C, Huen NY, Schlom J, Tsang KY. Strategies for cancer vaccine development. J Biomed Biotechnol 2010; 2010: pii: 596432.

56. Drake CG. Prostate cancer as a model for tumour immunotherapy. Nat Rev Immunol 2010; 10: 580–93.

57. Arlen PM, Kaufman HL, DiPaola RS. Pox viral vaccine approaches. Semin Oncol 2005; 32: 549–55.

58. Harrington LE, Most Rv R, Whitton JL, Ahmed R. Recombinant vaccinia virus-induced T-cell immunity: quantitation of the response to the virus vector and the foreign epitope. J Virol 2002; 76: 3329–37.

59. NCT01322490: A Trial of PROSTVAC +/- GM-CSF in Men With Asymptomatic or Minimally Symptomatic Metastatic Castrate-Resistant Prostate Cancer (mCRPC) (Prospect)(ClinicalTrials.gov).).

60. Amato RJ, Shingler W, Goonewardena M, et al. Vaccination of renal cell cancer patients with modified vaccinia Ankara delivering the tumor antigen 5T4 (TroVax) alone or administered in combination with interferon-alpha (IFN-alpha): a phase 2 trial. J Immunother 2009; 32: 765–72.

61. Acres B. Cancer immunotherapy: phase II clinical studies with TG4010 (MVA-MUC1-IL2). J BUON 2007; 12(Suppl 1): S71–5.

62. Pasquini S, Xiang Z, Wang Y, et al. Cytokines and costimulatory molecules as genetic adjuvants. Immunol Cell Biol 1997; 75: 397–401.

63. Conry RM, Curiel DT, Strong TV, et al. Safety and immunogenicity of a DNA vaccine encoding carcinoembryonic antigen and hepatitis B surface antigen in colorectal carcinoma patients. Clin Cancer Res 2002; 8: 2782–7.

64. Binder RJ, Srivastava PK. Peptides chaperoned by heat-shock proteins are a necessary and sufficient source of antigen in the cross-priming of CD8+ T cells. Nat Immunol 2005; 6: 593–9.

65. Best SR, Peng S, Juang CM, et al. Administration of HPV DNA vaccine via electroporation elicits the strongest CD8+ T cell immune responses compared to intramuscular injection and intradermal gene gun delivery. Vaccine 2009; 27: 5450–9.

66. Pavlenko M, Roos AK, Lundqvist A, et al. A phase I trial of DNA vaccination with a plasmid expressing prostate-specific antigen in patients with hormone-refractory prostate cancer. Br J Cancer 2004; 91: 688–94.

67. McNeel DG, Dunphy EJ, Davies JG, et al. Safety and immunological efficacy of a DNA vaccine encoding prostatic acid phosphatase in patients with stage D0 prostate cancer. J Clin Oncol 2009; 27: 4047–54.

68. Yamamoto A, Kormann M, Rosenecker J, Rudolph C. Current prospects for mRNA gene delivery. Eur J Pharm Biopharm 2009; 71: 484–9.
69. Pascolo S. Vaccination with messenger RNA. Methods Mol Med 2006; 127: 23–40.
70. CureVac GmbH: CureVac presents convincing data from the first ever Phase I/IIa clinical study with a mRNA based vaccine. Press Release, October 4, 2010.
71. Srivastava P. Roles of heat-shock proteins in innate and adaptive immunity. Nat Rev Immunol 2002; 2: 185–94.
72. Tamura Y, Peng P, Liu K, Daou M, Srivastava PK. Immunotherapy of tumors with autologous tumor-derived heat shock protein preparations. Science 1997; 278: 117–20.
73. Wood C, Srivastava P, Bukowski R, et al. An adjuvant autologous therapeutic vaccine (HSPPC-96; vitespen) versus observation alone for patients at high risk of recurrence after nephrectomy for renal cell carcinoma: a multicentre, open-label, randomised phase III trial. Lancet 2008; 372: 145–54.
74. Butts C, Murray N, Maksymiuk A, et al. Randomized phase IIB trial of BLP25 liposome vaccine in stage IIIB and IV non-small-cell lung cancer. J Clin Oncol 2005; 23: 6674–81.
75. Dranoff G, Jaffee E, Lazenby A, et al. Vaccination with irradiated tumor cells engineered to secrete murine granulocyte-macrophage colony-stimulating factor stimulates potent, specific, and long-lasting anti-tumor immunity. Proc Natl Acad Sci USA 1993; 90: 3539–43.
76. Jocham D, Richter A, Hoffmann L, et al. Adjuvant autologous renal tumour cell vaccine and risk of tumour progression in patients with renal-cell carcinoma after radical nephrectomy: phase III, randomised controlled trial. Lancet 2004; 363: 594–9.
77. Fishman M, Antonia S. Specific antitumour vaccine for renal cancer. Lancet 2004; 363: 583–4.
78. Kaehler KC, Piel S, Livingstone E, et al. Update on immunologic therapy with anti-CTLA-4 antibodies in melanoma: identification of clinical and biological response patterns, immune-related adverse events, and their management. Semin Oncol 2010; 37: 485–98.
79. Hodi FS, O'Day SJ, McDermott DF, et al. Improved survival with ipilimumab in patients with metastatic melanoma. N Engl J Med 2010; 363: 711–23.
80. Langer LF, Clay TM, Morse MA. Update on anti-CTLA-4 antibodies in clinical trials. Expert Opin Biol Ther 2007; 7: 1245–56.
81. O'Mahony D, Morris JC, Quinn C, et al. A pilot study of CTLA-4 blockade after cancer vaccine failure in patients with advanced malignancy. Clin Cancer Res 2007; 13: 958–64.
82. Fong L, Kwek SS, O'Brien S, et al. Potentiating endogenous antitumor immunity to prostate cancer through combination immunotherapy with CTLA4 blockade and GM-CSF. Cancer Res 2009; 69: 609–15.
83. Small EJ, Tchekmedyian NS, Rini BI, et al. A pilot trial of CTLA-4 blockade with human anti-CTLA-4 in patients with hormone-refractory prostate cancer. Clin Cancer Res 2007; 13: 1810–15.
84. Tollefson MK, Karnes RJ, Thompson RH, et al. A randomized phase II study of ipilimumab with androgen ablation compared with androgen ablation alone in patients with advanced prostate cancer. 2010 Genitourinary Cancers Symposium Abstract No: 168 (2010).
85. Slovin SF, Beer TM, Higano CS, Tejwani S. Initial phase II experience of ipilimumab (IPI) alone and in combination with radiotherapy (XRT) in patients with metastatic castration-resistant prostate cancer (mCRPC). J Clin Oncol 2009; 27 (suppl; abstract 5138): 15s.
86. Gerritsen W, van den Eertwegh AJ, de Gruijl T, et al. Expanded phase I combination trial of GVAX immunotherapy for prostate cancer and ipilimumab in patients with metastatic hormone-refractory prostate cancer (mHPRC). J Clin Oncol 2008 26 (May 20 suppl; abstract 5146).
87. NCT01057810:Randomized, Double-Blind, Phase 3 Trial to Compare the Efficacy of Ipilimumab vs Placebo in Asymptomatic or Minimally Symptomatic Patients With Metastatic Chemotherapy-Naïve Castration Resistant Prostate Cancer (ClinicalTrials.gov).
88. NCT00861614: A Randomized, Double-Blind, Phase 3 Trial Comparing Ipilimumab vs. Placebo Following Radiotherapy in Subjects With Castration Resistant Prostate Cancer That Have Received Prior Treatment With Docetaxel (ClinicalTrials.gov).
89. Hirano F, Kaneko K, Tamura H, et al. Blockade of B7-H1 and PD-1 by monoclonal antibodies potentiates cancer therapeutic immunity. Cancer Res 2005; 65: 1089–96.
90. Iwai Y, Terawaki S, Honjo T. PD-1 blockade inhibits hematogenous spread of poorly immunogenic tumor cells by enhanced recruitment of effector T cells. Int Immunol 2005; 17: 133–44.
91. Thompson RH, Gillett MD, Cheville JC, et al. Costimulatory B7-H1 in renal cell carcinoma patients: Indicator of tumor aggressiveness and potential therapeutic target. Proc Natl Acad Sci USA 2004; 101: 17174–9.

92. Brahmer JR, Drake CG, Wollner I, et al. Phase I study of single-agent anti-programmed death-1 (MDX-1106) in refractory solid tumors: safety, clinical activity, pharmacodynamics, and immunologic correlates. J Clin Oncol 2010; 28: 3167–75.

93. Shimizu J, Yamazaki S, Sakaguchi S. Induction of tumor immunity by removing CD25+CD4+ T cells: a common basis between tumor immunity and autoimmunity. J Immunol 1999; 163: 5211–18.

94. Sutmuller RP, van Duivenvoorde LM, van Elsas A, et al. Synergism of cytotoxic T lymphocyte-associated antigen 4 blockade and depletion of CD25(+) regulatory T cells in antitumor therapy reveals alternative pathways for suppression of autoreactive cytotoxic T lymphocyte responses. J Exp Med 2001; 194: 823–32.

95. Atchison E, Eklund J, Martone B, et al. A pilot study of denileukin diftitox (DD) in combination with high-dose interleukin-2 (IL-2) for patients with metastatic renal cell carcinoma (RCC). J Immunother 2010; 33: 716–22.

96. Tagawa ST, Beltran H, Vallabhajosula S, et al. Anti-prostate-specific membrane antigen-based radioimmunotherapy for prostate cancer. Cancer 2010; 116(4 Suppl): 1075–83.

97. Bander NH, Nanus DM, Milowsky MI, et al. Targeted systemic therapy of prostate cancer with a monoclonal antibody to prostate-specific membrane antigen. Semin Oncol 2003; 30: 667–76.

4 | Autologous cellular immunotherapy in late-stage prostate cancer: The development history of Sipuleucel-T (PROVENGE®)

David L. Urdal and Mark W. Frohlich

INTRODUCTION TO PROSTATE CANCER

Prostate cancer is the most common type of cancer in men living in developed countries and is the second most common type of cancer in men in North America. In 2010, there were expected to be over 217,000 new diagnoses of this disease (1).

Most men living in developed countries who are diagnosed with prostate cancer are in the early stage of the disease (approximately 80%) (2). Primary treatment options for men diagnosed with early-stage prostate cancer include surgery (radical prostatectomy), radiation therapy (external beam or brachytherapy), and cryotherapy to control the disease (3). Approximately 20–40% of men who have received primary therapy will have the recurrence of the disease (4). For those with disease recurrence, in approximately 85% of men, androgen deprivation therapy through surgical or medical castration will control the disease, by achieving castrate levels of testosterone and depriving hormone-sensitive tumor cells of one of the essential growth factors (5–8). While these secondary treatments can control the progression of the disease for months to years, the natural progression of prostate cancer leads to metastatic castrate-resistant prostate cancer (mCRPC) (9). Patients with mCRPC had few treatment options available until 2004 when the chemotherapy drug docetaxel was approved by the Food and Drug Administration (FDA) as the first drug to show a survival advantage for men in this setting (9). Then in 2010, the first autologous cellular immunotherapy drug, sipuleucel-T (Provenge®), was approved by the FDA after demonstrating one of the largest clinically meaningful survival advantages observed in men in this setting (10).

INTRODUCTION TO ACTIVE CELLULAR IMMUNOTHERAPY

To address the unmet medical need for additional prostate cancer treatments, a number of experimental approaches have been explored in the last several years, including both active and passive immunotherapy approaches (11). One active immunotherapeutic approach is active cellular immunotherapy (ACI), which targets antigen presenting cells (APCs) to stimulate a T-cell response to tumor-associated antigens. This approach had its origins in several experimental studies that started with the identification of the most potent APC, the dendritic cell, by Steinman and colleagues (12). This cell type plays a key role in initiating T-cell immune responses and is found in a variety of tissues including the peripheral blood. A number of methods have been developed that describe the isolation and culture of these cells, also define conditions under which they can be "loaded" ex vivo with antigens (13).

One approach isolated APCs from the peripheral blood by buoyant density centrifugation and was first tested clinically by Hsu and colleagues. They isolated APCs from the peripheral blood of patients with B-cell lymphoma and cultured them ex vivo with a patient-specific B-cell lymphoma idiotype antigen and then infused the idiotype-loaded APCs into the patient, resulting in the development of an anti-idiotype immune response and a preliminary evidence of clinical benefit (14). More recently, Lacy and colleagues provided a further evidence of the value of this approach in treating patients with multiple myeloma in a Phase II study with an ACI which used idiotype-loaded APCs isolated from the peripheral blood for treating post-transplant multiple myeloma patients during remission (15,16). Patients who had received this ACI appeared to have improved survival chances compared with historical controls.

Laus and colleagues advanced the potential of an ACI approach in the treatment of prostate cancer by demonstrating that APCs isolated from rat spleens and activated ex vivo with a fusion protein, which combined rat prostatic acid phosphatase (PAP) with rat granulocyte-macrophage colony-stimulating factor (GM-CSF) (rat PAP-rat GM-CSF), was then infused into normal rats to induce autoimmune prostatitis (16,17), a key mediator of which, appeared to be CD4+, but not CD8+ T-cells. Direct injection of the PAP-GM-CSF fusion antigen induced antibody responses in rats, but not autoimmune prostatitis; the infusion of rat APCs that had been cultured with a control antigen and GM-CSF did not induce inflammation in the prostate. Having a method by which autoimmune prostatitis could be consistently induced led to the notion that the infusion of APCs that had been activated ex vivo with a recombinant PAP-GM-CSF antigen might provide for a novel means by which cancer derived from the prostate might be treated.

In particular, PAP was chosen as the target antigen in prostate cancer based on these experimental results in rats and because its expression in humans is relatively specific to the prostate: it is expressed in both normal and cancerous prostate tissue and can be detected only at much lower levels in pancreatic islet cells, stomach parietal cells, kidney cells, liver cells, urethral glands, salivary glands, and rectal tissue (16,17). PAP is expressed at high levels in >95% of primary prostate adenocarcinoma, as well as in some non-prostate tumors (colorectal, islet cell, ovarian, breast, bladder, salivary, and lung adenomas or carcinomas) (17).

The demonstration of the induction of autoimmune prostatitis and immunity to PAP in the rat model subsequently led to the development of an analogous approach for human clinical trials. Sipuleucel-T is thus composed of autologous peripheral blood mononuclear cells (PBMCs), including APCs, cultured ex vivo with a recombinant fusion protein composed of human PAP linked to human GM-CSF (PAP-GM-CSF). The PBMCs are obtained by leukapheresis and the cellular composition of sipuleucel-T varies depending on the cells obtained from each leukapheresis procedure. It typically includes T-cells expressing the cell surface antigen CD3 (approximately 65%); APCs expressing CD54 and major histocompatibility class II (MHC class II) (approximately 18%), many of which are also CD14 positive (18,19). The final product also contains B cells expressing CD19 and natural killer (NK) cells expressing CD56 (16–18).

While the greatest source of variation in the composition of the product is due to the variation in the composition of the blood from one individual to another, there is a remarkable consistency in the response of cells to the culture with the recombinant PAP-GM-CSF. For example, studies performed to characterize the product include studies designed to identify and characterize the cells responsible for antigen presentation. Recombinant PAP-GM-CSF was fluorescently labeled and used to identify the cells in the culture that took up the antigen (19). Large CD54 positive cells expressing MHC class II were consistently shown to be responsible for antigen uptake (19). Using T-cell hybridomas that were specific to PAP peptide epitopes, it was demonstrated that the CD54+ cells were also the cells that developed the capacity to present antigen. These cells also were shown to express CD86 and CD40 molecules in addition to CD54 and MHC class II that play a role in the interaction between APCs and T-cells. It was also observed that the culture of the PBMCs with PAP-GM-CSF resulted in the upregulation of these markers, and thus the upregulation of CD54 is a measure of the activation of APCs and forms the basis for the potency assay for sipuleucel-T (19). Figure 4.1(A) summarizes the results of the potency assay across the first two sipuleucel-T Phase III studies (20). The results showed that CD54 was upregulated 5- to 6-fold at the first dose and 10- to 11-fold at the second and third dose, given two and four weeks after the first dose (21,22). Thus, CD54 upregulation had a pattern consistent with the idea that the first dose primes the patient and the second and third doses boost the response. Compelling evidence that measuring the upregulation of CD54 was a suitable measurement of product potency came with the advent of the survival results from the first Phase III trials which demonstrated a correlation between a higher cumulative CD54 upregulation and longer survival [Figure 4.1(B)] (20).

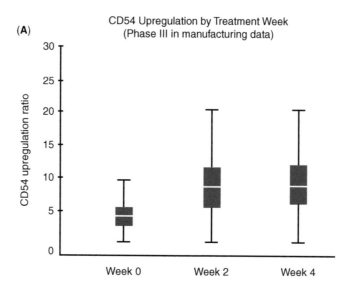

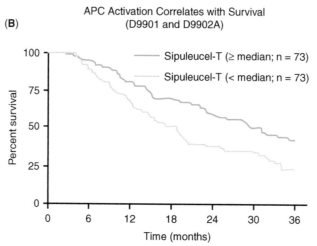

Figure 4.1 The CD54 upregulation ratio is the ratio of the average number of PBMCs post-culture with the recombinant fusion protein compared to the number of pre-culture cells. (**A**) describes the CD54 upregulation by treatment time (infusions at weeks 0, 2, and 4) and demonstrates an approximate 5-fold increase in CD54 expression over the mean after each infusion. The elevated CD54 upregulation is maintained at the second and third infusions and demonstrates an immunological prime-boost phenomenon. (**B**) demonstrates the correlation of APC activation capacity (cumulative CD54 upregulation) with overall survival in two Phase III studies (D9901 and D9902A).

CLINICAL DEVELOPMENT OF SIPULEUCEL-T AND REGULATORY MILESTONES
Clinical Efficacy of Sipuleucel-T
Phase I and II Clinical Studies

The Investigational New Drug application for sipuleucel-T was submitted in December 1996 for the treatment of prostate cancer (22). Several Phase I and II studies evaluated the safety and efficacy in men with CRPC (23,24). The immune response to PAP-GM-CSF was used to assess a number of different dosing regimens. The first study followed a dosing regimen pioneered by the B-cell lymphoma study conducted by Hsu and colleagues and examined the monthly dosing for three months followed by a boost at six months (14). The second study examined the priming of subjects with sipuleucel-T followed by boosting with the PAP-GM-CSF antigen subcutaneously (18). The results of all studies demonstrated that intravenous infusions of sipuleucel-T in subjects with prostate cancer were generally well tolerated with no dose-limiting toxicities observed. Prostate specific antigen (PSA) reductions of >50% were noted in approximately 10% of subjects. Three doses of sipuleucel-T resulted in substantial PA2024-specific immune responses and appeared to delay the time to disease progression (TTP) compared with historic controls. One subject showed a complete response to therapy (25).

Results of open-label Phase II trials in men with androgen-dependent prostate cancer also demonstrated that intravenous infusions of sipuleucel-T were generally well tolerated with no dose-limiting toxicities observed. Additionally, prolongation of PSA doubling time was observed in these uncontrolled studies (26). None of the Phase I or II studies of sipuleucel-T had a long-term survival follow-up.

After the completion of Phase I and II studies and feedback from the FDA, the Phase III clinical plan was initiated to evaluate the safety and efficacy of sipuleucel-T with two trials, D9901 and D9902, which were identical in original design (27,28). The trials were multi-centered, randomized, double-blind, controlled Phase III studies in subjects with asymptom-atic mCRPC. The primary endpoint was TTP. All subjects were to be followed for 36 months or until death, whichever occurred first.

Subjects eligible for these studies had histologically documented adenocarcinoma of the prostate with >25% of tumor cells staining positive for PAP by immunohistochemistry. Meta-static disease had to be evidenced by soft tissue and/or bony metastases. Finally, subjects were required to have castrate levels of testosterone (<50 ng/dL) by orchiectomy or luteinizing hormone-releasing hormone (LHRH)-agonist therapy.

The studies were each designed to randomize approximately 120 subjects in a 2:1 ratio to receive either sipuleucel-T or control. The treatment regimen consisted of sipuleucel-T or control infusions at week 0, 2, and 4. All subjects underwent leukapheresis and subjects assigned to receive control received one-third of their leukapheresis product (not cultured with the PAP-GM-CSF antigen). Two-thirds were cryopreserved for potential use in an open-label Phase II protocol that was available to eligible subjects in the control arm after they had reached the TTP endpoint.

Enrollment in D9901 began in January 2000 and in D9902 a few months later. In 2002, an analysis of the primary endpoint in the intent-to-treat (ITT) population of Study D9901 revealed that a progression had occurred much more rapidly than expected and while there appeared to be a trend toward a delay in TTP it did not achieve any statistical significance (28). Exploratory subgroup analyses suggested that sipuleucel-T subjects who had presented with more differenti-ated primary tumors (Gleason sum ≤7) had a more substantial delay in TTP treatment. Based on these data, enrolment in Study D9902 was discontinued early and the protocol was amended to change the entry criteria to restrict the enrolment to subjects with primary tumors with a Gleason sum of ≤7. The new trial was designated D9902B (also known as IMmunotherapy for Prostate AdenoCarcinoma Treatment, IMPACT) and the trial representing the subjects enrolled by the original criteria was designated D9902A (10). All subjects continued to be followed for survival.

In late 2004, the last subjects in D9901 and D9902A had completed their three-year follow-up for survival. Study D9901 revealed a striking survival benefit, a 41% reduction in the risk of death for subjects treated with sipuleucel-T compared with those assigned to receive control was observed (hazard ratio [HR] = 0.59 [95% confidence interval [CI]: 0.39, 0.88]; P = 0.01, log rank) in the ITT population. The improvement in median survival for sipuleucel-T subjects was 4.5 months (Table 4.1) (27). For Study D9902A, a trend toward an increased survival was seen, with an HR of 0.79 ([95% CI: 0.48, 1.28]; P = 0.33, log rank) and a 3.3-month increase in the median survival for sipuleucel-T (27).

A combined analysis of D9901 and D9902A studies showed a 33% reduction in the risk of death (HR = 0.67 [95% CI: 0.49, 0.91]; P = 0.011, log rank) (27). The survival benefit was also cor-related with product potency [Figure 4.1(B)]. The most common adverse events associated with

Table 4.1 Summary of Overall Survival (Phase III Studies)

	Study D9901[a] (N = 127)	Study D9902A[a] (N = 98)	Study D9902B[b] (N = 512)
Hazard Ratio	0.59	0.79	0.78
95% Confidence Interval	0.39, 0.88	0.48, 1.28	0.61, 0.98
P-value	0.01	0.33	0.03
Median Survival (months)			
Sipuleucel-T	25.9	19.0	25.8
Control	21.4	15.7	21.7
Median Survival Benefit (months)	4.5	3.3	4.1
36-month Survival Probability (%)			
Sipuleucel-T	34	33	32
Control	11	15	23

[a]Unadjusted Cox model and log rank as presented in the individual CSRs. Study D9902A was stratified by bisphosphonate use (27).
[b]Cox model adjusted for PSA and lactate dehydrogenase, as defined in the SAP (10).
[a,b]Data are published in Higano (27) and Kantoff (10) with the HRs >1, indicating a greater risk for subjects treated with control relative to sipuleucel-T. In contrast, data present in Table 4.1 and in the text are HRs <1, indicating a greater risk for subjects treated with sipuleucel-T relative to control.

treatment were chills, pyrexia, headache, asthenia, dyspnea, vomiting, and tremor and were typically Grade 1–2 and lasted about two days.

In September 2005, Dendreon had a meeting with the FDA's Center for Biologics Evaluation and Research to discuss a proposed Biologics License Application (BLA) submission for sipuleucel-T based on the results from Studies D9901 and D9902A (23). At this meeting, CBER agreed that the significant survival benefit observed in Study D9901 in combination with Study D9902A, and the low toxicity profile, were sufficient to serve as the clinical basis for the BLA filing. Furthermore, since the survival benefit was seen across all Gleason sum subgroups and was the most suitable and compelling endpoint for clinical trials in this setting, the D9902B trial was amended to elevate overall survival (OS) to the primary endpoint and to open trial enrolment to all Gleason sum categories (10). In addition, the eligibility criteria were amended to include minimally symptomatic subjects, in addition to asymptomatic subjects. The trial design and statistical parameters were agreed upon with the FDA under a Special Protocol Assessment.

Based on this discussion with the FDA, the first phase of a commercial manufacturing facility was built in 2006 and the BLA for sipuleucel-T was submitted later that year with clinical safety and efficacy data from Studies D9901 and D9902A (24). The application was accepted for review and in March 2007 the FDA Cellular, Tissue, and Gene Therapies Advisory Committee reviewed aspects of the dossier and was unanimous (17 yes, 0 no) in its opinion that the submitted data established sipuleucel-T as reasonably safe for the intended population, and a majority (13 yes, 4 no) voted that the submitted data provided substantial evidence for the efficacy of sipuleucel-T in subjects with asymptomatic mCRPC (29). The committee also expressed the sentiment that while the evidence of a survival benefit was compelling, they hoped that supportive evidence on the product's efficacy might be obtained from the ongoing D9902B trial. Following the FDA Advisory Committee vote, the FDA requested additional clinical data to support the efficacy claim.

IMPACT (D9902B) Study

These additional data were to come from the D9902B trial that was to complete its enrollment in the fall of 2007. Study D9902B (IMPACT) was a multi-center, double-blind, controlled Phase III trial conducted in 512 subjects with asymptomatic or minimally symptomatic mCRPC (10). Subjects were randomly assigned in a 2:1 ratio to receive either sipuleucel-T

(341 subjects) or control (171 subjects). The primary endpoint was overall survival, analyzed by means of a stratified Cox regression model adjusted for baseline levels of serum PSA and lactate dehydrogenase (LDH). Eligible men had mCRPC, an expected survival period of at least six months, serum PSA ≥5 ng/mL, an Eastern Cooperative Oncology Group performance status of 0 or 1, no visceral metastases (lung, liver, or brain), and a serum testosterone level of <50 ng/dL. Subjects with moderate or severe symptomatic metastatic disease, as defined by average weekly pain on a visual analog scale of 4 or more, or narcotic analgesics within 21 days prior to registration, were excluded.

Data from the IMPACT study were first reported in April 2009 and published in July 2010 (10). There was a 22% reduction in the risk of death in subjects who received sipuleucel-T compared with subjects in the control arm (HR=0.78 [95% CI: 061, 0.98]; P=0.03) (Figure 4.2(A), Table 4.1) (10). There was a 4.1-month median survival advantage. The treatment effect was also demonstrated with an unadjusted Cox model and log rank test analysis (HR = 0.77 [95% CI: 0.61, 0.97]; P = 0.02). There was no evidence that docetaxel administered following study treatment could explain the observed survival differences. Specifically, the treatment effect persisted in an analysis in which subjects were censored at the time of docetaxel initiation (HR = 0.65 [95% CI: 0.47, 0.90]; P = 0.01) [Figure 4.2(B)] and in an analysis adjusting for docetaxel as a time-dependent covariate (HR = 0.78 [95% CI: 0.62, 0.98]; P = 0.03). Consistent with the prior Phase III randomized studies, no significant difference in TTP could be demonstrated. Adverse events associated with treatment in this study were chills, fever, headache, influenza-like illness, myalgia, hypertension, hyperhidrosis, and groin pain and were similar to those observed in other Phase III studies (D9901 and D9902A) (10).

Cellular and humoral immune responses were assessed in the IMPACT study. Humoral responses (post-baseline titer >400) to the PAP-GM-CSF recombinant fusion protein were observed in 66.2% of sipuleucel-T and 2.9% of control subjects, whereas responses against PAP in these arms were 28.5% and 1.4%, respectively (10). T-cell proliferation responses at week 6 to sipuleucel-T were observed in 73.0% of sipuleucel-T subjects and 12.1% of control subjects. Sipuleucel-T-treated subjects with humoral responses to PAP-GM-CSF or PAP detected after baseline had improved survival; and while correlations between T-cell proliferation responses to either PAP-GM-CSF or PAP at week 6 and survival rate could not be demonstrated (10), subsequent analyses suggest that the magnitude of interferon gamma (IFNγ) enzyme-linked immunosorbent spot assay responses at 26 weeks and T-cell proliferation responses at 14 weeks may correlate with the survival rate (30).

These results are consistent with the immune response data that were collected during the Phase I and II clinical trials, with the preclinical rat studies and with the studies that were performed to characterize the product and understand its mechanism of action. In particular, the PAP-GM-CSF antigen is taken up by large CD54+, MHC class II+ APCs; the APCs are activated by the culture as reflected by the upregulation of CD54, MHC class II and other molecules; and the APCs present the PAP epitopes in an MHC class II restricted manner to PAP-specific T-cell hybridomas (19). The cumulative upregulation of CD54 on APC correlates with the overall survival (Figure 4.1) and displays a pattern reminiscent of the therapy priming the immune system with the first dose and boosting the response with the second and third infusions. Keeping in mind that sipuleucel-T is an autologous cellular immunotherapy product that is composed of PBMCs, including APCs, recent experiments have established that the other cells in the product are not just passive bystanders, but are actively involved in defining the character of the product. T-cell cytokines like interleukin-2 (IL-2), IFNγ, and IL-17, for example, have been found in the culture at the time of the preparation of the second and third doses at a minimum of approximately 50-fold higher compared with the first dose (21,22) further suggesting that the first dose of sipuleucel-T is priming the patient and engaging the T-cell compartment in ways that can be detected at the time of manufacture of the second and third doses. The activation of NK cells has also been seen consistently in the culture during the manufacture of the second dose of sipuleucel-T (interestingly, not during the manufacture of the first or the third dose) suggesting that both the adaptive and innate arms of the immune system are being engaged during the process of manufacturing and administering the three infusions of sipuleucel-T to patients.

Efficacy Conclusions of Phase III Studies of Sipuleucel-T

The IMPACT trial supported by the results of the Phase III Studies D9901 and D9902A (29) demonstrates that sipuleucel-T provides a clinically meaningful prolongation of overall survival. No significant differences have been observed in TTP. Potential explanations for the

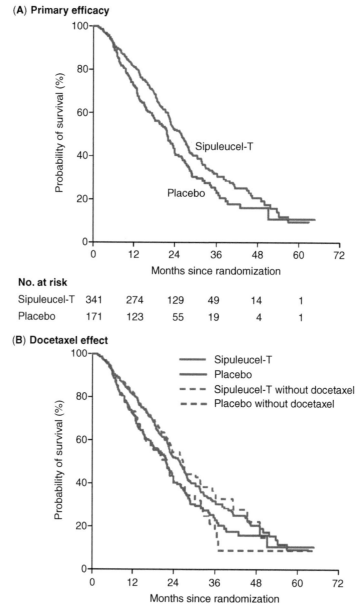

Figure 4.2 Kaplan–Meier estimates of overall survival. (**A**) shows the primary efficacy of treatment with sipuleucel-T compared to placebo. (**B**) shows the analysis with and without censoring at the time of the initiation of docetaxel therapy after sipuleucel-T treatment. *Source*: Ref. 10.

lack of effect of TTP include the fact that the immune response may not have had adequate time to provide an anti-tumor effect given the relatively rapid time to disease progression as defined in these trials. Furthermore, TTP has proved to be a challenging endpoint to assess in advanced prostate cancer, given the predominance of bony disease and the reliance on bone scans. Several agents have demonstrated an effect on one endpoint, but not the other (10).

Safety Conclusions of Phase III Studies of Sipuleucel-T

Sipuleucel-T is a treatment that can be administered in the outpatient setting. The most common adverse events reported in 601 prostate cancer patients in the sipuleucel-T group, who underwent at least one leukapheresis procedure in Phase III trials were chills, fatigue, fever, back pain, nausea, joint ache, and headache (10, 27) (Table 4.2). Most of these events were mild to moderate in severity, occurred within a day of infusion, and were transient, lasting approximately two days.

Regulatory Resolution

An amended BLA describing the efficacy, safety data, the chemistry, manufacturing, and controls for sipuleucel-T was filed in October 2009. FDA granted approval for sipuleucel-T on April 29, 2010.

Plans are under way to submit a marketing authorization application form to the European Medicines Agency (EMA) to obtain the approval for the distribution of sipuleucel-T in Europe. We are also evaluating different opportunities to explore the safety and efficacy of sipuleucel-T in other patient populations or in combination with other approved therapies.

Table 4.2 Incidence of Adverse Events Occurring in ≥5% of Subjects Randomized to Sipuleucel-T

Adverse Event[a]	Sipuleucel-T (N=601) N (%) 591 (98.3)	Control (N=303) N (%) 291 (96.0)
Chills	319 (53.1)	33 (10.9)
Fatigue	247 (41.1)	105 (34.7)
Fever	188 (31.3)	29 (9.6)
Back pain	178 (29.6)	87 (28.7)
Nausea	129 (21.5)	45 (14.9)
Joint ache	188 (19.6)	62 (20.5)
Headache	109 (18.1)	20 (6.6)
Citrate toxicity	89 (14.8)	43 (14.2)
Paresthesia	85 (14.1)	43 (14.2)
Vomiting	80 (13.3)	23 (7.6)
Anemia	75 (12.5)	34 (11.2)
Constipation	74 (12.3)	40 (13.2)
Pain	74 (12.3)	20 (6.6)
Oral paresthesia	74 (12.3)	43 (14.2)
Pain in extremity	73 (12.1)	40 (13.2)
Dizziness	71 (11.8)	34 (11.2)
Muscle ache	71 (11.8)	17 (5.6)
Asthenia	65 (10.8)	20 (6.6)
Diarrhea	60 (10.0)	34 (11.2)
Influenza-like illness	58 (9.7)	11 (3.6)
Musculoskeletal pain	54 (9.0)	31 (10.2)
Dyspnea	52 (8.7)	14 (4.6)
Peripheral edema	50 (8.3)	31 (10.2)

(Continued)

51

Table 4.2 (*Continued*) Incidence of Adverse Events Occurring in ≥5% of Subjects Randomized to Sipuleucel-T

Adverse Event[a]	Sipuleucel-T (N=601) N (%) 591 (98.3)	Control (N=303) N (%) 291 (96.0)
Hot flushes	49 (8.2)	29 (9.6)
Hematuria	46 (7.7)	18 (5.9)
Muscle spasms	46 (7.7)	17 (5.6)
Hypertension	45 (7.5)	0 (0.0)
Anorexia	39 (6.5)	3 (1.0)
Bone pain	38 (6.3)	3 (1.0)
Upper respiratory tract infection	38 (6.3)	0 (0.0)
Insomnia	37 (6.2)	1 (0.3)
Musculoskeletal chest pain	36 (6.0)	2 (0.7)
Cough	35 (5.8)	0 (0.0)
Neck pain	34 (5.7)	2 (0.7)
Weight loss	34 (5.7)	1 (0.3)
Urinary tract infection	33 (5.5)	2 (0.7)
Rash	31 (5.2)	0 (0.0)
Sweating	30 (5.0)	0 (0.0)
Tremor	30 (5.0)	0 (0.0)

[a]All grades of adverse events from Sipuleucel-T Prescribing Information. *Source*: http://www.provenge.com.

COMMERCIAL STEPS IN MANUFACTURING SIPULEUCEL-T

In parallel with the clinical development of sipuleucel-T, the manufacturing process and commercial supply chain for this autologous ACI were also established. Sipuleucel-T requires a patient-specific manufacturing process that collects and tracks each patient's sipuleucel-T dose from leukapheresis through activation, quality testing, and infusion (Figure 4.3) (21). Each dose of sipuleucel-T is the product of one patient's PBMCs collected from a single leukapheresis, activated with the PAP-GM-CSF antigen. A complete course of treatment comprises three infusions, each of which is preceded by a leukapheresis procedure.

Before each leukapheresis procedure, the patient's health condition is assessed for their ability to tolerate the procedure. If acceptable, they undergo a standard 1.5 to 2.0 blood volume leukapheresis to harvest PBMCs. After collection, the PBMCs are transported to a Dendreon manufacturing facility where they are aseptically processed and activated by culturing them with the recombinant fusion protein (PAP-GM-CSF); then the PBMCs are washed and prepared for shipment to the patient's physician site for infusion. The ex vivo culture yields activated, antigen-loaded APCs capable of presenting PAP epitopes to T-cells. Before and after activation, a series of quality tests is performed on each dose of sipuleucel-T to ensure the safety, purity, identity, and potency of the product, including the assessment of key product parameters such as total nucleated cell count, CD54 cell count, and CD54 upregulation of the patient's PBMCs following activation with PAP-GM-CSF. Each dose of sipuleucel-T contains a minimum of 50 million autologous CD54[+] cells and is sterile by Gram stain and endotoxin. Each step in the process of manufacturing sipuleucel-T must be performed within a specific period of time.

Results from the manufacturing specifications are reviewed to determine whether the final product can be ready for infusion into a patient. If the final product passes, it is approved and released for infusion. If the product is "rejected," the patient will be rescheduled for another leukapheresis procedure assuming they are able to continue treatment. After processing, the final infusion product is transported from the manufacturing facility to the clinical study center for infusion into the patient approximately three days after leukapheresis collection of PBMCs. Preservation of the chain of identity is the key for an autologous cellular immunotherapy to track patient identity through each step in the manufacturing process.

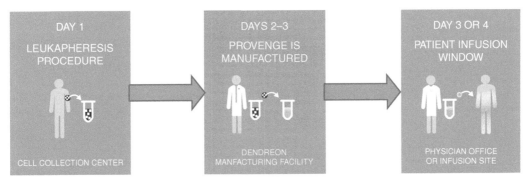

Figure 4.3 Sipuleucel-T is manufactured from PBMCs isolated approximately at weeks 0, 2, and 4 by leukapheresis. PBMCs are cultured ex vivo with PAP-GM-CSF for approximately 2 days, washed, quality tested, and infused into the patient. A course of sipuleucel-T treatment comprises 3 infusions.

THE FUTURE OF ACTIVE IMMUNOTHERAPY IN PROSTATE CANCER

With the approval of sipuleucel-T, the first autologous cellular immunotherapy, a new paradigm in prostate cancer treatment has become a reality. A number of other approaches to active immunotherapy for prostate cancer have been tried (11) and some look promising (31). We and others have learned that time to disease progression is a challenging endpoint to measure in this disease and with this form of therapy; progression occurs relatively quickly and it takes time for an effector immune response to be engendered, potentially resulting in a delayed effect of the therapy. This means the endpoint of overall survival will provide the most compelling evidence of the activity of this important new modality of active immunotherapy. While overall survival takes longer to measure in a clinical trial, it remains the gold standard clinical endpoint for oncology studies.

The overall survival benefit of sipuleucel-T is accompanied by a side effect profile that consists primarily of fever and chills that persist for 24 to 48 hours following product infusion. The full course of therapy is approximately one month, facilitating the use of potential subsequent therapies and/or future drug combinations. The year 2010 was a good year for men with prostate cancer—whereas docetaxel was the only drug known to have an effect on survival from prostate cancer at the beginning of the year, the year ended with the approval of sipuleucel-T for men with asymptomatic or minimally symptomatic mCRPC and of cabazitaxel (32) as a second-line chemotherapy for the treatment of men who had failed docetaxel treatment, as well as with positive Phase III data for the hormonal agent abiraterone in men previously treated with docetaxel (33).

The year 2010 might also be recorded as the year of immunotherapy. The approval of sipuleucel-T was a milestone that has invigorated the discovery and development of other active immunotherapy agents. The results from the evaluation of ipilimumab in metastatic melanoma (34) showed an overall survival benefit for the first time in metastatic melanoma, and demonstrated that a patient's immune system was effectively harnessed to fight the disease. At Dendreon, the approval of sipuleucel-T has reignited the development of other ACIs in our pipeline with the advance of our product candidate directed to HER2/neu into Phase II clinical studies in invasive bladder cancer. There is much more to come and exciting times are ahead.

REFERENCES

1. Jemal A, Siegel R, Xu J, Ward E. Cancer statistics, 2010. CA Cancer J Clin 2010; 60: 277–300.
2. Tannock IF, de Wit R, Berry WR, et al. Docetaxel plus prednisone or mitoxantrone plus prednisone for advanced prostate cancer. N Engl J Med 2004; 351: 1502–12.

3. Fizazi K, Sternberg CN, Fitzpatrick JM, Watson RW, Tabesh M. Role of targeted therapy in the treatment of advanced prostate cancer. BJU Int 2010; 105: 748–67.
4. Ward JF, Moul JW. Rising prostate-specific antigen after primary prostate cancer therapy. Nat Clin Pract Urol 2005; 2: 174–82.
5. Crawford ED, Eisenberger MA, McLeod DG, et al. A controlled trial of leuprolide with and without flutamide in prostatic carcinoma. N Engl J Med 1989; 321: 419–24.
6. Schellhammer PF, Venner P, Haas GP, et al. Prostate specific antigen decreases after withdrawal of antiandrogen therapy with bicalutamide or flutamide in patients receiving combined androgen blockade. J Urol 1997; 157: 1731–5.
7. Scher HI, Kelly WK. Flutamide withdrawal syndrome: its impact on clinical trials in hormone-refractory prostate cancer. J Clin Oncol 1993; 11: 1566–72.
8. Small EJ, Srinivas S. The antiandrogen withdrawal syndrome. Experience in a large cohort of unselected patients with advanced prostate cancer. Cancer 1995; 76: 1428–34.
9. Petrylak DP, Tangen CM, Husain MH, et al. Docetaxel and estramustine compared with mitoxantrone and prednisone for advanced refractory prostate cancer. N Engl J Med 2004; 351: 1513–20.
10. Kantoff PW, Higano CS, Shore ND, et al. Sipuleucel-T immunotherapy for castration-resistant prostate cancer. N Engl J Med 2010; 363: 411–22.
11. Drake CG. Prostate cancer as a model for tumour immunotherapy. Nat Rev Immunol 2010; 10: 580–93.
12. Steinman RM, Cohn ZA. Identification of a novel cell type in peripheral lymphoid organs of mice. I. Morphology, quantitation, tissue distribution. J Exp Med 1973; 137: 1142–62.
13. Palucka AK, Ueno H, Fay J, Bancherow J. Dendritic cells: a critical player in cancer therapy? J Immunother 2008; 31: 793–805.
14. Hsu FJ, Benike C, Fagnoni F, et al. Vaccination of patients with B-cell lymphoma using autologous antigen-pulsed dendritic cells. Nat Med 1996; 2: 52–8.
15. Lacy MQ, Mandrekar S, Dispenzieri A, et al. Idiotype-pulsed antigen-presenting cells following autologous transplantation for multiple myeloma may be associated with prolonged survival. Am J Hematol 2009; 84: 799–802.
16. Valone FH, Small FH, Mackenzie M, et al. Dendritic cell-based treatment of cancer: closing in on a cellular therapy. Cancer J 2001; 7(Suppl 2): S53–61.
17. Laus R, Yang DM, Ruegg CL, et al. Dendritic cells immunotherapy of prostate cancer: Preclinical models and early clinical experience. Cancer Res Ther Control 2001; 11: 1–10.
18. Burch PA, Breen JK, Buckner JC, et al. Priming tissue-specific cellular immunity in a Phase I trial of autologous dendritic cells for prostate cancer. Clin Cancer Res 2000; 6: 2175–82.
19. Sheikh NA, Jones LA. CD54 is a surrogate marker of antigen presenting cell activation. Cancer Immunol Immunother 2008; 57: 1381–90.
20. Urdal D. Sipuleucel-T: Autologous Cellular Immunotherapy for the Treatment of Men with Asymptomatic or Minimally Symptomatic Metastatic Castrate Resistant Prostate Cancer. 2010: 8th Annual Meeting, Cellular Immunotherapy (CIMT).
21. Wesley JD, Chadwick E, Kuan LY, et al. Characterization of antigen specific T-cell activation and cytokine expression induced by sipuleucel-T. 2010: International Society for Biological Therapy of Cancer (iSTBC).
22. Sheikh NA, dela Rosa C, Frohlich MW, Urdal DL, Provost NM. Sipuleucel-T treatment results in sequential ex vivo activation of APCs and T cells during the culture step - evidence for in vivo immunological priming. 2010: American Association for Cancer Research, 101st Annual Meeting.
23. (FDA), F.a.D.A., BLA Number: STN #125197.000, Dendreon Corporation (sipuleucel-T), Pharm/Tox Module Reviewed by Center: April 11, Editor. 2007.
24. (FDA), F.a.D.A., Sipuleucel-T Briefing Document (BLA STN 125197/0). Dendreon Corporation. 2010.
25. Burch PA, Croghan GA, Gastineau DA, et al. Immunotherapy (APC8015, Provenge®) targeting prostatic acid phosphatase can induce durable remission of metastatic androgen-independent prostate cancer: a Phase 2 trial. Prostate 2004; 60: 197–204.
26. Rini BI, Weinberg V, Fong L, Conry S, Hershberg RM, Small EJ. Combination immunotherapy with prostatic acid phosphatase pulsed antigen-presenting cells (Provenge) plus bevacizumab in patients with serologic progression of prostate cancer after definitive local therapy. Cancer 2005; 107: 67–74.
27. Higano CS, Schellhammer PF, Small EJ, Burch PA, Nemuaitis J, Yuh L, Provost N, Frohlich MW. Integrated data from 2 randomized double-blind, placebo-controlled, Phase 3 trials of active cellular immunotherapy with sipuleucel-T in advanced prostate cancer. Cancer 2009; 115: 3670–79.
28. Small EJ, Schellhammer PF, Higano CS, Redfern CH, Nemunaitis JJ, Valone FH, Verjee SS, Jones LA, and Hershberg RM. Placebo-controlled Phase III trial of immunological therapy with sipuleucel-T

(APC8015) in patients with metastatic, asymptomatic hormone refractory prostate cancer. J Clin Oncol 2006; 24: 3089–94.

29. Administration, F.a.D., Biologics License Application (BLA) Medical Review, Submission Number: BLA125197, FDA. p. [Available from: www.fda.gov/downloads/BiologicsBloodVaccines/CellularGeneTherapyProducts/AprpovedProducts/UCM214560.pdf].

30. Frohlich MW. Sipuleucel-T product potency parameters and correlation with overall survival. 2010: International Society for Biological Therapy of Cancer.

31. Kantoff PW, Schuetz TJ, Blumenstein BA, et al. Overall survival analysis of a Phase II randomized controlled trial of a Poxviral-based PSA-targeted immunotherapy in metastatic castration-resistant prostate cancer. J Clin Oncol 2010; 28: 1099–105.

32. Sartor O, Halstead M, Katz L. Improving outcomes with recent advances in chemotherapy for castrate-resistant prostate cancer. Clin Genitourin Cancer 2010; 8: 23–8.

33. Pal SK, Sartor O. Phase III data for abiraterone in an evolving landscape for castration-resistant prostate cancer. Maturitas 2011; 68: 103–5.

34. Yuan J, Page DB, Ku GY, et al. Correlation of clinical and immunological data in a metastatic melanoma patient with heterogeneous tumor responses to ipilimumab therapy. Cancer Immun 2010; 10: 1.

5 | Design, development, and translation of poxvirus-based vaccines for cancer

Benedetto Farsaci, Anna Kwilas, and James W. Hodge

INTRODUCTION

Rapidly emerging achievements in the areas of molecular biology and immunology have led to the development of many safe and effective viral vectors that are currently in late-stage clinical trials for the treatment of numerous types of cancer. This chapter outlines the strategies and successes of poxviral-based vaccines, including PANVAC, PROSTVAC, TroVax, TG4010, and ALVAC. The identification of an efficient dosing schedule, the selection of appropriate target tumor antigens, and the combination of vaccine with current chemotherapy and radiation treatment regimens are described, along with completed, ongoing, and planned clinical trials. The chapter closes with a discussion of the future of poxviral-mediated immunotherapy for the treatment of cancer.

Viral vectors are among the more flexible means of enhancing the presentation of tumor antigens to the immune system. Viruses can be engineered to express entire tumor antigen genes and, often, multiple genes. Recombinant viruses can be produced more easily than whole tumor cell or dendritic cell (DC) vaccines, and in many cases are able to infect professional antigen-presenting cells (APCs), which aids their ability to induce an effective antitumor immune response (Fig. 5.1). Poxviruses are attractive as viral vaccine vectors due to their ability to incorporate large quantities of DNA (including multiple transgenes), their natural immuno-stimulatory qualities, and their ability to express their transgenes in professional APCs, specifically DCs (1–4).

Of the poxviruses, vaccinia virus is the most commonly used for cancer immunotherapy. Vaccinia virus is a double-stranded DNA virus with a linear genome of ~190 kb, encoding about 250 genes. Vaccinia virus is best known as the live vaccine, successfully administered to over one billion people, resulting in the eradication of smallpox (5). As with all poxviruses, vaccinia virus replicates and transcribes its genome in the cytoplasm of the host cell. Vaccinia virus vectors efficiently infect mammalian cells, replicating for ~7 days before the infected cell is eliminated by the immune system (4). In addition to vaccinia virus, modified vaccinia virus Ankara (MVA) and avipox viruses, including canarypox and fowlpox, have also been used as viral cancer vaccine vectors. MVA is a highly attenuated strain of vaccinia virus that was generated by more than 500 serial passages of a smallpox vaccine from Ankara, Turkey, in chick embryo fibroblasts, resulting in a loss of ~10% of the vaccinia virus genome. MVA can infect mammalian cells and synthesize its encoded proteins, but is unable to produce infectious viruses. Canarypox and fowlpox can be pathogenic in many species of wild and captive birds, but are unable to productively infect primates and humans (6). Avipox viruses can infect mammalian cells and express their encoded transgenes for 14–21 days, but are unable to complete their life cycle and generate infectious viruses (7,8).

STRATEGIES TO IMPROVE POXVIRAL CANCER IMMUNOTHERAPY
Diversified Prime and Boost

Transgenes expressed by vaccinia virus are highly immunogenic, more so than if the antigens are administered with adjuvant (9,10). This phenomenon is attributed to the proinflammatory environment produced by the expression of vaccinia virus proteins. This characteristic makes vaccinia virus a good choice for inducing anti-tumor immune responses. However, because vaccinia virus so efficiently induces a host antivirus immune response, it can only be administered 1–2 times before the generation of neutralizing antibodies makes it unable to productively infect a host and further induce an immune response against its transgene (11). In order to induce and support a sufficient immune response to eradicate

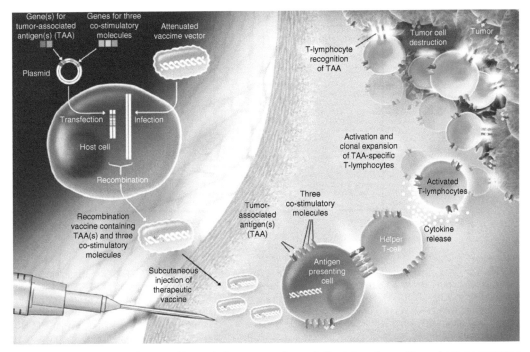

Figure 5.1 Construction of a recombinant viral cancer vaccine and stimulation of an antitumor immune response. Recombinant poxviral vectors are constructed and grown in vitro. When administered to a patient, these vectors infect many cell types, including APCs, leading to the expression of their transgenes and the APC-mediated activation of T cells against the expressed TAA. TAA-specific T cells then attack tumor cells that express the vector-encoded TAA.

tumor cells expressing weak tumor antigens, a cancer vaccine must be administered multiple times. For this reason, a diversified prime-boost strategy has been suggested in which a vaccinia virus vaccine vector is given as the priming vaccination and a recombinant fowlpox vaccine vector, encoding the same tumor antigen, is used in subsequent booster vaccinations (12–14). Vaccinia virus vectors can induce robust T-cell responses in their encoded transgenes during the priming phase; then fowlpox vectors can strengthen this response upon subsequent administration. Fowlpox vectors can continue to be administered mainly because neutralizing antibodies are not generated against them (15). In patients, this vaccination strategy has produced greater immune responses to the encoded tumor antigen than with vaccinia alone, or fowlpox alone, or fowlpox followed by vaccinia (12,16,17). The diversified prime and boost strategy has also led to improved survival rates in patients with diverse carcinomas (Fig. 5.2) (17).

Use of Multiple Costimulatory Molecules

In order for the immune system to mount an effective antitumor response, an adequate number of functional T cells specific for the antigens expressed by the malignancy must be activated. While poxvirus vectors alone are able to induce an immune response to weak tumor antigens, this response is often not sufficient to eradicate tumor cells. Induction of a successful T-cell response requires at least two signals between APCs and naïve T cells. The first is the antigen presentation in a peptide–MHC complex on the surface of an APC that interacts with the T-cell receptor (signal 1); the second is delivered via the interaction of T-cell co-stimulatory molecules on the surface of the APC with their ligands on the interacting

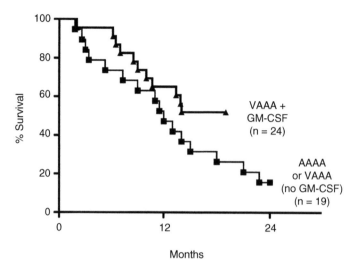

Figure 5.2 A diversified prime–boost regimen with poxviruses expressing CEA-TRICOM administered with GM-CSF results in improved patient survival. Patients were given either monthly doses of rF-CEA/TRICOM or primed with rV-CEA/TRICOM, then given monthly doses of rF-CEA/TRICOM without GM-CSF (■), or patients were primed with rV-CEA/TRICOM, then given monthly doses of rF-CEA/TRICOM with GM-CSF administered during and after each vaccination (▲). Patients on the diversified prime–boost dosing schedule with GM-CSF exhibited an increased survival rate. *Abbreviations*: CEA, carcinoembryonic antigen; GM-CSF, granulocyte macrophage colony-stimulating factor; TRICOM, TRIad of COstimulatory Molecules. *Source*: Ref. 17.

T cell (signal 2) (18). The outcome of signal 1 is greatly dependent on signal 2. One hurdle in targeting tumor antigens is that, since they are normally expressed in the body, they are considered part of the "self" antigen repertoire. Therefore, to induce an immune response against these self antigens, an immunotherapy must override immune tolerance. In the presence of a weak signal 1, such as that generated by a weak tumor antigen, T-cell co-stimulation is especially important (19).

One way that tumor cells can evade the immune system is if insufficient levels of co-stimulatory (signal 2) molecules are expressed to stimulate T-cell activation (20,21). To improve the immunostimulatory effect of poxviral vectors, the co-stimulatory molecule B7-1 was included in the vectors along with transgenes for the tumor antigen (22,23). It was soon discovered that adding two more co-stimulatory molecules, namely intercellular adhesion molecule 1 (ICAM-1) and leukocyte function-associated antigen 3 (LFA-3), further improved the immunostimulatory capacity of the poxviral vectors (18,24). These co-stimulatory molecules work synergistically to improve the immune response generated by the poxviral vectors, not only by increasing the interaction time between the APC and the T cell but also by priming unique signaling pathways in the stimulated T cells (25). Recombinant poxviral vectors expressing B7-1, ICAM-1, and LFA-3 were designated TRICOM, for TRIad of COstimulatory Molecules. TRICOM has demonstrated an ability to activate T cells to a much greater degree than that seen with vectors containing any of the molecules alone (13,24,26–28). In addition to increasing the quantity of T cells generated, an inclusion of TRICOM in the poxviral vectors improves the quality of the resulting activated T cells by increasing their avidity (19,29). High-avidity T cells kill their target cells more efficiently, especially in the presence of low levels of antigen, and are thus believed to play a pivotal role in antitumor immunity (30). It has been shown that tumor antigens can be rendered more immunogenic either by altering their mode of presentation or by using immunostimulants, both of which can be accomplished by poxviral TRICOM vectors.

POXVIRAL-BASED VACCINES AS MONOTHERAPY
PANVAC

The goal of cancer immunotherapy is to elicit an immune response against a tumor antigen, thereby triggering T cells to attack and kill the tumor. Therefore, when creating a viral immunotherapy vector, it is important to choose both an effective virus and an appropriate target tumor antigen. Tumor-associated antigens (TAAs) are selectively expressed or overexpressed in tumors. Examples include the oncofetal antigen, carcinoembryonic antigen (CEA), and mucin-1 (MUC-1). CEA and MUC-1 are overexpressed in a variety of carcinomas (lung, breast, colorectal, pancreatic and ovarian) compared to normal healthy adult tissues and so these were two of the antigens included in poxviral immunotherapy vectors. Specific agonist epitopes were mutated in both CEA and MUC-1 to improve their interaction with MHC molecules and T-cell receptors (31,32). Recombinant vaccinia virus expressing the optimized CEA and MUC-1, as well as TRICOM, is identified as PANVAC-V; recombinant fowlpox expressing these genes is identified as PANVAC-F. Preclinical studies have demonstrated the efficacy of PANVAC in infecting cultured DCs and inducing both CEA- and MUC1-specific cytotoxic T lymphocyte (CTL) responses in vitro (33). In vivo studies using a CEA-transgenic mouse model, where levels of CEA expression are similar to those of advanced colorectal cancer patients, demonstrated that vaccination with a regimen of rV-CEA/TRICOM and rF-CEA/TRICOM, the precursors to PANVAC-V/F, resulted in anti-CEA immune responses and improved survival among tumor-bearing mice (13). The addition of granulocyte macrophage colony-stimulating factor (GM-CSF) to the vaccination regimen further improved the anti-CEA immune response. These results were very indicative of the improved immune responses and survival observed in patients after administering the diversified prime/boost regimen of rV-CEA/TRICOM and rF-CEA/TRICOM and GM-CSF (Table 5.1, Fig. 5.2) (17).

The first clinical study evaluating the efficacy of PANVAC was conducted in 25 patients with various types of metastatic carcinomas (colorectal, gastric, ovarian, lung, breast, etc.; Table 5.1) (34). Patients received a priming dose of PANVAC-V followed by three biweekly boosts with PANVAC-F, then monthly doses of PANVAC-F. GM-CSF was administered with each vaccination and once daily for three days following each vaccination. Over half (9 of 16) of the evaluable patients developed T-cell responses to CEA, MUC-1, or both. Multiple previous chemotherapy treatments and a short time since the most recent chemotherapy treatment correlated with a lack of an immune response. The vaccines were well tolerated, and three patients in this trial had prolonged stable disease or improvement. One patient with metastatic gastric cancer had stable disease for five months, while another patient with metastatic breast cancer had a 24% reduction in the volume of liver metastases at 6 months. The third patient with metastatic clear cell ovarian cancer had a complete resolution of symptomatic ascites and disease stabilization for >12 months. In addition to those mentioned above, a number of patients had prolonged survival after coming off the trial, and several patients had improved clinical responses to subsequent therapies (34).

In a separate set of trials, PANVAC was evaluated in patients with stage III and IV pancreatic cancer (Table 5.1). A slight increase in survival in this initial trial led to a trial testing the efficacy of PANVAC in patients with advanced pancreatic cancer (35,36). In that trial, PANVAC therapy was compared with the second-line chemotherapy in patients who had failed the first-line chemotherapy with gemcitabine. The trial, however, did not meet its primary end point of improving survival in this patient population (37). Currently, a new phase I trial is being conducted to evaluate the efficacy of PANVAC in patients with advanced or metastatic pancreatic cancer that cannot be removed surgically (38).

An ongoing phase II trial is evaluating the performance of PANVAC in patients with colorectal cancer after a complete resection of liver or lung metastases, comparing the efficacy of the vaccine to that of ex vivo cultured DCs infected with the same vectors (Table 5.1) (39). These patients must also have received at least two months of postoperative chemotherapy. Patients in the PANVAC arm will receive a priming dose of PANVAC-V accompanied by GM-CSF, followed by three monthly doses of PANVAC-F also accompanied by GM-CSF.

Table 5.1 Clinical Trials of Poxviral Vaccines Being Evaluated as Monotherapy

Carcinoma	Target Antigen	Vector	Comment	Clinical Trial Phase	Clinical Outcome
Breast	HER2	MVA-BN-HER2		I (73)	66% of patients developed humoral and/or cellular responses
	HER2	MVA-BN-HER2 (mod)		I (74,126)	HER-2 specific antibodies in >50% of patients Ongoing
Colorectal	CEA, MUC-1	PANVAC	With GM-GSF	II (39)	Ongoing
	5T4	TroVax	Patients undergoing liver metastasis resection	I/II (61)	5/17 had disease stabilization for 3–18 mo
				I/II (62)	18/19 patients developed humoral and/or cellular responses
Melanoma	none	ALVAC	Vector expressed IL-12	I (80)	1/9 complete responses
			Vector expressed IL-2	I (79)	3/8 achieved partial regression
					5/8 achieved disease stabilization (3 for >191 days and 2 for >400 days)
			Vector expressed GM-CSF		8/8 achieved disease stabilization (2 for >27 days and 6 for >400 days)
	MAGE		With GM-GSF	II (81)	1/30 partial responses
					2/30 achieved disease stabilization for >2 years
	GP100		With IL-2	II (138)	Ongoing
	MART-1			II (139)	Ongoing
Pancreatic	CEA, MUC-1	PANVAC	With GM-GSF	I (35,36)	Trend towards increased survival
					One-year survival was 33% versus 30%
				III (37)	Did not meet primary endpoint of increased survival
				I (38)	Ongoing

	Antigen	Vaccine	Combination	Phase (ref)	Immunologic responses
Prostate	PSA, PAP	MVA-BN-PRO		I (76,77)	
	PSA	PROSTVAC	With GM-CSF	II (51)	66% of patients had >6 months progression-free survival & patients experienced increased PSA doubling time (pretreatment versus treatment p=0.002)
				II (54)	Survival advantage of 14.6 mo over predicted
				II (53)	Survival advantage of 8.5 mo over controls
	MUC-1	TG4010 (also expressing IL-2)		II (69)	8/40 had PSA stabilization ≥8 months 13/40 had increased PSA doubling time
	5T4	TroVax	With GM-GSF	II (67)	24/27 patients achieved disease stabilization for 2->10 months
Renal Cell	MUC-1	TG4010 (also expressing IL-2)	With IFN-α	II (70)	6/20 patients had stable disease for >6 months 5/27 patients had stable disease for >6 months
	5T4	TroVax	With high-dose IL-2	II (63)	No improvement in objective response over IL-2 alone
		TroVax	With low-dose IL-2	II (64)	2 complete responses for >24 months 1 partial response for >12 months; 6/25 had stable disease for 6–21 mo
	5T4	TroVax	With IFN-α	II (66)	1 partial response for >7 mo 14/28 had stable disease for 1.73–9.6mo
			With IFN-α	I/II (65)	Improved time to progression over IFN-α alone

Abbreviations: IFN-α, interferon-α;; CEA, carcinoembryonic antigen; MUC-1, mucin-1; PSA, prostate-specific antigen; PAP, prostatic acid phosphatase; GM-GSF, granulocyte macrophage colony-stimulating factor; IL, interleukin; MAGE, melanoma-associated antigen; MART-1, melanoma antigen recognized by T cells-1.

Patients in the DC/PANVAC arm will receive a priming dose of DCs infected with PANVAC-V, followed by three monthly doses of DCs infected with PANVAC-F. Immune responses and disease states will be evaluated within a month of finishing the initial vaccination course and every three months thereafter for patients who have not progressed. Two-year disease-free survival rates will be compared between the two vaccination strategies.

In addition to the trials described above, PANVAC therapy is being investigated in combination with standard-of-care chemotherapy for the treatment of breast cancer, as described later in this chapter.

PROSTVAC

Prostate cancer is the third most common cause of death from cancer in men of all ages and the most common cause of death from cancer in men over age 75 (40). Several unique TAAs are overexpressed in prostate cancer cells, such as prostate-specific antigen (PSA) (41,42), prostatic acid phosphatase (PAP) (43,44), and prostate-specific membrane antigen (PSMA) (45,46). As an added benefit, tumor cell lysis generated by a vaccine that targets one of these antigens, such as PSA, may expose the immune system to additional TAAs, such as PSMA, PAP, and MUC-1, leading to an immune response against TAAs not targeted specifically by the vaccine. This phenomenon, known as antigen spreading or antigen cascade, may ultimately result in an immune targeting of tumor cells via multiple TAAs (47,48).

Therapeutic cancer vaccines have been proved effective in treating prostate cancer. In fact, a recent phase III trial of the sipuleucel-T vaccine (Provenge; Dendreon Corp., Seattle, WA) showed a significant survival advantage in patients with metastatic prostate cancer, leading to its approval by the FDA as a standard of care in 2010 (49). Another therapeutic cancer vaccine in advanced testing is PROSTVAC, a recombinant poxviral vaccine targeting PSA and containing TRICOM. Recombinant vaccinia virus expressing PSA as well as TRICOM is identified as PROSTVAC-V, while recombinant fowlpox virus expressing these genes is identified as PROSTVAC-F. PROSTVAC has been investigated in both early- (castration-sensitive) and late-stage (castration-resistant) disease.

A phase I study in patients with metastatic castration-resistant prostate cancer (mCRPC) demonstrated that PROSTVAC was tolerated well. Moreover, patients treated with PROSTVAC had increased levels of PSA-specific T cells, and 9 of 15 patients had decreased PSA velocity after vaccination (Table 5.1) (50). A subsequent phase II Eastern Cooperative Oncology Group (ECOG) trial evaluated PROSTVAC in patients with metastatic, clinically localized prostate cancer with elevated blood PAP levels (stage D0; Table 5.1) (51). Patients were treated with an initial dose of PROSTVAC-V, then monthly PROSTVAC-F for two months followed by PROSTVAC-F every three months until PSA progression. After six months, 66% of patients had a >6-month PSA progression-free survival. In addition, the median on-study PSA doubling time increased from 4.4 months to 7.7 months, suggesting that the vaccine may delay the disease progression.

Two additional phase II studies have demonstrated the clinical potential of PROSTVAC in patients with mCRPC (Table 5.1). In a phase II trial, 125 patients with mCRPC and Gleason scores of ≤7 were randomized to receive either PROSTVAC in a diversified prime/boost dosing schedule with monthly boosts or an empty vector placebo. Although there was no benefit in terms of time to progression, there was a long-term survival benefit for patients treated with PROSTVAC. Indeed, an initial analysis showed a median overall survival of 24.4 months for patients treated with the vaccine, compared with 16.3 months for patients in the control arm (52). A final analysis confirmed this survival advantage, demonstrating an 8.5-month increase in overall survival among patients treated with PROSTVAC over patients treated with placebo (Fig. 5.3A) (53). A second trial of PROSTVAC conducted at the National Cancer Institute in 32 patients with mCRPC provided evidence of a tumor-specific immune response in vaccinated patients. All patients were vaccinated with PROSTVAC, resulting in declines in PSA (38% of patients) and PSA velocity (47% of patients). Immune analysis indicated a >2-fold increase in PSA-specific T cells in 45% of patients, 38% of whom had a >6-fold increase in PSA-specific T cells. Increased immune

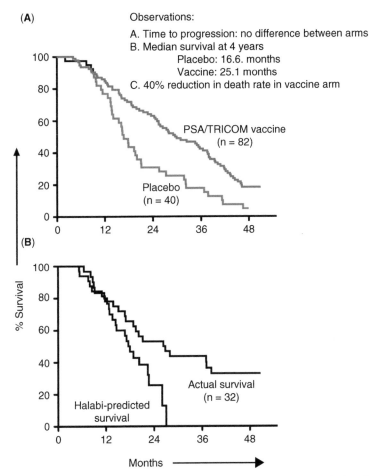

Figure 5.3 A survival analysis of two phase II trials with PROSTVAC. **(A)** Overall survival analysis of a phase II, randomized, placebo-controlled trial of PROSTVAC in patients with CRPC. Graphs indicate the Kaplan–Meier estimator for vaccine (blue) and control (red) arms. Vertical ticks indicate censoring times. **(B)** Overall survival analysis of another phase II study of PROSTVAC in patients with CRPC. The Kaplan–Meier curve for all 32 patients enrolled demonstrates a median Halabi-predicted survival of 17.4 months and a median actual survival of 26.6 months. *Abbreviation*: CRPC, castration-resistant prostate cancer. *Source*: Refs. 53,54.

response was associated with a trend toward improved overall survival. Median overall survival among all patients was 26.6 months (Table 5.1) (54). Since all patients were treated with vaccine, overall survival was compared to predicted survival based on the Halabi nomogram. The Halabi nomogram was developed from the survival outcomes of 1101 patients with mCRPC, treated between 1991 and 2001 in CALGB clinical trials with chemotherapy or second-line hormonal manipulation. The nomogram employs seven baseline characteristics to assess disease volume and aggressiveness to predict survival time (55). For all patients in the NCI trial, the Halabi-predicted survival was 17.4 months, compared with the actual observed median survival of 26.6 months (Fig. 5.3B) (54). This trial also provided insight into the type of patients best suited to treatment with vaccines, since a more striking outcome was seen among patients with more indolent disease characteristics. Patients with a Halabi-predicted survival of <18 months showed no significant improvement after treatment with PROSTVAC (median survival: 14.6 months; Halabi-predicted survival: 12.3 months). Patients with a Halabi-predicted survival of ≥18 months, however, had the greatest benefit, with a median overall survival that will meet or exceed

37.3 months (predicted survival: 20.9 months) (56). These data suggest that, in addition to using overall survival as an endpoint, future trials employing poxviral vaccine immunotherapy alone should be conducted primarily in patients with a more indolent disease. Follow-up studies are currently in development to further evaluate this hypothesis. PROSTVAC is also being evaluated in clinical trials in combination with numerous standard-of-care therapies and investigational new treatments. These trials will be discussed in later sections of this chapter.

TroVax

TroVax, a recombinant MVA virus expressing the oncofetal TAA 5T4, has also entered clinical trials. 5T4 is normally expressed in the placenta and at low levels in some gastrointestinal tissues, but is highly expressed in most breast, kidney, gastrointestinal, prostate, and ovarian cancers (57,58). In preclinical mouse models of colorectal cancer and melanoma, TroVax has demonstrated preventative and therapeutic efficacy (59,60). TroVax has been examined clinically for the treatment of colorectal, renal cell, and prostate cancers.

In an initial trial in patients with metastatic colorectal cancer, three monthly doses of TroVax were administered with an optional two additional vaccinations (Table 5.1) (61). The vaccine was safe and tolerated well, and it was demonstrated that a 5T4 immune response could be boosted in the presence of MVA neutralizing antibodies. Five of 22 patients in this trial experienced disease stabilization for 3–18 months, and there was a correlation between 5T4 antibody levels and increased survival or time to progression. In a second trial in patients with metastatic colorectal cancer, TroVax was administered twice (two weeks apart) before and twice after the surgical resection of liver metastases (Table 5.1) (62). In this trial, a trend toward improved survival was associated with the magnitude of the 5T4 immune response. Additional trials have evaluated TroVax in combination with the standard-of-care chemotherapy for the treatment of colorectal cancer, as discussed later in this chapter.

Clinical trials evaluating TroVax for the treatment of renal cell carcinoma have combined the vaccine with either interleukin 2 (IL-2; Table 5.1) or interferon-α (IFN-α). When high-dose IL-2 was combined with the vaccine, the IL-2 was administered the same day as the second dose of TroVax and for the next five days, with all patients receiving at least two cycles of IL-2 (63). On this therapeutic regimen, 12 of 25 patients had stable disease, but the addition of TroVax did not improve the objective response obtained over IL-2 therapy alone. When the combination included low-dose IL-2, TroVax was administered two weeks prior to the start of IL-2 therapy, and the vaccine and IL-2 were never given simultaneously (64). Two patients in this trial had complete objective responses for >24 months, while another had a partial response that lasted >12 months. An additional six patients had stable disease for 6–21 months. Statistical analysis determined that there was a significant correlation between the magnitude of 5T4 antibody response and progression-free and overall survivals. Of the two trials combining TroVax with IFN-α, one suggested an improved time to disease progression with the combination therapy (65). The other reported that 14 of 28 patients achieved disease stabilization while on combination therapy, and that one patient achieved a partial response for >7 months (66).

A trial assessing the efficacy of TroVax in patients with hormone-refractory prostate cancer has been completed. In this trial, TroVax was administered every two weeks with or without GM-CSF, which was given for 14 days following vaccination (Table 5.1). After the first five vaccinations, TroVax was administered monthly for three months, then every other month for six months (67). No patients in this trial exhibited an objective clinical response, but improved disease stabilization was observed in the 24 patients who developed a 5T4 antibody response. It was also determined that the administration of GM-CSF had no additional benefit in these patients.

TG4010

Another MVA-based cancer vaccine that has entered clinical trials is TG4010, a recombinant MVA vector expressing the TAA MUC-I and cytokine IL-2. TG4010 has been tested in patients with prostate and renal cell cancers. An initial phase I study demonstrated that TG4010 was safe and well tolerated, and also suggested that TG4010 may have clinical benefit in patients with non-small–cell lung cancer (Table 5.1) (68).

TG4010 was first tested in patients with non-metastatic prostate cancer and biochemical failure (rising PSA levels) (69). These patients received either weekly injections of TG4010 for 6 weeks then one injection every three weeks, or injections of TG4010 every three weeks from the beginning of the trial (Table 5.1). Thirteen of 40 patients had a >two-fold improvement in PSA doubling time, and eight patients had stable PSA levels for at least eight months. Though not statistically significant, patients receiving the initial weekly schedule of vaccination had longer periods of PSA stabilization. Therefore, when TG4010 was evaluated in patients with renal cell carcinoma, it was given weekly for six weeks, then every three weeks until disease progression, at which time TG4010 treatment was continued but in combination with IL-2 and IFN-α (70). During their time on TG4010 alone, 5 of 27 evaluable patients had stable disease for >6 months. Upon progression and addition of cytokine therapy, 6 of 20 evaluable patients had stable disease for >6 months.

MVA-BN-HER2 & MVA-BN-Pro

Two additional MVA-based cancer vaccines have entered clinical testing. MVA-BN-HER2 expresses a modified form of the Her-2 protein expressed by 20–30% of breast cancer patients. Her2 contains the extracellular domains of Her-2, but lacks the intracellular domains and also encodes two tetanus toxoid T-cell epitopes to facilitate the stimulation of an immune response to Her-2 (71). MVA-BN-Pro expresses two prostate-specific antigens: PSA and PAP. In preclinical testing in Her-2 transgenic mice, MVA-BN-HER2 induced anti-Her-2 immune responses resulting in an antitumor activity (71). In two clinical trials evaluating the safety and efficacy of this vaccine, MVA-BN-HER2 was administered at three-week intervals to metastatic breast cancer patients with Her-2+ tumors after treatment with first- or second-line chemotherapy (Table 5.1) (72,73). MVA-BN-HER2 was well tolerated and induced a humoral and/or cellular immune response to Her-2 in most patients. Recently, a new, more immunogenic version of MVA-BN-HER2 was created (74). This MVA-BN-HER2 is more efficacious in the HER-2 transgenic mouse model and is currently being tested in breast cancer patients with nonmetastatic Her-2+ tumors following adjuvant or neoadjuvant chemotherapy (74,75). MVA-BN-Pro has also shown promising results in preclinical studies (76). Monthly treatments with 1, 2, or 4 injections of MVA-BN-Pro are being tested in patients with nonmetastatic, hormone-insensitive prostate cancer (77). Preliminary results indicate that MVA-BN-Pro induces immune responses to both PSA and PAP in this patient population (76).

ALVAC

In addition to MVA, canarypox-based cancer immunotherapy vectors have also entered into clinical trials. A group of canarypox vectors collectively known as ALVAC, expressing various TAAs and immunomodulatory molecules, has been tested for the treatment of melanoma and colorectal cancer. An initial trial utilizing ALVAC expressing CEA and B7-1 in patients with CEA-expressing adenocarcinomas demonstrated that monthly administration was safe and well tolerated (Table 5.1) (78). In this trial, stable disease was established in 3 of 18 patients (two with colorectal cancer and one with pancreatic cancer), all of whom developed CEA-specific T cells.

ALVAC vectors expressing multiple transgenes have also been tested in patients with melanoma. In two separate trials, biweekly intratumoral injection of ALVAC expressing either IL-12, or IL-2, or GM-CSF was evaluated in metastatic melanoma patients (Table 5.1) (79,80). One of the nine patients receiving ALVAC IL-12 had a complete response in the injected lesions (80). Stable disease was observed in the eight lesions receiving ALVAC GM-CSF, and three of eight lesions receiving ALVAC IL-2 underwent partial regression (79). In another trial, ALVAC was engineered to express two antigenic peptides of melanoma-associated antigen (MAGE; Table 5.1) (81). Patients received four injections of ALVAC three weeks apart, followed by three vaccinations with MAGE peptides alone, also three weeks apart. Of the 30 patients, one achieved a partial objective response and two had stable disease. Two ongoing trials are utilizing ALVAC in melanoma patients. One combines ALVAC expressing gp100 (a peptide from the melanoma antigen glycoprotein 100) with patient-derived anti-gp100 cells. The other combines ALVAC expressing MART-1 (melanoma antigen recognized by T cells-1) with patient-derived anti-MART-1 F5 cells (Table 5.1) (82,83).

THE NEXT FRONTIER: POXVIRUS-BASED VACCINES IN COMBINATION THERAPY

Though encouraging results have come from the trials evaluating poxviral immunotherapy vectors alone, improved long-term anti-tumor outcomes from the use of these vectors will likely require combination therapy with current standard of care radiation or chemotherapy.

In preclinical studies, poxviral vectors have shown increased efficacy when combined with current chemotherapy agents and radiation, which target additional components of tumor development. Chemotherapy or radiation-induced cell death could serve as a potential source of tumor antigen to boost the immune response and both have been shown to modulate the gene expression of tumor cells rendering them better T-cell targets. In vitro studies have shown that exposing tumor cells to sublethal doses of radiation alters their phenotype by upregulating a number of genes such as Fas, MHC I and II, ICAM-1, and TAAs such as CEA and MUC-1. As a consequence, these tumor cells become more susceptible to T-cell-mediated killing (83–88). In murine studies, local irradiation of tumors or the use of radiolabeled antibodies after priming with rV-CEA/TRICOM and before boosting with rF-CEA/TRICOM showed a synergistic effect resulting in increased anti-tumor efficacy as compared with either modality alone (89,90). Chemotherapeutic agents, such as cyclophosphamide, cisplatin, 5-fluorouracil, and docetaxel, are also capable of upregulating multiple surface molecules on tumor cells rendering them more immunogenic (91–101). Docetaxel is one of the most widely used chemotherapeutic agents for cancer therapy. In tumor-bearing mice, the administration of docetaxel with the CEA/TRICOM vaccine platform resulted in an improved immune response to CEA and decreased tumor burden more so than if either treatment was used alone (47). This increased efficacy was only observed, however, when docetaxel was given seven days after the last booster vaccination and not prior to or during the vaccination regimen, highlighting the importance of proper scheduling of chemotherapeutic and immunotherapeutic treatments.

CLINICAL EXPERIENCE OF VACCINES IN COMBINATION WITH CHEMOTHERAPY

An ongoing trial is assessing the effectiveness of combining docetaxel with PANVAC for the treatment of metastatic breast cancer (Table 5.2) (102,103). Patients are eligible if they have received unlimited prior chemotherapy regimens, including prior docetaxel treatment, as long as their treatment was at least 12 months prior to enrollment in the study. Patients in the PAN-VAC plus docetaxel arm will receive a prime of PANVAC-V with monthly boosts of PANVAC-F. Patients will receive weekly docetaxel with dexamethasone for three weeks in each four-week cycle. Patients in the docetaxel-alone arm will receive no vaccine, but will receive weekly docetaxel with dexamethasone for three weeks in each four-week cycle. Patients will be assessed for disease progression and progression-free survival. Currently, three of the four patients in this study who have received PANVAC plus docetaxel have had measurable disease improvement (104). One patient had a 50% reduction in the diameter of a chest wall lesion, another on study for 12 months showed improvement on bone scan, and another achieved a partial response by Response Evaluation Criteria in Solid Tumors (RECIST) criteria. While combining PANVAC with docetaxel does seems to provide some clinical benefit in patients with metastatic breast cancer, confirming these results and evaluating progression-free survival will require additional patient enrollment and follow-up studies.

Docetaxel is the standard of care therapy for patients with mCRPC (105,106). An early trial evaluating the combination of a poxviral vaccine targeting PSA with docetaxel determined that PSA-specific T cells could be elicited in the presence of docetaxel, and that a combination therapy or vaccination prior to docetaxel therapy may lead to improved outcomes (107). Currently,

Table 5.2 Clinical Trials of Poxviral Vaccines Being Evaluated in Combination

Carcinoma	Target Antigen	Vector	Combination Therapy	Clinical Trial Phase	Clinical Outcome
Breast	HER2	MVA-BN-HER2	Trastuzumab or Lapatinib	II (73)	1 complete response 1 partial response
Colorectal	CEA, MUC-1	PANVAC	Docetaxel	II (102)	Ongoing
	CEA	ALVAC (also expressing B7-1)	FOLFIRI	II (115)	No differences in clinical response with respect to vaccine timing
	5T4	TroVax	FOLFOX	II (111)	1/11 complete responses 5/11 partial responses 1/11 achieved stable disease
			FOLFIRI	II (110)	1/19 complete responses 6/19 partial responses 5/19 achieved stable disease
Non-small-cell lung	MUC-1	TG4010 (also expressing IL-2)	Cisplatin and vinorelbine upon progression	II (116)	2/14 had stable disease (vaccine alone) 1/14 complete responses (combo) 1/14 partial responses (combo) 1-yr survival rate=60%
			Cisplatin and vinorelbine upfront		13/37 partial responses 1-yr survival rate=53%
Prostate	PSA	Vaccinia (admixed w/vaccinia expressing B7-1)	Docetaxel	II (107)	38% of patients experienced a decline in PSA 47% of them experienced an increased PSA-doubling time Increased survival of 2.4 mo compared with historical control
			External beam radiation	II (48)	13/17 patients developed a PSA-specific T-cell response of ≥3-fold
			Nilutamide	II (122,123)	Increased time to progression when vaccine is given prior to nilutamide (6.2 vs. 3.7 yrs)
	5T4	TroVax	Docetaxel	II (109)	Ongoing
	PSA	PROSTVAC	Docetaxel	II (108)	Ongoing
			Sm-153	II (119)	Ongoing
			Flutamide	II (124)	Ongoing
			Ipilimumab	I (125)	Overall increase in PSA doubling time 47% of patients experienced a decline in PSA

Abbreviations: CEA, carcinoembryonic antigen; FOLFIRI, 5-fluorouracil, leucovorin, and irinotecan; FOLFOX, 5-fluorouracil, leucovorin, and oxaliplatin; IL, interleukin; MUC-1, mucin-1; PSA, prostate-specific antigen.

a randomized phase II ECOG study is investigating the combination of docetaxel and prednisone with PROSTVAC (Table 5.2) (108). In this trial, patients with mCRPC will receive PROSTVAC-V with four boosts of PROSTVAC-F prior to docetaxel therapy, or docetaxel therapy alone. The overall survival of these patients will be evaluated, as will the association between PSA-specific immune responses and time to progression. Another ongoing phase II trial in this patient population is testing the efficacy of docetaxel in combination with TroVax (109). In this trial, patients will receive either docetaxel therapy alone or in combination with TroVax vaccination. The primary endpoint of this trial is to determine if this combination of therapies has an effect on the length of progression-free survival in these patients.

Two trials in patients with metastatic colorectal cancer have tested the efficacy of TroVax in combination with two different chemotherapy regimens: 5-fluorouracil, leucovorin, and oxaliplatin (FOLFOX), or 5-fluorouracil, leucovorin, and irinotecan (FOLFIRI; Table 5.2) (110,111). Of the 11 patients in the TroVax/FOLFOX trial, 1 exhibited stable disease, 5 had a partial response, and 1 had a complete objective response. Of the 19 evaluable patients in the TroVax/FOLFIRI trial, 5 had stable disease, 6 had a partial response, and 1 had a complete response. A phase III trial testing the efficacy of TroVax in patients with metastatic renal cell carcinoma undergoing standard chemotherapy was discontinued because the primary endpoint of improved progression-free survival and overall survival would not be met (112). However, a subset analysis of the patients in this trial found that those receiving TroVax plus IL-2 exhibited a survival advantage (113). Also, there was a trend toward improved survival for patients who mounted a 5T4 antibody response and had low pre-vaccination platelet levels, suggesting that TroVax may be more effective in certain patient populations. Based on the promising results in the TroVax-alone study, a clinical trial is currently being planned to evaluate the efficacy of TroVax in combination with docetaxel in prostate cancer patients (Table 5.2) (114).

Like TroVax, ALVAC-CEA/B7-1 has been tested in combination with the FOLFIRI chemotherapy regimen in metastatic colorectal patients (115). Patients in this trial received ALVAC-CEA/B7-1 prior to and during chemotherapy, ALVAC-CEA/B7-1 vaccination with tetanus toxoid as an adjuvant prior to and during chemotherapy, or chemotherapy prior to ALVAC-CEA/B7-1 vaccination. No differences in clinical response were observed among the groups, and some patients experienced grade 3 and 4 toxicities.

Following initial promising results with TG4010 in non-small-cell lung cancer, a trial was conducted to evaluate the use of TG4010 in combination with cisplatin and vinorelbine in this patient population (Table 5.2). Patients were given either TG4010 alone until disease progression, at which point TG4010 was combined with cisplatin and vinorelbine, or given TG4010 in combination with cisplatin and vinorelbine from the beginning of the trial (116). In both treatment arms, TG4010 was administered weekly for 6 weeks, then once every three weeks. Two of the 21 patients who received TG4010 alone achieved stable disease for >6 months. The addition of cisplatin and vinorelbine resulted in one complete and one partial objective response among 14 evaluable patients in this group. Thirteen of 37 evaluable patients receiving TG4010 in combination with cisplatin and vinorelbine from the beginning of the treatment period achieved a partial objective response. TG4010 is continuing to be evaluated in this patient population (103).

CLINICAL EVALUATION OF VACCINES IN COMBINATION WITH RADIOTHERAPY

A randomized phase II clinical trial involving a first-generation poxviral vaccine expressing PSA provided clinical proof of concept of the synergy between external beam radiation and immunotherapy. Thirty patients with localized prostate cancer were treated with standard radiation therapy; two-thirds of these patients received vaccine as well. For patients receiving both, radiation was administered between the fourth and sixth booster vaccinations (Table 5.2). Of the patients receiving radiation plus vaccine, 89% had a ≥3-fold increase in PSA-specific T cells after radiation, compared with no change in T-cell levels in patients treated with radiation alone (48). A follow-up study confirmed a similar magnitude of T-cell responses in a similar proportion of patients (117).

The early clinical trials described above, as well as several preclinical studies, provided the basis for an ongoing randomized phase II study of samarium-153 (Sm-153) with and without vaccine in patients with CRPC. Sm-153 is an FDA-approved radionuclide for palliation of bone pain in metastatic cancer patients (Table 5.2) (85,89,118). This study is designed to evaluate whether PROSTVAC in combination with Sm-153 can improve time to progression in patients with CRPC metastatic predominantly to bone, compared with Sm-153 alone. The study will also evaluate the effects of low-level local radiation on patients' ability to generate specific immunologic responses (119).

VACCINES IN COMBINATION WITH OTHER THERAPEUTIC AGENTS
Vaccines and Hormonal Therapy

Hormonal therapy may also work synergistically with therapeutic cancer vaccines for the treatment of prostate cancer. Flutamide, an FDA-approved androgen receptor antagonist commonly used as a second-line hormonal agent, diminishes the antiproliferative effects of testosterone on T cells (120). Androgen-deprivation therapy may also have broader effects on the immune system by enlarging the thymus, enriching the T-cell repertoire, and minimizing immune tolerance to prostate TAAs, which in turn could enhance the immune response to therapeutic cancer vaccines (46,121). Early trials of poxviral vaccines targeting PSA in combination with hormonal therapy have suggested the clinical benefit of combining these two therapeutic modalities. In one trial, 42 patients with nonmetastatic CRPC were randomized to treatment with nilutamide, an FDA-approved androgen receptor antagonist, or a poxviral vaccine, with the option of receiving the combination treatment upon disease progression (Table 5.2) (122). Preliminary findings suggested an improved clinical benefit with the combination therapy (especially when vaccine was started earlier in the disease process), which was confirmed in a recent overall survival analysis (123). It was also observed that patients who received the vaccine before nilutamide had improved survival compared with patients who received hormone therapy prior to vaccine. These data support the hypothesis that patients with more indolent disease may derive greater clinical benefit from vaccine alone or vaccine given prior to second-line hormone therapy compared with hormone therapy alone or hormone therapy followed by vaccine (122). An additional trial is currently accruing patients to extend these findings. In this study, nonmetastatic CRPC patients will be treated with either a combination of flutamide and PROSTVAC or flutamide alone (Table 5.2). The primary endpoint is time to progression, but immune parameters will also be evaluated (124).

VACCINES AND BIOLOGIC RESPONSE MODIFIERS

Clinical trials have also evaluated PROSTVAC in combination with emerging biologic response modifiers such as anti-CTLA-4, a monoclonal antibody (mAb) that binds to the CTLA-4 molecule of the T cell, potentially enhancing cytolytic T-cell activity. A phase I trial combining PROSTVAC with escalating doses of ipilimumab (Yervoy, Medarex, Princeton, NJ), an anti-CTLA-4 mAb, has been carried out (Table 5.2). Although autoimmune side effects typical of CTLA-4 blockade were seen, clinical benefits included declines in PSA in 47% of patients and increased PSA doubling time. Immunologic analyses showed that 56% of evaluable patients had 2.5- to 5-fold increases in PSA-specific T cells (125). This study provided preliminary evidence of the efficacy of this combination.

MVA-BN-HER2 has also been evaluated in combination with biologic response modifiers. In one of the two clinical trials evaluating MVA-BN-HER2, one treatment arm received vaccine concurrently with either trastuzumab, a Her-2/neu mAb, or lapatinib, a tyrosine kinase inhibitor (126) (Table 5.2). In this group of patients there was one complete and one partial objective response (72).

PERSPECTIVES ON THE FUTURE OF POXVIRAL-BASED IMMUNOTHERAPY

Since the approval of sipuleucel-T by the FDA in 2010 for treatment of patients with mCRPC who have progressed on docetaxel-based therapy, immunotherapy for cancer treatment has become an approved clinical alternative (49). Furthermore, poxvirus-based vaccines have been shown to be a valid alternative to DC-based vaccine platforms (127). Even though sipuleucel-T and the alternate poxviral-based vaccine platforms discussed above can improve overall survival with low toxicity, a major concern about the benefits of immunotherapy is the lack of effect on time to disease progression (Fig. 5.3A and B). Mathematical tumor growth models have helped to show that immunologic therapies act by slowing tumor growth, thus prolonging survival (128). This differs from most standard-of-care therapies, which cause initial tumor shrinkage due to the sensitivity of cancer cells to the therapy. This period of shrinkage, however, is followed by a rebound of tumor growth velocity, when tumors become resistant to the treatment. The finding that tumor growth rates measured during clinical trials correlate with overall survival provides a novel strategy for evaluating clinical trial data (128,129). More importantly, tumor regression and growth rates determined in five intramural NCI prostate cancer trials confirmed that the growth rate constant could be a valid indicator of therapeutic efficacy, suggesting that the effectiveness of immunotherapy can be better determined by improved overall survival rather than by time to disease progression (130).

In addition to aiding the generation of an immune response, combination therapy may also allow clinical benefits to be achieved with lower drug concentrations. This is a significant consideration, since toxicities from chemotherapy or radiotherapy are the major causes of dose reduction or treatment interruption in cancer patients (131). Validating the safety and efficacy of combination therapy will support the practice of administering vaccines earlier in the disease process, as does the fact that better results are seen in patients with a more indolent disease (54).

As discussed, a number of preclinical and clinical reports have shown that conventional chemotherapies, radiotherapies, or small-molecule inhibitors can synergistically potentiate vaccine-mediated immune attack against tumor cells. The direct antitumor effect mediated by cytotoxic therapies can decrease tumor volume, diminishing tumor-produced immune suppression and leaving a smaller tumor mass for the immune system to attack. The destruction of tumor cells by these therapies can also lead to exposure of additional TAAs (18), with the consequence of a larger antigen pool that leads, in turn, to a more robust immune response. The immunomodulatory properties of some new investigational agents can also be exploited in combination with immunotherapy. Low-dose GX15-070, a BCL-2 small molecule inhibitor, has been shown in animal models to selectively affect the number of immunosuppressive T-regulatory lymphocytes, resulting in improved antitumor responses (132,133). The inhibitory effect of the anti-angiogenetic agent sunitinib on myeloid-derived suppressor cells in patients with renal cell carcinoma has been the rationale for preclinical studies of this drug combined with immunotherapy (134–136). In addition, concurrent vaccination with multiple distinct vaccine platforms that target the same antigen but generate phenotypically and functionally distinct T-cell populations may prove to be a viable cancer treatment option (137). Just as regimens utilizing multiple chemotherapy agents targeting different aspects of tumor growth are now used in combination, in the future, vaccine platforms may be combined to generate a more robust and effective antitumor immune response.

As a therapeutic modality, cancer vaccines are unique in their ability to initiate a dynamic process of immune system activation, along with low toxicity and the potential for combination with low-dose chemotherapy or radiotherapy. Ongoing phase II and planned phase III trials could establish the flexibility and efficacy of poxviral-based cancer vaccines, alone and in combination, and support their use as standard-of-care therapy for numerous types of cancer.

ACKNOWLEDGMENTS

The authors thank Bonnie L. Casey for editorial assistance in the preparation of this chapter.

REFERENCES

1. Bonini C, Lee SP, Riddell SR, Greenberg PD. Targeting antigen in mature dendritic cells for simultaneous stimulation of CD4+ and CD8+ T cells. J Immunol 2001; 166: 5250–7.
2. Brown M, Davies DH, Skinner MA, et al. Antigen gene transfer to cultured human dendritic cells using recombinant avipoxvirus vectors. Cancer Gene Ther 1999; 6: 238–45.
3. Drillien R, Spehner D, Bohbot A, Hanau D. Vaccinia virus-related events and phenotypic changes after infection of dendritic cells derived from human monocytes. Virology 2000; 268: 471–81.
4. Moss B. Genetically engineered poxviruses for recombinant gene expression, vaccination, and safety. Proc Natl Acad Sci USA 1996; 93: 11341–8.
5. Fenner F, Henderson DA, Arita I, et al. Smallpox and Its Eradication. Geneva, Switzerland: World Health Organization, 1988.
6. Pastoret PP, Vanderplasschen A. Poxviruses as vaccine vectors. Comp Immunol Microbiol Infect Dis 2003; 26: 343–55.
7. Aarts WM, Schlom J, Hodge JW. Vector-based vaccine/cytokine combination therapy to enhance induction of immune responses to a self-antigen and antitumor activity. Cancer Res 2002; 62: 5770–7.
8. Somogyi P, Frazier J, Skinner MA. Fowlpox virus host range restriction: gene expression, DNA replication, and morphogenesis in nonpermissive mammalian cells. Virology 1993; 197: 439–44.
9. Arlen PM, Kaufman HL, DiPaola RS. Pox viral vaccine approaches. Semin Oncol 2005; 32: 549–55.
10. Kass E, Schlom J, Thompson J, et al. Induction of protective host immunity to carcinoembryonic antigen (CEA), a self-antigen in CEA transgenic mice, by immunizing with a recombinant vaccinia-CEA virus. Cancer Res 1999; 59: 676–83.
11. Tsang KY, Zaremba S, Nieroda CA, et al. Generation of human cytotoxic T cells specific for human carcinoembryonic antigen epitopes from patients immunized with recombinant vaccinia-CEA vaccine. J Natl Cancer Inst 1995; 87: 982–90.
12. Hodge JW, McLaughlin JP, Kantor JA, Schlom J. Diversified prime and boost protocols using recombinant vaccinia virus and recombinant non-replicating avian pox virus to enhance T-cell immunity and antitumor responses. Vaccine 1997; 15: 759–68.
13. Grosenbach DW, Barrientos JC, Schlom J, Hodge JW. Synergy of vaccine strategies to amplify antigen-specific immune responses and antitumor effects. Cancer Res 2001; 61: 4497–505.
14. Kudo-Saito C, Schlom J, Hodge JW. Intratumoral vaccination and diversified subcutaneous/intratumoral vaccination with recombinant poxviruses encoding a tumor antigen and multiple costimulatory molecules. Clin Cancer Res 2004; 10: 1090–9.
15. Taylor J, Paoletti E. Fowlpox virus as a vector in non-avian species. Vaccine 1988; 6: 466–8.
16. Marshall JL, Hoyer RJ, Toomey MA, et al. Phase I study in advanced cancer patients of a diversified prime-and-boost vaccination protocol using recombinant vaccinia virus and recombinant nonreplicating avipox virus to elicit anti-carcinoembryonic antigen immune responses. J Clin Oncol 2000; 18: 3964–73.
17. Marshall JL, Gulley JL, Arlen PM, et al. Phase I study of sequential vaccinations with fowlpox-CEA(6D)-TRICOM alone and sequentially with vaccinia-CEA(6D)-TRICOM, with and without granulocyte-macrophage colony-stimulating factor, in patients with carcinoembryonic antigen-expressing carcinomas. J Clin Oncol 2005; 23: 720–31.
18. Garnett CT, Greiner JW, Tsang KY, et al. TRICOM vector based cancer vaccines. Curr Pharm Des 2006; 12: 351–61.
19. Oh S, Hodge JW, Ahlers JD, et al. Selective induction of high avidity CTL by altering the balance of signals from APC. J Immunol 2003; 170: 2523–30.
20. Gregory CD, Murray RJ, Edwards CF, Rickinson AB. Downregulation of cell adhesion molecules LFA-3 and ICAM-1 in Epstein-Barr virus-positive Burkitt's lymphoma underlies tumor cell escape from virus-specific T cell surveillance. J Exp Med 1988; 167: 1811–24.
21. Hellstrom KE, Hellstrom I, Linsley P, Chen L. On the role of costimulation in tumor immunity. Ann NY Acad Sci 1993; 690: 225–30.
22. Zajac P, Schutz A, Oertli D, et al. Enhanced generation of cytotoxic T lymphocytes using recombinant vaccinia virus expressing human tumor-associated antigens and B7 costimulatory molecules. Cancer Res 1998; 58: 4567–71.
23. Kaufman HL, Deraffele G, Mitcham J, et al. Targeting the local tumor microenvironment with vaccinia virus expressing B7.1 for the treatment of melanoma. J Clin Invest 2005; 115: 1903–12.
24. Hodge JW, Sabzevari H, Yafal AG, et al. A triad of costimulatory molecules synergize to amplify T-cell activation. Cancer Res 1999; 59: 5800–7.

25. Wingren AG, Parra E, Varga M, et al. T cell activation pathways: B7, LFA-3, and ICAM-1 shape unique T cell profiles. Crit Rev Immunol 1995; 15: 235–53.

26. Zhu M, Terasawa H, Gulley J, et al. Enhanced activation of human T cells via avipox vector-mediated hyperexpression of a triad of costimulatory molecules in human dendritic cells. Cancer Res 2001; 61: 3725–34.

27. Hodge JW, Rad AN, Grosenbach DW, et al. Enhanced activation of T cells by dendritic cells engineered to hyperexpress a triad of costimulatory molecules. J Natl Cancer Inst 2000; 92: 1228–39.

28. Hodge JW, Grosenbach DW, Aarts WM, Poole DJ, Schlom J. Vaccine therapy of established tumors in the absence of autoimmunity. Clin Cancer Res 2003; 9: 1837–49.

29. Hodge JW, Chakraborty M, Kudo-Saito C, Garnett CT, Schlom J. Multiple costimulatory modalities enhance CTL avidity. J Immunol 2005; 174: 5994–6004.

30. Yang S, Tsang KY, Schlom J. Induction of higher-avidity human CTLs by vector-mediated enhanced costimulation of antigen-presenting cells. Clin Cancer Res 2005; 11: 5603–15.

31. Tsang KY, Palena C, Gulley J, Arlen P, Schlom J. A human cytotoxic T-lymphocyte epitope and its agonist epitope from the nonvariable number of tandem repeat sequence of MUC-1. Clin Cancer Res 2004; 10: 2139–49.

32. Zaremba S, Barzaga E, Zhu M, et al. Identification of an enhancer agonist cytotoxic T lymphocyte peptide from human carcinoembryonic antigen. Cancer Res 1997; 57: 4570–7.

33. Tsang KY, Palena C, Yokokawa J, et al. Analyses of recombinant vaccinia and fowlpox vaccine vectors expressing transgenes for two human tumor antigens and three human costimulatory molecules. Clin Cancer Res 2005; 11: 1597–607.

34. Gulley JL, Arlen PM, Tsang KY, et al. Pilot study of vaccination with recombinant CEA-MUC-1-TRI-COM poxviral-based vaccines in patients with metastatic carcinoma. Clin Cancer Res 2008; 14: 3060–9.

35. Schuetz TKH, Marshall J, Safran H. Extended survival in second-line pancreatic cancer after theraputic vaccination. J Clin Oncol 2005; 23: 2576.

36. Schuetz TMJ, Kaufman H, Safran H, Panicali D. Two Phase I studies of prime-boost vaccinations with vaccinia-fowlpox vaccines expressing CEA, MUC-1 and TRICOM costimulatory molecules (B7.1/ICAM-1/LFA-3) in patients with advanced pancreatic cancer. J Clin Oncol 2004; 22: 2564.

37. Therion Biologics Announces Conclusion of PANVAC-VF Phase 3 Trial. 2006. [Available from: http://www.medicalnewstoday.com/medicalnews.php?newsid=46137].

38. Vaccine Therapy and GM-CSF in Treating Patients with Locally Advanced or Metastatic Pancreatic Cancer That Cannot Be Removed By Surgery. [updated January 28, 2011February 2011]; Phase II clinical trial]. [Available from: www.clinicaltrials.gov/ct2/show/NCT00669734?term=PANVAC&rank=1].

39. Lou E, Marshall J, Aklilu M, et al. A phase II study of active immunotherapy with PANVAC or autologous, cultured dendritic cells infected with PANVAC after complete resection of hepatic metastases of colorectal carcinoma. Clin Colorectal Cancer 2006; 5: 368–71.

40. Prostate cancer. U.S. National Library of Medicine, National Institutes of Health; 2010. [Available from: http://www.ncbi.nlm.nih.gov/pubmedhealth/PMH0001418].

41. Madan RA, Gulley JL, Arlen PM. PSA-based vaccines for the treatment of prostate cancer. Expert Rev Vaccines 2006; 5: 199–209.

42. Oesterling JE. Prostate specific antigen: a critical assessment of the most useful tumor marker for adenocarcinoma of the prostate. J Urol 1991; 145: 907–23.

43. Vihko P, Virkkunen P, Henttu P, et al. Molecular cloning and sequence analysis of cDNA encoding human prostatic acid phosphatase. FEBS Lett 1988; 236: 275–81.

44. Veeramani S, Yuan TC, Chen SJ, et al. Cellular prostatic acid phosphatase: a protein tyrosine phosphatase involved in androgen-independent proliferation of prostate cancer. Endocr Relat Cancer 2005; 12: 805–22.

45. Murphy GP, Elgamal AA, Su SL, Bostwick DG, Holmes EH. Current evaluation of the tissue localization and diagnostic utility of prostate specific membrane antigen. Cancer 1998; 83: 2259–69.

46. Wright GL Jr, Grob BM, Haley C, et al. Upregulation of prostate-specific membrane antigen after androgen-deprivation therapy. Urology 1996; 48: 326–34.

47. Garnett CT, Schlom J, Hodge JW. Combination of docetaxel and recombinant vaccine enhances T-cell responses and antitumor activity: effects of docetaxel on immune enhancement. Clin Cancer Res 2008; 14: 3536–44.

48. Gulley JL, Arlen PM, Bastian A, et al. Combining a recombinant cancer vaccine with standard definitive radiotherapy in patients with localized prostate cancer. Clin Cancer Res 2005; 11: 3353–62.

49. Kantoff PW, Higano CS, Shore ND, et al. Sipuleucel-T immunotherapy for castration-resistant prostate cancer. N Engl J Med 2010; 363: 411–22.

50. DiPaola RS, Plante M, Kaufman H, et al. A phase I trial of pox PSA vaccines (PROSTVAC-VF) with B7-1, ICAM-1, and LFA-3 co-stimulatory molecules (TRICOM) in patients with prostate cancer. J Transl Med 2006; 4: 1.

51. DiPaola RS, Chen Y, Bubley GJ, et al. A Phase II study of PROSTVAC-V (vaccinia)/TRICOM and PROSTVAC-F (fowlpox)/TRICOM with GM-CSF in patients with PSA progression after local therapy for prostate cancer: results of ECOG 9802 [abstract]. 2009 Genitourinary Cancers Symposium. 2009.

52. Kantoff PW, Glode LM, Tannenbaum SI, Bilhartz DL, Pittman WG, Schuetz TJ, editors. Randomized, double-blind, vector-controlled study of targeted immunotherapy in patients (pts) with hormone-refractory prostate cancer (HRPC). 2006 ASCO Annual Meeting Proceedings Part I; 2006: J Clin Oncol.

53. Kantoff PW, Schuetz TJ, Blumenstein BA, et al. Overall survival analysis of a phase II randomized controlled trial of a Poxviral-based PSA-targeted immunotherapy in metastatic castration-resistant prostate cancer. J Clin Oncol 2010; 28: 1099–105.

54. Gulley JL, Arlen PM, Madan RA, et al. Immunologic and prognostic factors associated with overall survival employing a poxviral-based PSA vaccine in metastatic castrate-resistant prostate cancer. Cancer Immunol Immunother 2010; 59: 663–74.

55. Halabi S, Small EJ, Kantoff PW, et al. Prognostic model for predicting survival in men with hormone-refractory metastatic prostate cancer. J Clin Oncol 2003; 21: 1232–7.

56. Madan RA, Gulley JL, Dahut WL, Tsang KY, Steinberg SM, Schlom J, et al., editors. Overall survival (OS) analysis of a phase II study using a pox viral-based vaccine, PSA-TRICOM, in the treatment of metastatic, castrate-resistant prostate cancer (mCRPC): Implications for clinical trial design [Abstract]. 2008 ASCO Annual Meeting Proceedings; 2008: J Clin Oncol.

57. Hole N, Stern PL. A 72 kD trophoblast glycoprotein defined by a monoclonal antibody. Br J Cancer 1988; 57: 239–46.

58. Southall PJ, Boxer GM, Bagshawe KD, et al. Immunohistological distribution of 5T4 antigen in normal and malignant tissues. Br J Cancer 1990; 61: 89–95.

59. Harrop R, Ryan MG, Myers KA, et al. Active treatment of murine tumors with a highly attenuated vaccinia virus expressing the tumor associated antigen 5T4 (TroVax) is CD4+ T cell dependent and antibody mediated. Cancer Immunol Immunother 2006; 55: 1081–90.

60. Mulryan K, Ryan MG, Myers KA, et al. Attenuated recombinant vaccinia virus expressing oncofetal antigen (tumor-associated antigen) 5T4 induces active therapy of established tumors. Mol Cancer Ther 2002; 1: 1129–37.

61. Harrop R, Connolly N, Redchenko I, et al. Vaccination of colorectal cancer patients with modified vaccinia Ankara delivering the tumor antigen 5T4 (TroVax) induces immune responses which correlate with disease control: a phase I/II trial. Clin Cancer Res 2006; 12: 3416–24.

62. Elkord E, Dangoor A, Drury NL, et al. An MVA-based vaccine targeting the oncofetal antigen 5T4 in patients undergoing surgical resection of colorectal cancer liver metastases. J Immunother 2008; 31: 820–9.

63. Kaufman HL, Taback B, Sherman W, et al. Phase II trial of Modified Vaccinia Ankara (MVA) virus expressing 5T4 and high dose Interleukin-2 (IL-2) in patients with metastatic renal cell carcinoma. J Transl Med 2009; 7: 2.

64. Amato RJ, Shingler W, Naylor S, et al. Vaccination of renal cell cancer patients with modified vaccinia ankara delivering tumor antigen 5T4 (TroVax) administered with interleukin 2: a phase II trial. Clin Cancer Res 2008; 14: 7504–10.

65. Hawkins RE, Macdermott C, Shablak A, et al. Vaccination of patients with metastatic renal cancer with modified vaccinia Ankara encoding the tumor antigen 5T4 (TroVax) given alongside interferon-alpha. J Immunother 2009; 32: 424–9.

66. Amato RJ, Shingler W, Goonewardena M, et al. Vaccination of renal cell cancer patients with modified vaccinia Ankara delivering the tumor antigen 5T4 (TroVax) alone or administered in combination with interferon-alpha (IFN-alpha): a phase 2 trial. J Immunother 2009; 32: 765–72.

67. Amato RJ, Drury N, Naylor S, et al. Vaccination of prostate cancer patients with modified vaccinia ankara delivering the tumor antigen 5T4 (TroVax): a phase 2 trial. J Immunother 2008; 31: 577–85.

68. Rochlitz C, Figlin R, Squiban P, et al. Phase I immunotherapy with a modified vaccinia virus (MVA) expressing human MUC1 as antigen-specific immunotherapy in patients with MUC1-positive advanced cancer. J Gene Med 2003; 5: 690–9.

69. Dreicer R, Stadler WM, Ahmann FR, et al. MVA-MUC1-IL2 vaccine immunotherapy (TG4010) improves PSA doubling time in patients with prostate cancer with biochemical failure. Invest New Drugs 2009; 27: 379–86.

70. Oudard S, Rixe O, Beuselinck B, et al. A phase II study of the cancer vaccine TG4010 alone and in combination with cytokines in patients with metastatic renal clear-cell carcinoma: clinical and immunological findings. Cancer Immunol Immunother 2011; 60: 261–71.

71. Mandl SJ, Delcayre A, Curry D, et al. MVA-BN-HER2: A Novel Vaccine for the Treatment of Breast Cancers Which Overexpress HER-2. J Immunother 2006; 29: 652 10.1097/01.cji.0000211343.73588.59.

72. A. Guardino MC, T. Pienkowski, S. Radulovic, F. Legrand, A. Nguyen, L. Fernandez, J. Coutts, N. Moore, O. Hwang, B. Trieger, L. Brand, L. Reiner, A. Delcayre and W. Godfrey Treatment - Her2-Targeted Therapy Results of Two Phase I Clinical Trials of MVA-BN®-HER2 in HER-2 Overexpressing Metastatic Breast Cancer Patients. Cancer Research: December 15, 2009; Volume 69, Issue 24, Supplement 3 doi: 101158/0008-5472SABCS-09-5089 Abstracts: Thirty-Second Annual CTRC-AACR San Antonio Breast Cancer Symposium--Dec 10-13,2009; San Antonio, TX. [Abstract]. 2009; 69: Supplement 3.

73. Guardino A, Cassidy M, Pienkowski T, et al. Treatment - Her2-Targeted Therapy Results of Two Phase I Clinical Trials of MVA-BN®-HER2 in HER-2 Overexpressing Metastatic Breast Cancer Patients. Cancer Research: December 15, 2009; Volume 69, Issue 24, Supplement 3 doi: 101158/0008-5472SABCS-09-5089 Abstracts: Thirty-Second Annual CTRC-AACR San Antonio Breast Cancer Symposium-- Dec 10-13, 2009; San Antonio, TX. [Abstract]. 2009; 69: Supplement 3.

74. Bavarian-Nordic. MVA-BN® HER2. [cited 2011 02/27/11]; [Available from: http://www.bavarian-nordic.com/pipeline/mva-bn-her2.aspx].

75. ImmunoTherapeutics B. A Safety and Immunology Study of a Modified Vaccinia Vaccine for HER-2(+) Breast Cancer After Adjuvant Therapy. 2011 [updated February 7, 2011; cited 2011 02/27/11]; [Available from: http://clinicaltrials.gov/ct2/show/NCT01152398].

76. Bavarian-Nordic. MVA-BN® PRO. [cited 2011 02/27/11]; [Available from: http://www.bavarian-nordic.com/pipeline/mva-bn-pro.aspx].

77. A Safety Trial of MVA-BN®-PRO in Men With Androgen-Insensitive Prostate Cancer (BNIT-PR-001). [updated May 13, 2009 02/27/11]; [Available from: http://clinicaltrials.gov/ct2/show/NCT00629057].

78. Horig H, Lee DS, Conkright W, et al. Phase I clinical trial of a recombinant canarypoxvirus (ALVAC) vaccine expressing human carcinoembryonic antigen and the B7.1 co-stimulatory molecule. Cancer Immunol Immunother 2000; 49: 504–14.

79. Hofbauer GF, Baur T, Bonnet MC, et al. Clinical phase I intratumoral administration of two recombinant ALVAC canarypox viruses expressing human granulocyte-macrophage colony-stimulating factor or interleukin-2: the transgene determines the composition of the inflammatory infiltrate. Melanoma Res 2008; 18: 104–11.

80. Triozzi PL, Strong TV, Bucy RP, et al. Intratumoral administration of a recombinant canarypox virus expressing interleukin 12 in patients with metastatic melanoma. Hum Gene Ther 2005; 16: 91–100.

81. van Baren N, Bonnet MC, Dreno B, et al. Tumoral and immunologic response after vaccination of melanoma patients with an ALVAC virus encoding MAGE antigens recognized by T cells. J Clin Oncol 2005; 23: 9008–21.

82. Quarmby S, Hunter RD, Kumar S. Irradiation induced expression of CD31, ICAM-1 and VCAM-1 in human microvascular endothelial cells. Anticancer Res 2000; 20: 3375–81.

83. Sheard MA, Vojtesek B, Janakova L, Kovarik J, Zaloudik J. Up-regulation of Fas (CD95) in human p53wild-type cancer cells treated with ionizing radiation. Int J Cancer 1997; 73: 757–62.

84. Santin AD, Hermonat PL, Hiserodt JC, et al. Effects of irradiation on the expression of major histocompatibility complex class I antigen and adhesion costimulation molecules ICAM-1 in human cervical cancer. Int J Radiat Oncol Biol Phys 1997; 39: 737–42.

85. Garnett CT, Palena C, Chakraborty M, et al. Sublethal irradiation of human tumor cells modulates phenotype resulting in enhanced killing by cytotoxic T lymphocytes. Cancer Res 2004; 64: 7985–94.

86. Chakraborty M, Abrams SI, Camphausen K, et al. Irradiation of tumor cells up-regulates Fas and enhances CTL lytic activity and CTL adoptive immunotherapy. J Immunol 2003; 170: 6338–47.

87. Hareyama M, Imai K, Kubo K, et al. Effect of radiation on the expression of carcinoembryonic antigen of human gastric adenocarcinoma cells. Cancer 1991; 67: 2269–74.

88. Friedman EJ. Immune modulation by ionizing radiation and its implications for cancer immunotherapy. Curr Pharm Des 2002; 8: 1765–80.

89. Chakraborty M, Abrams SI, Coleman CN, et al. External beam radiation of tumors alters phenotype of tumor cells to render them susceptible to vaccine-mediated T-cell killing. Cancer Res 2004; 64: 4328–37.

90. Chakraborty M, Gelbard A, Carrasquillo JA, et al. Use of radiolabeled monoclonal antibody to enhance vaccine-mediated antitumor effects. Cancer Immunol Immunother 2008; 57: 1173–83.

91. Aquino A, Prete SP, Greiner JW, et al. Effect of the combined treatment with 5-fluorouracil, gamma-interferon or folinic acid on carcinoembryonic antigen expression in colon cancer cells. Clin Cancer Res 1998; 4: 2473–81.

92. Prete SP, Aquino A, Masci G, et al. Drug-induced changes of carcinoembryonic antigen expression in human cancer cells: effect of 5-fluorouracil. J Pharmacol Exp Ther 1996; 279: 1574–81.

93. Eckert K, FuhrmannSelter T, Maurer HR. Docetaxel enhances the expression of E-cadherin and carcinoembryonic antigen (CEA) on human colon cancer cell lines in vitro. Anticancer Res 1997; 17: 7–12.

94. Grunberg E, Eckert K, Maurer HR. Docetaxel treatment of HT-29 colon carcinoma cells reinforces the adhesion and immunocytotoxicity of peripheral blood lymphocytes in vitro. Int J Oncol 1998; 12: 957–63.

95. Sundelin K, Roberg K, Grenman R, Hakansson L. Effects of cisplatin, alpha-interferon, and 13-cis retinoic acid on the expression of Fas (CD95), intercellular adhesion molecule-1 (ICAM-1), and epidermal growth factor receptor (EGFR) in oral cancer cell lines. J Oral Pathol Med 2007; 36: 177–83.

96. Mizutani Y, Wu XX, Yoshida O, Shirasaka T, Bonavida B. Chemoimmunosensitization of the T24 human bladder cancer line to Fas-mediated cytotoxicity and apoptosis by cisplatin and 5-fluorouracil. Oncol Rep 1999; 6: 979–82.

97. Bergmann-Leitner ES, Abrams SI. Treatment of human colon carcinoma cell lines with anti-neoplastic agents enhances their lytic sensitivity to antigen-specific CD8+ cytotoxic T lymphocytes. Cancer Immunol Immunother 2001; 50: 445–55.

98. AbdAlla EE, Blair GE, Jones RA, Sue-Ling HM, Johnston D. Mechanism of synergy of levamisole and fluorouracil: induction of human leukocyte antigen class I in a colorectal cancer cell line. J Natl Cancer Inst 1995; 87: 489–96.

99. Chan OT, Yang LX. The immunological effects of taxanes. Cancer Immunol Immunother 2000; 49: 181–5.

100. Fisk B, Ioannides CG. Increased sensitivity of adriamycin-selected tumor lines to CTL-mediated lysis results in enhanced drug sensitivity. Cancer Res 1998; 58: 4790–3.

101. Matsuzaki I, Suzuki H, Kitamura M, et al. Cisplatin induces fas expression in esophageal cancer cell lines and enhanced cytotoxicity in combination with LAK cells. Oncology 2000; 59: 336–43.

102. Arlen PM, Pazdur M, Skarupa L, Rauckhorst M, Gulley JL. A randomized phase II study of docetaxel alone or in combination with PANVAC-V (vaccinia) and PANVAC-F (fowlpox) in patients with metastatic breast cancer (NCI 05-C-0229). Clin Breast Cancer 2006; 7: 176–9.

103. Immunotherapy With TG4010 in Patients With Advanced Non-Small Cel Lung Cancer. [updated September 2, 2010March, 2011]; [Available from: http://clinicaltrials.gov/ct2/show/NCT00415818?term=tg4010&rank=1].

104. M. Mohebtash RAM, J. L. Gulley, J. Jones, M. Pazdur, M. Rauckhorst, J. Schlom, P. M. Arlen PANVAC vaccine alone or with docetaxel for patients with metastatic breast cancer. J Clin Oncol [2008 ASCO Annual Meeting]. 2008; 26.

105. Petrylak DP, Tangen CM, Hussain MH, et al. Docetaxel and estramustine compared with mitoxantrone and prednisone for advanced refractory prostate cancer. N Engl J Med 2004; 351: 1513–20.

106. Tannock IF, de Wit R, Berry WR, et al. Docetaxel plus prednisone or mitoxantrone plus prednisone for advanced prostate cancer. N Engl J Med 2004; 351: 1502–12.

107. Arlen PM, Gulley JL, Parker C, et al. A randomized phase II study of concurrent docetaxel plus vaccine versus vaccine alone in metastatic androgen-independent prostate cancer. Clin Cancer Res 2006; 12: 1260–9.

108. Phase II Randomized Study of Docetaxel and Prednisone With Versus Without Vaccine Therapy Comprising Vaccinia-PSA(L155)-TRICOM and Fowlpox-PSA(L155)-TRICOM in Patients With Castration-Resistant Metastatic Prostate Cancer. NCI Clinical Trials (PDQ); [February 2011]; Phase II clinical trial]. [Available from: http://www.cancer.gov/clinicaltrials/search/view?cdrid=675173&version=HealthProfessional&protocolsearchid=8856309].

109. TroVax In Subjects With Hormone Refractory Prostate Cancer (HRPC). [updated January 20, 2011March, 2011]; [Available from: http://clinicaltrials.gov/ct2/show/NCT01194960?term=Trovax&rank=5].

110. Harrop R, Drury N, Shingler W, et al. Vaccination of colorectal cancer patients with TroVax given alongside chemotherapy (5-fluorouracil, leukovorin and irinotecan) is safe and induces potent immune responses. Cancer Immunol Immunother 2008; 57: 977–86.

111. Harrop R, Drury N, Shingler W, et al. Vaccination of colorectal cancer patients with modified vaccinia ankara encoding the tumor antigen 5T4 (TroVax) given alongside chemotherapy induces potent immune responses. Clin Cancer Res 2007; 13: 4487–94.

112. Amato RJ, Hawkins RE, Kaufman HL, et al. Vaccination of metastatic renal cancer patients with MVA-5T4: a randomized, double-blind, placebo-controlled phase III study. Clin Cancer Res 2010; 16: 5539–47.

113. Kim DW, Krishnamurthy V, Bines SD, Kaufman HL. TroVax, a recombinant modified vaccinia Ankara virus encoding 5T4: Lessons learned and future development. Hum Vaccin 2010; 6: 12–19.

114. Amato RJ. 5T4-modified vaccinia Ankara: progress in tumor-associated antigen-based immunotherapy. Expert Opin Biol Ther 2010; 10: 281–7.

115. Kaufman HL, Lenz HJ, Marshall J, et al. Combination chemotherapy and ALVAC-CEA/B7.1 vaccine in patients with metastatic colorectal cancer. Clin Cancer Res 2008; 14: 4843–9.

116. Ramlau R, Quoix E, Rolski J, et al. A phase II study of Tg4010 (Mva-Muc1-Il2) in association with chemotherapy in patients with stage III/IV Non-small cell lung cancer. J Thorac Oncol 2008; 3: 735–44.

117. Lechleider RJ, Arlen PM, Tsang KY, et al. Safety and immunologic response of a viral vaccine to prostate-specific antigen in combination with radiation therapy when metronomic-dose interleukin 2 is used as an adjuvant. Clin Cancer Res 2008; 14: 5284–91.

118. Kudo-Saito C, Schlom J, Camphausen K, Coleman CN, Hodge JW. The requirement of multimodal therapy (vaccine, local tumor radiation, and reduction of suppressor cells) to eliminate established tumors. Clin Cancer Res 2005; 11: 4533–44.

119. 153Sm-EDTMP With or Without a PSA/TRICOM Vaccine To Treat Men With Androgen-Insensitive Prostate Cancer. NCI Clinical Trials (PDQ); [February 2011]; Phase II clinical trial]. [Available from: http://www.cancer.gov/clinicaltrials/search/view?cdrid=535561&version=HealthProfessional&protocolsearchid=8813434].

120. Mercader M, Bodner BK, Moser MT, et al. T cell infiltration of the prostate induced by androgen withdrawal in patients with prostate cancer. Proc Natl Acad Sci USA 2001; 98: 14565–70.

121. Sharifi N, Gulley JL, Dahut WL. Androgen deprivation therapy for prostate cancer. JAMA 2005; 294: 238–44.

122. Madan RA, Gulley JL, Schlom J, et al. Analysis of overall survival in patients with nonmetastatic castration-resistant prostate cancer treated with vaccine, nilutamide, and combination therapy. Clin Cancer Res 2008; 14: 4526–31.

123. Arlen PM, Gulley JL, Todd N, et al. Antiandrogen, vaccine and combination therapy in patients with nonmetastatic hormone refractory prostate cancer. J Urol 2005; 174: 539–46.

124. Vaccine Therapy With PROSTVAC/TRICOM and Flutamide Versus Flutamide Alone to Treat Prostate Cancer. NCI Clinicla Trials (PDQ); [February 2011]; [Available from: http://www.cancer.gov/clinicaltrials/search/view?cdrid=535593&version=HealthProfessional&protocolsearchid=8813434].

125. Mohebtash M, Madan RA, Arlen PM, et al. Phase I trial of targeted therapy with PSA-TRICOM vaccine (V) and ipilimumab (ipi) in patients (pts) with metastatic castration-resistant prostate cancer (mCRPC). [abstract]. 2009 ASCO Annual Meeting J Clin Oncol; 2009.

126. A Safety and Immunology Study of a Modified Vaccinia Vaccine for HER-2(+) Breast Cancer After Adjuvant Therapy. [updated February 7, 201102/27/11]; [Available from: http://clinicaltrials.gov/ct2/show/NCT01152398].

127. Gilbert PA, McFadden G. Poxvirus cancer therapy. Recent Pat Antiinfect Drug Discov 2006; 1: 309–21.

128. Stein WD, Figg WD, Dahut W, et al. Tumor growth rates derived from data for patients in a clinical trial correlate strongly with patient survival: a novel strategy for evaluation of clinical trial data. Oncologist 2008; 13: 1046–54.

129. Stein WD, Yang J, Bates SE, Fojo T. Bevacizumab reduces the growth rate constants of renal carcinomas: a novel algorithm suggests early discontinuation of bevacizumab resulted in a lack of survival advantage. Oncologist 2008; 13: 1055–62.

130. Stein WD, Gulley JL, Schlom J, et al. Tumor Regression and Growth Rates Determined in Five Intramural NCI Prostate Cancer Trials: The Growth Rate Constant as an Indicator of Therapeutic Efficacy. Clin Cancer Res 2011; 17: 907–17.

131. Eng C. Toxic effects and their management: daily clinical challenges in the treatment of colorectal cancer. Nat Rev Clin Oncol 2009; 6: 207–18.

132. Lutsiak ME, Semnani RT, De Pascalis R, et al. Inhibition of CD4(+)25+ T regulatory cell function implicated in enhanced immune response by low-dose cyclophosphamide. Blood 2005; 105: 2862–8.

133. Farsaci B, Sabzevari H, Higgins JP, et al. Effect of a small molecule BCL-2 inhibitor on immune function and use with a recombinant vaccine. Int J Cancer 2010; 127: 1603–13.

134. Ko JS, Zea AH, Rini BI, et al. Sunitinib mediates reversal of myeloid-derived suppressor cell accumulation in renal cell carcinoma patients. Clin Cancer Res 2009; 15: 2148–57.

135. Ozao-Choy J, Ma G, Kao J, et al. The novel role of tyrosine kinase inhibitor in the reversal of immune suppression and modulation of tumor microenvironment for immune-based cancer therapies. Cancer Res 2009; 69: 2514–22.

136. Bose A, Taylor JL, Alber S, et al. Sunitinib facilitates the activation and recruitment of therapeutic anti-tumor immunity in concert with specific vaccination. Int J Cancer 2010.

137. Boehm AL, Higgins J, Franzusoff A, Schlom J, Hodge JW. Concurrent vaccination with two distinct vaccine platforms targeting the same antigen generates phenotypically and functionally distinct T-cell populations. Cancer Immunol Immunother 2010; 59: 397–408.

138. Anti-gp100 Cells Plus ALVAC gp100 Vaccine to Treat Advanced Melanoma. [updated Jan 11, 2011Feb 16, 2011]; [Available from: http://www.clinicaltrials.gov/ct2/show/NCT00610311?term=ALVAC+cancer&rank=2].

139. Anti-MART-1 F5 Cells Plus ALVAC MART-1 Vaccine to Treat Advanced Melanoma. [updated January 11, 2011; cited 2011]; [Available from: http://www.clinicaltrials.gov/ct2/show/NCT00612222?term=ALVAC+cancer&rank=1].

6 | Of mice and men (and dogs!): The first approved cancer therapy vaccine

Philip J. Bergman and Jedd D. Wolchok

INTRODUCTION

The most common oral malignancy in dogs is melanoma (1–4). Oral melanoma is most commonly diagnosed in Scottish terriers, golden retrievers, poodles, and dachshunds (2,5). Oral melanoma is primarily a disease of older dogs without gender predilection, but may be seen in younger dogs (5–7). Melanomas in dogs have extremely diverse biologic behaviors depending on a large variety of factors. A greater understanding of these factors significantly helps the clinician to delineate in advance the appropriate staging, prognosis, and treatments. The primary factors which determine the biologic behavior of an oral melanoma in a dog are site, size, stage, and histologic parameters (5–9). Unfortunately, even with a comprehensive understanding of all of these factors, there are melanomas which have an unreliable biologic behavior; hence the need for additional research into this relatively common, heterogeneous, but a frequently extremely malignant tumor. Molecular biological aspects of canine melanoma have been previously reviewed (10,11).

BIOLOGIC BEHAVIOR

The biologic behavior of canine oral melanoma is extremely variable and best characterized based on anatomic site, size, stage, and histologic parameters. On divergent ends of the spectrum would be a low-grade 0.5 cm haired-skin melanoma, which is highly likely to be cured with simple surgical extirpation, in comparison to a 5.0 cm high-grade malignant oral melanoma with a poor to grave prognosis. Similar to the development of a rational staging, two primary questions must be answered while making a prognostic and therapeutic plan for any tumor: what is the local invasiveness of the tumor and what is the metastatic propensity? The answers to these questions will determine the prognosis, and to be discussed later, the premise of this chapter, which is treatment with local tumor control and a therapeutic DNA vaccine.

The anatomic site of melanoma is highly, though not completely, predictive of local invasiveness and metastatic propensity. Melanomas involving the haired skin, which are not in proximity to mucosal margins, often behave in a benign manner (1,12). Surgical extirpation through a lumpectomy is often curative, but histopathologic examination is imperative for the delineation of margins as well as the description of cytologic features. Oral and/or mucosal melanoma has been routinely considered an extremely malignant tumor with a high degree of local invasiveness and high metastatic propensity (2,5–8). This biologic behavior is extremely similar to that of human oral and/or mucosal melanoma (1,13). Melanoma is the most common oral tumor in dogs; additional neoplastic differentials include squamous cell carcinoma, fibrosarcoma, epulides/odontogenic tumors, and others (1,2,4,14–16). Melanomas in the oral cavities of dogs are found in the following locations by order of decreasing frequency: gingiva, lips, tongue, and hard palate. While most melanomas are pigmented, amelanotic oral melanomas are noted clinically and have been previously reported (17).

SIZE AND STAGE

For dogs with oral melanoma, primary tumor size has been found to be extremely prognostic. The WHO staging scheme for dogs with oral melanoma is based on size and metastasis, with stage I being less than 2 cm diameter tumor, stage II measuring 2 cm to <4 cm diameter tumor, stage III of 4 cm or greater tumor and/or lymph node metastasis, and stage IV equaling distant metastasis (Fig. 6.1). MacEwen and colleagues reported median survival times (MSTs) for dogs with oral melanoma treated with surgery to be approximately 17–18, 5–6 and 3 months with

T: Primary tumor

        T1   Tumor <2 cm in diameter

        T2   Tumor 2–4 cm in diameter

        T3   Tumor >4 cm in diameter

N: Regional lymph nodes

        N0   No evidence of regional node involvement

        N1   Histologic/cytologic evidence of regional node involvement

        N2   Fixed nodes

M: Distant metastasis

        M0   No evidence of distant metastasis

        M1   Evidence of distant metastasis

Stage I = T1 N0 M0

Stage II = T2 N0 M0

Stage III = T2 N1 M0 or T3 N0 M0

Stage IV = any T, any N and M1

Figure 6.1   Traditional, World Health Organization TNM-based staging scheme for dogs with oral melanoma.

stage I, II, and III disease, respectively (6). More recent reports suggest stage I oral melanoma treated with standardized therapies including surgery, radiation and/or chemotherapy have an MST of approximately 12–14 months, with most dogs dying of distant metastatic disease, not local recurrence (18,19). Other investigators have found dogs with stage I oral melanoma to have a median progression-free survival time of 19 months similar to the original MacEwen et al. report (20).

STAGING

The staging of dogs with melanoma is relatively straightforward. A minimum database should include a thorough history and physical examination, complete blood count and platelet count, biochemical profile, urinalysis, 3-view chest films, and local lymph node aspiration with cytology as to whether lymphadenomegaly is present or not. Williams and Packer reported that ~70% of dogs with oral melanoma had metastasis when lymphadenomegaly was present, but more importantly ~40% had metastasis when no lymphadenomegaly was present (21). Additional considerations should be made for abdominal compartment testing (e.g. abdominal ultrasound) in all cases of canine malignant melanoma (CMM), especially in cases with potentially moderately to highly metastatic anatomic sites such as the oral cavity, feet, or mucosal surface of the lips, as melanoma may metastasize to the abdominal lymph nodes, liver, adrenal glands, and other sites. The use of sentinel lymph node mapping and lymphadenectomy has been proved to be of diagnostic, prognostic, and clinical benefit in human melanoma (22). Relatively few investigations have been reported to date for sentinel lymph node mapping and/or excision for dogs with malignancies (23–26) and these authors strongly encourage additional investigation in this area and specifically with canine melanoma.

TREATMENT

The treatment for dogs with melanoma without distant metastatic disease on staging starts with local tumor control. This is generally best completed through surgical extirpation due to its speed, increased curative intent, and reduced cost compared to other modalities. The dose of surgery is generally based on the anatomic site of the melanoma, with cutaneous melanomas usually requiring lumpectomy and all other sites requiring more aggressive and wide excision. While large resections such as partial mandibulectomy or maxillectomy carry an inherent level of morbidity, owner satisfaction rates are routinely considered high. The importance of complete staging cannot be overstated while contemplating larger resections; the presence of distant metastatic disease would attenuate the use of more radical surgical procedures and convert the patient to medical and/or palliative care options.

Radiation therapy (RT) plays a role in the treatment of canine melanoma when the tumor is not surgically resectable, when the tumor has been removed with incomplete margins, and/or the melanoma has metastasized to local lymph nodes without further distant metastasis. The use of smaller fractions of RT (e.g. 3–4 Gy) given daily to every other day can allow for a greater total dose and fewer chronic RT reactions; however, melanoma appears comparatively resistant to these types of fractionation schemes (19,27). Coarse fractionation schemes for canine melanoma using 6–9 Gy of RT weekly to every other week to a total dose of 24–36 Gy have been reported by a variety of investigators with complete remission rates of 53–69% and partial remission rates of 25–30% (18–20,28,29). Unfortunately, recurrence and/or distant metastasis were common in all of these studies. Other modalities reported for local tumor control as case reports and/or case series have included intralesional cisplatin implants, intralesional bleomycin with electronic pulsing and many others, but widespread use has not been reported to date (30–32).

In dogs with melanoma in the aforementioned anatomic sites predicted to have a moderate to high metastatic propensity, or dogs with cutaneous melanoma with a high tumor score and/or increased proliferation index through increased Ki-67 expression, systemic therapies are warranted. Rassnick and colleagues reported an overall response rate of 28% using carboplatin for dogs with malignant melanoma (33). Unfortunately, only one dog had a minimally durable complete response (~150 days), and the rest were nondurable partial responses. Similarly, Boria et al. reported an 18% response rate and a median survival time of 119 days with cisplatin and piroxicam in canine oral melanoma (34). Other reports using single agent dacarbazine, melphalan, or doxorubicin suggest poor to dismal activity (35–37). More recently and importantly, two studies suggest that chemotherapy plays an insignificant role in the adjuvant treatment of canine melanoma (19,38). While it can be argued that the studies performed to date to evaluate the activity of chemotherapy in an adjuvant setting for canine melanoma have been suboptimal due to a variety of reasons, the extensive human literature in this specific setting suggests melanoma is an extremely chemotherapy-resistant tumor (39). It is clear that new approaches to the systemic treatment of this disease are desperately needed.

Immunotherapy represents one potential logical systemic therapeutic strategy for melanoma. A variety of immunotherapeutic strategies for the treatment of human melanoma have been reported previously, with typically poor outcomes due to a lack of breaking tolerance. Immunotherapy strategies to date in canine melanoma have used autologous tumor cell vaccines (with or without transfection with immunostimulatory cytokines and/or melanosomal differentiation antigens), allogeneic tumor cell vaccines transfected with interleukin 2 or granulocyte macrophage colony-stimulating factor (GM-CSF), liposomal-encapsulated non-specific immunostimulators (e.g. L-MTP-PE), intralesional Fas ligand DNA, bacterial super-antigen approaches with GM-CSF or interleukin 2 as immune adjuvants, and lastly canine dendritic cell vaccines loaded with melanosomal differentiation antigens (6,40–46). Although these approaches have produced some clinical anti-tumor responses, the methodologies for the generation of these products are expensive, time consuming, sometimes dependent on patient tumor samples being established into cell lines and fraught with the difficulties of consistency, reproducibility, and other quality control issues.

The advent of DNA vaccination circumvents many of the previously encountered hurdles in vaccine development. DNA is relatively inexpensive and simple to purify in large quantities. The antigen of interest is cloned into a bacterial expression plasmid with a constitutively active promoter. The plasmid is introduced into the skin or muscle with an intradermal or intramuscular injection. Once in the skin or muscle, professional antigen- presenting cells, particularly dendritic cells, are able to present the transcribed and translated antigen in the proper context of major histocompatibility complex and co-stimulatory molecules. Although DNA vaccines have induced immune responses to viral proteins, vaccinating against tissue-specific self proteins on cancer cells is clearly a more difficult problem. One way to induce immunity against a tissue-specific differentiation antigen on cancer cells is to vaccinate with xenogeneic (different species) antigen or DNA that is homologous to the cancer antigen. As outlined in a cartoon form in Figure 6.2, vaccination with DNA encoding cancer differentiation antigens is ineffective when self-DNA is used, but tumor immunity can be induced by orthologous DNA from another species (47).

We have chosen to target defined melanoma differentiation antigens of the tyrosinase family. Tyrosinase is a melanosomal glycoprotein, essential in melanin synthesis. Immunization with xenogeneic human DNA encoding tyrosinase family proteins induced antibodies and cytotoxic T-cells against syngeneic B16 melanoma cells in C57BL/6 mice, but immunization with mouse tyrosinase-related DNA did not induce detectable immunity (48). In particular, xenogeneic DNA vaccination induced tumor protection from syngeneic melanoma challenge and autoimmune hypopigmentation. Thus, xenogeneic DNA vaccination could break tolerance against a self tumor differentiation antigen, inducing antibody, T-cell, and anti-tumor responses.

From April 2000 to June 2007, approximately 500 dogs with previously histologically confirmed spontaneous malignant melanoma were treated at the Animal Medical Center with xenogeneic DNA vaccinations. Pre-trial evaluation included complete physical examination, a complete blood count and platelet count, serum chemistry profile, urinalysis, lactate dehydrogenase, antinuclear antibody, and three-dimensional measurements of the primary tumor if present (or maximal tumor size from medical records if patient was treated prior to pre-trial considerations). For evaluation of metastatic disease, three-view radiographs of the thorax were obtained and regional lymph nodes were evaluated with fine needle aspiration/cytology and/or biopsy/histopathology. All dogs were clinically staged according to the WHO staging

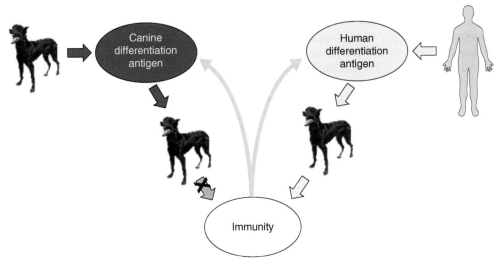

Figure 6.2   A cartoon outlining the xenogeneic DNA vaccination concept.

system of stage I (tumor <2 cm diameter), stage II (tumor 2–4 cm diameter, negative nodes), stage III (tumor >4 cm and/or positive nodes) or stage IV (distant metastatic disease). The numbers of previous treatments with surgery, radiation, and/or chemotherapy were recorded. Dogs with WHO stage II, III, or IV histologically confirmed malignant melanoma were included in the studies due to the lack of effective available systemic treatments. Due to a strong safety profile, dogs with stage I melanoma were enrolled in the study with the Institutional Review Board approval from 2005 on. Additional entry criteria were an estimated life expectancy of six weeks or more, free of clinically detectable brain metastases, no previous therapy (surgery, radiation, and/or chemotherapy) for at least three weeks, and no serious intercurrent medical illnesses. A written consent for entry into this trial was obtained from each dog's owner prior to the study; this consent included request for necropsy upon death due to any reason. These studies were performed under the approval of Animal Medical Center Institutional Review Board.

Cohorts of three dogs each received increasing doses of xenogeneic plasmid DNA encoding either human tyrosinase (huTyr; 100, 500, or 1500 mcg), murine GP75 (muGP75; 100, 500, or 1500 mcg), murine tyrosinase (muTyr; 5 dogs at 100 mcg, or 500 mcg each), or muTyr ± HuGM-CSF (9 dogs at 50 mcg muTyr, 3 dogs each at 100, 400, or 800 mcg HuGM-CSF, or 3 dogs each at 50 mcg muTyr with 100, 400, or 800 mcg HuGM-CSF) intramuscularly biweekly for a total of 4 vaccinations in the left caudal thigh with a Biojector® 2000 (Bioject Medical Technologies, Inc., Tualatin, OR) jet delivery device with #3 (intramuscular) Bioject syringes. The Biojector 2000 is a carbon dioxide-powered jet delivery device which is FDA approved for administration of intramuscular injections and has been used in DNA vaccine clinical investigations. Dogs with confirmed malignant melanoma not on the aforementioned official trials (due to a number of factors such as residence outside the approved study radius, timing of presentation, etc.) received 50 mcg MuTyr as outlined above except the device used in this case was a Vitajet spring-loaded needle-free injection device. Subjective pain level responses and postvaccinal presence of a wheal or other reaction were assessed and recorded by the veterinarian administering the DNA vaccination. The dogs did not receive any concomitant systemic anti-cancer treatments during the course of vaccination.

The signaling in dogs in these studies was similar to that in previously reported CMM studies. No toxicity was seen in any dogs receiving the aforementioned vaccines with the exception of minimal to mild pain responses on vaccination; one muGP75 dog experienced a mild aural depigmentation; and one muTyr dog experienced a moderate foot pad vitiligo. Dogs with stage I–III loco-regionally controlled CMM across the xenogeneic vaccine studies have a Kaplan–Meier (KM) MST of >1075 days (median not yet reached) whereas those dogs with stage I–III CMM without local tumor control have a KM MST of 553 days (P = 0.0002). The KM MST for stage II–IV dogs in the phase I trials of huTyr, muGP75, and muTyr are 389, 153, and 224 days, respectively. The KM MST for stage II–IV dogs treated with 50 mcg MuTyr, 100/400/800 mcg HuGM-CSF, or a combination MuTyr of HuGM-CSF are 242, 148, and >900 days (median not reached), respectively. In dogs which received any melanoma vaccine except for dogs on the MuTyr ± GM-CSF trial (i.e., HuTyr, MuTyr and MuGP75), the KM MST for stage I, II, III, and IV CMM was >939 days (median not reached with 92.8% survival), >908 days (median not reached, 79% alive at 1 year, 63% alive at 2 years), >1646 days (median not reached, 77%, 65%, 57% alive at 1, 2, 3 years), and 239 days (40.5% and 18.8% alive at 1 and 2 years), respectively (49,50). The results from dogs vaccinated with huTyr were published in 2003 (51).

We have investigated the humoral responses of dogs receiving HuTyr as a potential explanation for the long-term survivals seen in some of the dogs in this study. Using standard ELISA with a mammalian-expressed purified human tyrosinase protein as the target of interest (a kind gift of C Andreoni & JC Audonnet, Merial, Inc.), we have found 3/9 dogs with 2–5-fold postvaccinal humoral responses compared with pre-immune sera. We have confirmed these findings through a flow-cytometry-based assay of pre- and postvaccinal sera in permeabilized human SK-MEL melanoma cells expressing endogenous human tyrosinase. Interestingly, the three dogs with postvaccinal anti-HuTyr humoral responses are dogs with unexpected long-term tumor control (52). Co-investigators have also determined that normal dogs receiving the HuTyr-based melanoma vaccine develop Ag-specific IFN-γ T cells (53).

The results of these trials demonstrate that xenogeneic DNA vaccination in CMM is (*i*) safe, (*ii*) develops specific anti-tyrosinase immune responses, (*iii*) potentially therapeutic with particularly exciting results in stage II/III local-regional–controlled disease, and (*iv*) an attractive candidate for further evaluation in an adjuvant, minimal residual disease phase II setting for CMM. A safety and efficacy United States Department of Agriculture (USDA) licensure multi-institutional trial investigating HuTyr in dogs with locally controlled stage II/III oral melanoma was initiated in April 2006 across five sites (P. Bergman, Animal Medical Center, New York City; K. Meleo, Seattle; MK Klein, Tucson, Phoenix; S. Susaneck, Houston; P. Hess, North Carolina State University).

In late March 2007, we received conditional licensure from the USDA-CVB (Center for Veterinary Biologics) for the HuTyr-based canine melanoma vaccine and it became commercially available for use by US-based veterinary oncologists in June 2007. This represented the first US government-approved vaccine for the treatment of cancer. Based on the results of the aforementioned 5-site efficacy trial documenting a statistically significant improvement in survival for vaccinates versus controls (Am J Vet Res, in press), we received full licensure for the HuTyr-based canine melanoma vaccine from USDA-CVB in December 2009. This allowed our industrial partner to continue to have the product available commercially in addition to name the product as Oncept (MERIAL Limited, Duluth, GA). As of January 2011, approximately 5000 dogs with malignant melanoma have received the commercially available canine melanoma vaccine, and approximately 2000 dogs are entered into the internet-based Merial melanoma vaccine follow-up database by their respective veterinary oncologists (personal communication, Dr. Robert Menardi, Merial Ltd.). Subsequently, we have investigated the efficacy of local tumor control and use of MuTyr-based DNA vaccination in dogs with digit melanoma. These investigations have found an improvement in survival compared with historical outcomes with digit amputation only and also documented a decreased prognosis for dogs with an advanced stage disease and/or an increased time from digit amputation to the start of vaccination (54).

A similar approach has been used in human patients with metastatic melanoma in the minimal residual disease setting. Although no clinical response data are available since these patients did not have measurable disease, several phase I trials of xenogeneic DNA vaccines have been completed. Across studies of tyrosinase and gp100 DNA immunization, approximately 40% of patients develop quantifiable CD8+ T cell responses to the syngeneic human target antigen (55–57).

In summary, CMM is a more clinically faithful therapeutic model for HM when compared with more traditional mouse systems as both human and canine diseases are chemoresistant, radio-resistant, share similar metastatic phenotypes/site selectivity, and occur spontaneously in an outbred, immunocompetent scenario. In addition, this chapter also verifies that veterinary cancer centers and human cancer centers can work productively together to benefit veterinary and human patients afflicted with cancer. It is hoped in the future that this same vaccine may also play roles in the treatment of melanoma in other species (e.g., horses, cats, humans, etc.) due to its xenogeneic origins, and in melanoma prevention once the genetic determinants of melanoma risk in dogs are further defined. It is easy to see how the veterinary oncology profession is uniquely able to greatly contribute to advances in both canine as well as human melanoma, in addition to many other cancers with similar comparative aspects across species. These authors believe that the xenogeneic DNA vaccine platform holds promise with other antigen targets. To this end we have recently completed a phase I study of murine CD20 DNA vaccination in dogs with B-cell non-Hodgkin's lymphoma. We also have phase I and phase II studies initiating shortly, that will use murine CD20 and rat HER2 DNA vaccination across the BrightHeart Veterinary Center's network. These authors and the fields of veterinary tumor immunotherapy and veterinary oncology are greatly indebted to the tireless work and seeds laid by the late Dr. Greg MacEwen; he is greatly missed.

ACKNOWLEDGMENTS

The authors would like to sincerely thank (*i*) the clinicians, pathologists, post-docs, residents, interns, and technical staff from the Animal Medical Center and Memorial Sloan-Kettering Cancer Center that supported these efforts, (*ii*) the clients and patients entrusted to our care which received the melanoma vaccinations, (*iii*) Drs. Robert Nordgren, Tim Leard, Robert Menardi, and other investigators from Merial, Ltd., (*iv*) Dr. Alan Houghton from MSKCC for his expert guidance, support, and mentorship of the development of this program and (*v*) Dr. Rick Stout from Bioject, Inc.

REFERENCES

1. Smith SH, Goldschmidt MH, McManus PM. A comparative review of melanocytic neoplasms. Vet Pathol 2002; 39: 651–78.
2. Goldschmidt MH. Benign and malignant melanocytic neoplasms of domestic animals. Am J Dermato-pathol 1985; 7(Suppl): 203–12.
3. Todoroff RJ, Brodey RS. Oral and pharyngeal neoplasia in the dog: a retrospective survey of 361 cases. J Am Vet Med Assoc 1979; 175: 567–71.
4. Wallace J, Matthiesen DT, Patnaik AK. Hemimaxillectomy for the treatment of oral tumors in 69 dogs. Vet Surg 1992; 21: 337–41.
5. Hahn KA, DeNicola DB, Richardson RC, Hahn EA. Canine oral malignant melanoma: Prognostic utility of an alternative staging system. J Small Anim Pract 1994; 35: 251–6.
6. MacEwen EG, Patnaik AK, Harvey HJ, Hayes AA, Matus R. Canine oral melanoma: comparison of surgery versus surgery plus Corynebacterium parvum. Cancer Invest 1986; 4: 397–402.
7. Harvey HJ, Macewen EG, Braun D, et al. Prognostic criteria for dogs with oral melanoma. J Am Vet Med Assoc 1981; 178: 580–2.
8. Bostock DE. Prognosis after surgical excision of canine melanomas. Vet Pathol 1979; 16: 32–40.
9. Spangler WL, Kass PH. The histologic and epidemiologic bases for prognostic considerations in canine melanocytic neoplasia. Vet Pathol 2006; 43: 136–49.
10. Modiano JF, Ritt MG, Wojcieszyn J. The molecular basis of canine melanoma: pathogenesis and trends in diagnosis and therapy. J Vet Intern Med 1999; 13: 163–74.
11. Sulaimon SS, Kitchell BE. The basic biology of malignant melanoma: molecular mechanisms of disease progression and comparative aspects. J Vet Intern Med 2003; 17: 760–72.
12. Goldschmidt MH. Pigmented lesions of the skin. Clin Dermatol 1994; 12: 507–14.
13. Vail DM, Macewen EG. Spontaneously occurring tumors of companion animals as models for human cancer. Cancer Invest 2000; 18: 781–92.
14. Bradley RL, Macewen EG, Loar AS. Mandibular resection for removal of oral tumors in 30 dogs and 6 cats. J Am Vet Med Assoc 1984; 184: 460–3.
15. Harvey HJ. Oral tumors. Vet Clin North Am Small Anim Pract 1985; 15: 493–500.
16. Kosovsky JK, Matthiesen DT, Marretta SM, Patnaik AK. Results of partial mandibulectomy for the treatment of oral tumors in 142 dogs. Vet Surg 1991; 20: 397–401.
17. Choi C, Kusewitt DF. Comparison of tyrosinase-related protein-2, S-100, and Melan A immunoreactivity in canine amelanotic melanomas. Vet Pathol 2003; 40: 713–18.
18. Freeman KP, Hahn KA, Harris FD, King GK. Treatment of dogs with oral melanoma by hypofractionated radiation therapy and platinum-based chemotherapy (1987–1997). J Vet Intern Med 2003; 17: 96–101.
19. Proulx DR, Ruslander DM, Dodge RK, et al. A retrospective analysis of 140 dogs with oral melanoma treated with external beam radiation. Vet Radiol Ultrasound 2003; 44: 352–9.
20. Theon AP, Rodriguez C, Madewell BR. Analysis of prognostic factors and patterns of failure in dogs with malignant oral tumors treated with megavoltage irradiation. J Am Vet Med Assoc 1997; 210: 778–84.
21. Williams LE, Packer RA. Association between lymph node size and metastasis in dogs with oral malignant melanoma: 100 cases (1987–2001). J Am Vet Med Assoc 2003; 222: 1234–6.
22. Leong SP, Accortt NA, Essner R, et al. Impact of sentinel node status and other risk factors on the clinical outcome of head and neck melanoma patients. Arch Otolaryngol Head Neck Surg 2006; 132: 370–3.
23. Herring ES, Smith MM, Robertson JL. Lymph node staging of oral and maxillofacial neoplasms in 31 dogs and cats. J Vet Dent 2002; 19: 122–6.

24. Nwogu CE, Kanter PM, Anderson TM. Pulmonary lymphatic mapping in dogs: use of technetium sulfur colloid and isosulfan blue for pulmonary sentinel lymph node mapping in dogs. Cancer Invest 2002; 20: 944–7.

25. Yudd AP, Kempf JS, Goydos JS, Stahl TJ, Feinstein RS. Use of sentinel node lymphoscintigraphy in malignant melanoma. Radiographics 1999; 19: 343–53.

26. Wells S, Bennett A, Walsh P, Owens S, Peauroi J. Clinical usefulness of intradermal fluorescein and patent blue violet dyes for sentinel lymph node identification in dogs. Vet Comp Oncol 2006; 4: 114–22.

27. Banks WC, Morris E. Results of radiation treatment of naturally occurring animal tumors. J Am Vet Med Assoc 1975; 166: 1063–4.

28. Bateman KE, Catton PA, Pennock PW, Kruth SA. 0-7-21 radiation therapy for the treatment of canine oral melanoma. J Vet Intern Med 1994; 8: 267–72.

29. Blackwood L, Dobson JM. Radiotherapy of oral malignant melanomas in dogs. J Am Vet Med Assoc 1996; 209: 98–102.

30. Kitchell BE, Brown DM, Luck EE, et al. Intralesional implant for treatment of primary oral malignant melanoma in dogs. J Am Vet Med Assoc 1994; 204: 229–36.

31. Theon AP, Madewell BR, Moore AS, Stephens C, Krag DN. Localized thermo-cisplatin therapy: a pilot study in spontaneous canine and feline tumours. Int J Hyperthermia 1991; 7: 881–92.

32. Spugnini EP, Dragonetti E, Vincenzi B, et al. Pulse-mediated chemotherapy enhances local control and survival in a spontaneous canine model of primary mucosal melanoma. Melanoma Res 2006; 16: 23–7.

33. Rassnick KM, Ruslander DM, Cotter SM, et al. Use of carboplatin for treatment of dogs with malignant melanoma: 27 cases (1989–2000). J Am Vet Med Assoc 2001; 218: 1444–8.

34. Boria PA, Murry DJ, Bennett PF, et al. Evaluation of cisplatin combined with piroxicam for the treatment of oral malignant melanoma and oral squamous cell carcinoma in dogs. J Am Vet Med Assoc 2004; 224: 388–94.

35. Page RL, Thrall DE, Dewhirst MW, et al. Phase I study of melphalan alone and melphalan plus whole body hyperthermia in dogs with malignant melanoma. Int J Hyperthermia 1991; 7: 559–66.

36. Ogilvie GK, Reynolds HA, Richardson RC, et al. Phase II evaluation of doxorubicin for treatment of various canine neoplasms. J Am Vet Med Assoc 1989; 195: 1580–3.

37. Aigner K, Hild P, Breithaupt H, et al. Isolated extremity perfusion with DTIC. An experimental and clinical study. Anticancer Res 1983; 3: 87–93.

38. Murphy S, Hayes AM, Blackwood L, et al. Oral malignant melanoma - the effect of coarse fractionation radiotherapy alone or with adjuvant carboplatin therapy. Vet Comp Oncol 2005; 3: 222–9.

39. O'Day S, Boasberg P. Management of metastatic melanoma 2005. Surg Oncol Clin N Am 2006; 15: 419–37.

40. Alexander AN, Huelsmeyer MK, Mitzey A, et al. Development of an allogeneic whole-cell tumor vaccine expressing xenogeneic gp100 and its implementation in a phase II clinical trial in canine patients with malignant melanoma. Cancer Immunol Immunother 2006; 55: 433–42.

41. Hogge GS, Burkholder JK, Culp J, et al. Preclinical development of human granulocyte-macrophage colony-stimulating factor-transfected melanoma cell vaccine using established canine cell lines and normal dogs. Cancer Gene Ther 1999; 6: 26–36.

42. MacEwen EG, Kurzman ID, Vail DM, et al. Adjuvant therapy for melanoma in dogs: results of randomized clinical trials using surgery, liposome-encapsulated muramyl tripeptide, and granulocyte macrophage colony-stimulating factor. Clin Cancer Res 1999; 5: 4249–58.

43. Bianco SR, Sun J, Fosmire SP, et al. Enhancing antimelanoma immune responses through apoptosis. Cancer Gene Ther 2003; 10: 726–36.

44. Dow SW, Elmslie RE, Willson AP, et al. In vivo tumor transfection with superantigen plus cytokine genes induces tumor regression and prolongs survival in dogs with malignant melanoma. J Clin Invest 1998; 101: 2406–14.

45. Gyorffy S, Rodriguez-Lecompte JC, Woods JP, et al. Bone marrow-derived dendritic cell vaccination of dogs with naturally occurring melanoma by using human gp100 antigen. J Vet Intern Med 2005; 19: 56–63.

46. Helfand SC, Soergel SA, Modiano JF, Hank JA, Sondel PM. Induction of lymphokine-activated killer (LAK) activity in canine lymphocytes with low dose human recombinant interleukin-2 in vitro. Cancer Biother 1994; 9: 237–44.

47. Guevara-Patino JA, Turk MJ, Wolchok JD, Houghton AN. Immunity to cancer through immune recognition of altered self: studies with melanoma. Adv Cancer Res 2003; 90: 157–77.

48. Weber LW, Bowne WB, Wolchok JD, et al. Tumor immunity and autoimmunity induced by immunization with homologous DNA. J Clin Invest 1998; 102: 1258–64.

49. Bergman PJ, Camps-Palau MA, McKnight JA, et al. Development of a xenogeneic DNA vaccine program for canine malignant melanoma at the Animal Medical Center. Vaccine 2006; 24: 4582–5.
50. Bergman PJ. Cancer immunotherapy. Vet Clin North Am Small Anim Pract 2010; 40: 507–18.
51. Bergman PJ, McKnight J, Novosad A, et al. Long-term survival of dogs with advanced malignant melanoma after DNA vaccination with xenogeneic human tyrosinase: a phase I trial. Clin Cancer Res 2003; 9: 1284–90.
52. Liao JC, Gregor P, Wolchok JD, et al. Vaccination with human tyrosinase DNA induces antibody responses in dogs with advanced melanoma. Cancer Immun 2006; 6: 8.
53. Goubier A, Fuhrmann L, Forest L, et al. Superiority of needle-free transdermal plasmid delivery for the induction of antigen-specific IFNgamma T cell responses in the dog. Vaccine 2008; 26: 2186–90.
54. Manley CA, Leibman NF, Wolchok JD, et al. Xenogeneic murine tyrosinase DNA vaccine for malignant melanoma of the digit of dogs. J Vet Intern Med 2011; 25: 94–9.
55. Wolchok JD, Yuan J, Houghton AN, et al. Safety and immunogenicity of tyrosinase DNA vaccines in patients with melanoma. Mol Ther 2007; 15: 2044–50.
56. Yuan J, Ku GY, Gallardo HF, et al. Safety and immunogenicity of a human and mouse gp100 DNA vaccine in a phase I trial of patients with melanoma. Cancer Immun 2009; 9: 5.
57. Ginsberg BA, Gallardo HF, Rasalan TS, et al. Immunologic response to xenogeneic gp100 DNA in melanoma patients: comparison of particle-mediated epidermal delivery with intramuscular injection. Clin Cancer Res 2010; 16: 4057–65.

7 | Recombinant protein vaccination for antigen-specific cancer immunotherapy

Pedro de Sousa Alves and Vincent Brichard

INTRODUCTION

Cancer immunotherapy is aimed at harnessing the host immune system to recognize the neoplastic lesions, at manipulating the tumor's microenvironment, and to avoiding the deleterious effects of cancer cells on immune effector function.

Intense research in recent decades has demonstrated that cancer is recognized by the host immune system, thus showing that tumors are antigenic and immunogenic (1). Tumor cells have been revealed to be actors in the customization of their microenvironment, secreting and expressing a wide variety of molecules that favor neoplastic development (2). In parallel with this, several immune system cell types have been shown to be deleterious to the anti-tumor effector function (3). It is thus apparent that therapeutic interventions, in order to attain the expected therapeutic success, should target not only cancer cells but also the host immune system.

Approaches to cancer immunotherapy can be divided into two groups: active and passive. Active immunotherapy aims to manipulate the host immune system, teaching it to identify the tumor cells and to act against them. Examples of such approaches are immunization with peptide and protein vaccines and with autologous dendritic cells loaded with a variety of antigens, DNA and live-vector vaccinations, allogenic tumor-cell vaccinations; and adoptive T-cell therapies. In contrast, passive immunotherapy aims either (*i*) to act directly against the tumor by activating, inhibiting, or interfering in the function of receptors expressed on the target tumor cells, or (*ii*) to act indirectly against the tumor by influencing the effector or regulatory cellular components of the immune system. Examples of such passive approaches are trastuzumab (*Herceptin*®, Genentech, South San Francisco, CA; an antibody against Her2/neu) and the recently developed antibodies interfering with cytotoxic T-lymphocyte antigen-4 (CTLA-4) (4) and programmed death 1 (PD1) (5).

The variety of approaches developed in recent decades highlights the complex interactions that tumor cells and the host immune system play following the onset of neoplastic progression, but also the disappointingly poor success of immunotherapeutic interventions in the clinical setting. Experimentally, in vivo, it has been demonstrated convincingly that the tumor–host interaction evolves with time (6). The tumor passes three major landmarks which stake out the path to the collapse of the host: elimination, equilibrium, and escape. All these steps, too, have been shown experimentally to be susceptible to targeting and manipulation (7). However, success in patients has been much less clearly evident (8,9).

Nevertheless, we are now reaching a potential turning point. As never before, researchers have unearthed many sources of relevant information (from genomics, transcriptomics, and proteomics), and never has our knowledge of the tumor–host interaction been so detailed or so deep. Consequently, many potentially promising immunotherapies have reached late stage of clinical development (4,5) and for the first time an active immunotherapy has been accepted by governmental authorities, for the indication of prostate cancer (10,11).

In this review we will describe the past, present, and potential future clinical development of recombinant microarray and gene expression-A3 (MAGE-A3), an active immunotherapy which is currently in phase III of clinical development.

RECOMBINANT PROTEINS IN CANCER IMMUNOTHERAPY

Belonging to the realm of active immunotherapy, the recombinant protein vaccination has several recognized advantages which have important implications for clinical development. First of all, by vaccinating with full-length protein both humoral and cellular immunity can be targeted, leading to the development of antibodies directed at diverse domains of the antigen, as well as inducing the activation and expansion of CD4[+] and CD8[+] T-cell responses to processed epitopes (both known and currently unknown) of the target antigen. The induction of both CD4[+] and CD8[+] T cells from the same antigen is beneficial for the diversity and breadth of the overall response in regard to both antibodies and T cells (12,13). Secondly, a recombinant full-length protein resembles a native antigen expressed by target cells and is therefore potentially more liable to generate relevant immune responses; in this way, account is taken of the complex proteomic machinery and antigen presentation routes that are present in eukaryotic cells (14). Thirdly, vaccination with a full-length protein allows the targeting of a wider patient population, as human leukocyte antigen (HLA) restriction is not an issue—in contrast to peptide vaccination, which is only applicable to the individuals who express the HLA allele(s) that present(s) the selected peptide(s).

Recombinant full-length tumor antigens have been applied in immunotherapeutic approaches. Well-established examples are NY-ESO-1 (a cancer–germline tumor antigen) and prostate-specific antigen (PSA; a prostate differentiation tumor antigen).

NY-ESO-1 is a tumor antigen expressed with high frequency in human cancer lesions (15,16) and it demonstrates a strong immunogenic profile, as demonstrated by (*i*) the detection of strong humoral responses, (*ii*) the identification of a wide number of epitopes in vaccinated patients in several clinical settings, and (*iii*) the detection of naturally occurring immune responses in unvaccinated cancer patients (17,18). Clinically, a full-length NY-ESO-1 has been combined with adjuvants, leading to the detection of CD4[+] and CD8[+] T-cell responses in resected NY-ESO-1-positive melanoma (19,20) and esophageal cancer (21). In the melanoma phase II study, a trend toward a reduction in the risk of relapse was observed in the cohort vaccinated with the antigen in the presence of an adjuvant, compared with patients vaccinated only with the antigen or placebo (20). The phase I study in esophageal cancer showed positive clinical responses (22).

PSA, a kallikrein-like serine protease, is expressed almost exclusively in the prostate epithelium; it can be detected in the majority of prostate cancers and is thus classified as a differentiation tumor antigen of prostate. This antigen is widely used as a marker of prostate cancer diagnosis and progression (23). Numerous T-cell epitopes have been described in the literature (24) and a full-length antigen has been employed in several clinical trials, with the detection of humoral and adaptive antigen-specific responses when adjuvants were co-delivered with the antigen (25,26).

While T-cell immunity was detected in most of these trials, clinical responses were rare but, together with the safety profile of these approaches, justifies the evaluation of recombinant protein immunotherapy approaches in additional clinical trials.

ANTIGEN SELECTION

The aim of immunotherapeutic approaches is to target neoplastic cells while leaving normal cells untouched. To achieve this objective, a careful selection of the antigen target is of prime importance. Cancer antigens fall into one of the following categories (27): cancer–germline shared tumor-specific antigens, also known as cancer–testis tumor-specific antigens, (e.g., MAGE-A, NY-ESO-1); overexpressed shared tumor antigens (e.g., MUC1, HER2/neu, PRAME, WT1); differentiation tumor antigens (e.g. Melan-A, PSA); viral antigens (e.g. *Human papilloma* virus); and mutated antigens (e.g. CD4K, caspase-8, p53, K-RAS). Although the latter are the most common antigens expressed by tumor cells (28–30) and are ideally specific, they are often particular to a given individual and to the particular time point of the neoplastic development, such as the rate that such mutations occur in tumor cells. In most situations, these facts detract from their possible application for immunotherapy in a wide patient population. However, the most relevant proofs of cancer immunotherapy have arisen from demonstrations of mutation-antigen targeting (31–36).

Consequently, the best alternative antigens for a wide targeting of cancer cells are cancer–germline tumor antigens, because of their tumor specificity, tumor diversity, frequent expression, immunogenicity, undetected expression in normal somatic adult tissues, and association with poor prognosis in different cancer settings (37–39).

MAGE-A3 is a member of the cancer–germline shared tumor-specific antigens, and is expressed solely in cancer cells. As is the case for other members of the MAGE-A group, the only exception to this pattern of expression found so far has been their detection on germline cells of human gonads, which are cells that do not express major histocompatibility complex molecules and are therefore unable to be targets for effector T lymphocytes (40). MAGE-A3 is commonly expressed in various histological cancer types, among which the most prevalent examples are melanoma, lung, bladder, and head-and-neck cancer (41–43).

The above-listed characteristics have been exploited in several phase I exploratory clinical trials in metastatic melanoma and have demonstrated that MAGE-A3 is of immunogenic and clinical interest (Fig. 7.1). A first clinical study, in which MAGE-A3-derived peptides were used for immunization, achieved tumor regression in three out of six melanoma patients (44). This first clinical evidence was again observed in a trial where 7 out of 25 patients (who received the entire vaccination schedule of HLA-A1-restricted MAGE-A3 peptide) showed tumor regression, in some cases persisting for more than two years (45). Among the limited number of patients analyzed (four), none presented detectable T-cell responses, although two of the four patients showed a complete tumor regression. Both these phase I studies have demonstrate that the immunogenic characteristics of MAGE-A3 are challenging, and are apparently related to the low T-cell frequencies detected in healthy human donors and in cancer patients (46,47). Importantly, neither of the two studies employing oligopeptides showed any significant toxicities or side effects (44,48). Although these studies demonstrated the potential clinical benefit of MAGE-A3 peptide vaccination, the striking lack of detectable T-cell responses in the blood of vaccinated patients prompted the investigation of immunostimulant (incomplete Freund's adjuvant) along with a helper major histocompatibility complex class II peptide (PADRE) and an HLA-A1-restricted MAGE-A3 peptide (49). In this trial, 18 patients with resected stage III and IV melanomas were enrolled. Of the 14 patients assessed, a major impairment of the immune effector function was reported, which raised concern about the immune fitness of the patients. However, five patients showed cytotoxic activity and eight revealed antigen-specific interferon -gamma production (49).

Subsequent studies aimed to improve these results by employing (*i*) a strong immunostimulant and (*ii*) a different route of immunization (intra-muscular) that was less prone to reactogenicity than the subcutaneous or intradermal route previously used, and (*iii*) a full-length recombinant MAGE-A3 sequence fused to a bacterial sequence—a lipidated protein D derived from *Haemophilus influenzae*, to improve immunogenicity and to provide bystander help. This fusion protein is termed ProtD-MAGE-A3 or recMAGE-A3 (the latter term is used hereinafter). The adjuvant was composed of monophosphoryl lipid A (MPL) (bacterial wall component) and QS21 (saponin). In a phase I/II study a total of 33 metastatic melanoma patients expressing MAGE-A3 were vaccinated. Of these, five showed clinically relevant responses (including two objective responses) after four vaccinations. No significant safety issues were reported (50). Antibody responses specific to MAGE-A3 were detected in a substantial majority (twenty-three) of the patients vaccinated (51).

In another phase II study, recombinant MAGE-A3 was administrated subcutaneously and intradermally with an immunostimulant in metastatic melanoma patients without visceral lesions. Of the 32 patients vaccinated, six clinical responses were reported. Tumor regressions were reported after long-term vaccination (>1 year), supporting the idea that a continuous administration of the vaccine might be important for clinical efficacy (52).

IMPORTANCE OF IMMUNOSTIMULANTS IN ANTIGEN VACCINATION

Recombinant MAGE-A3 was also applied to non-small-cell lung cancer (NSCLC). In a phase II clinical trial conducted in patients with resected MAGE-A3-positive lesions, recMAGE-A3 was administered to patients with or without the AS02$_B$ – a proprietary Adjuvant System developed

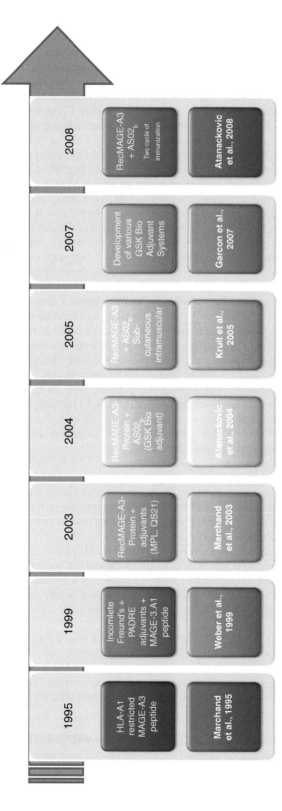

Figure 7.1 Evolution of clinical trials using MAGE-A3 tumor antigen as target for immunotherapy. *Abbreviations*: MAGE-A3, microarray and gene expression-A3; MPL, monophosphoryl lipid A; QS21, Saponin. AS02B (MPL, QS21, oil in water, emulsion-based Adjuvant System).

by GlaxoSmithKline Biologicals. The results demonstrated the potential importance of adding an immunostimulant to the recMAGE-A3 antigen in the induction of immune responses, as humoral responses and cytotoxic activity were only barely detected in the cohort vaccinated with recMAGE-A3 alone, in clear contrast to the responses observed in the cohort where the antigen and immunostimulant were administered to the patients (53). Clinically, in most of the patients who completed the immunization schedule with the recombinant MAGE-A3 plus the Adjuvant System, no evidence of disease was reported (54).

In addition to the immunogenicity and safety profile of recMAGE-A3 reported (52,53), the characterization of memory responses induced showed that the addition of an Adjuvant System to the antigen is indeed critical for the breadth of the recall responses to the antigen vaccinated (54): a single recall boost administered to patients vaccinated three years earlier with recMAGE-A3 and AS02$_B$ led to the attainment of the peak antibody responses previously reported, in contrast to patients who had been vaccinated with recMAGE-A3 only. Adaptive T-cell responses followed the same trend and were also characterized in the cohort recMAGE-A3/AS02$_B$, with a widening of the T-cell repertoire specific for MAGE-A3 (54).

These observations emphasize the importance of immunostimulants in immunization with self antigens. Indeed, immunostimulants are developed and associated with antigens with specific aims such as improvement of humoral and adaptive T-cell responses toward the antigen induction of long-term antigen-specific memory responses (54); overcoming immune impairment of the patient; breaking antigen-related tolerance (49); and allowing immunomodulation of the immune responses (55). The improvement of immunostimulant components led to the development of a new generation of immunostimulants that can be tailored to the antigens involved. Against this background, GlaxoSmithKline Biologicals has developed a series of Adjuvant Systems characterized by highly defined components, with characterized immune features and specific formulation techniques, which are well tolerated and have effective immunogenicity features (56).

Two Adjuvant Systems have been developed and applied in cancer settings by GlaxoSmithKline Biologicals: AS02$_B$ and AS15.

AS02$_B$ is the combination of an oil-in-water emulsion with MPL and QS21. MPL is derived from cell-wall lipopolysaccharide of Gram-negative bacteria and is detoxified and purified. MPL has demonstrated remarkable reduced reactogenicity features, in comparison to those of the parent lipopolysaccharide, while preserving adjuvant activity (56). MPL is a known TLR4 agonist (57). QS21 is a saponin with a demonstrated impact on the antigen presentation and the cytotoxicity of effector T cells (58). AS15 is a liposome-based adjuvant that includes MPL and QS21 and also CpG 7909, which is a known TLR9 agonist (59), and is currently employed in GSK Biologicals phase III cancer clinical trials.

FROM POC TO LATE-STAGE DEVELOPMENT

The strategy developed by GlaxoSmithKline Biologicals called Antigen-Specific Cancer Immunotherapeutics (ASCI) is characterized by the use of well-defined, recombinant, tumor antigens in cancer therapy.

The early clinical studies sponsored by GSK paved the way for the proof of concept (PoC) of MAGE-A3 immunotherapy in cancer patients and, later, for the development of large phase III clinical trials in melanoma and NSCLC (Figs. 7.2, 7.3A and B). Fundamentally, four main messages were obtained from the early phase I trials: first of all, that recMAGE-A3 is immunogenic (52,53); secondly, that vaccination with MAGE-A3 is well tolerated (50,52,53); thirdly, that Adjuvant Systems are required for enhanced immunogenicity and long-term memory (54); and fourthly, that reduced tumor burden might be beneficial for the success of immunotherapeutic recombinant protein approaches, as clinical responders were found in the patient population that did not have visceral metastatic disease (50). On the basis of these observations, GSK Biologicals' strategy for cancer immunotherapy focuses on the adjuvant treatment of patients who are still at high risk of relapse after conventional surgical treatment (60). The aim is to target patients with a minimal tumor burden or minimal residual disease, thus limiting the potential negative immunomodulatory effects induced directly by cancer on the host immune system (61,2). This is in line with the current thoughts about new cancer vaccination paradigms, which suggest the definition of clear endpoints and defined populations in an adjuvant setting—or without a rapidly progressive disease in a metastatic setting— to allow the vaccines adequate time to induce biological activity (62).

Selecting MAGE-A3 as the first target of the ASCI class, a phase II clinical PoC trial was started in 2002 (Fig. 7.2). An adjuvant therapy in NSCLC was selected as the clinical setting because of the recognized unmet medical need. According to various health organizations, lung cancer is the most common cancer type in the world, responsible for an estimated 1.5 million new cases each year and accounting for 12% of all cancer diagnoses. NSCLC is also the leading cause of global cancer mortality, resulting in 1.35 million deaths each year. The expected 5-year survival is only 15% for patients in the United States and Europe, comparing poorly with other cancers such as breast and prostate, which have 5-year survival rates above 80% (63). At the time of study design, treatment options for NSCLC were restricted to surgery at early stages of neoplastic development, followed by radiotherapy and/or chemotherapy for later NSCLC stages (III and IV). Following the principles described above, the PoC study was designed as double-blind, randomized (2:1), placebo-controlled phase II to evaluate the vaccination of patients with the recombinant MAGE-A3 associated with $AS02_B$ Adjuvant System. One hundred and eighty-two NSCLC patients were enrolled; all had MAGE-A3-positive, stage IB and II resected lesions and had not previously received an adjuvant therapy. Although the difference was not statistically significant, a relative reduction in risk of cancer recurrence of 25% was observed in the group receiving the recMAGE-A3

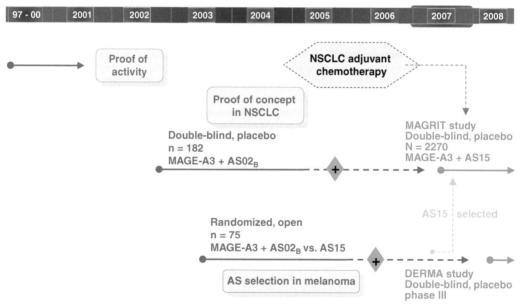

Figure 7.2 MAGE-A3 ASCI clinical development. The phase II trial performed in NSCLC patients (NCT00290355) has defined the proof-of-concept of the MAGE-A3 ASCI immunization. In parallel to this study, another phase II study in melanoma patients (NCT00086866) has been designed to evaluate in parallel two different Adjuvant Systems, $AS02_B$ and AS15, each one combined with MAGE-A3 protein. The main outcome of this study was the selection of AS15 as the immunostimulant for the development of large phase III trials (currently ongoing in NSCLC [NCT00480025] and in melanoma [NCT00796445]). *Abbreviations*: ASCI, Antigen-Specific Cancer Immunotherapeutics; MAGE-A3, microarray and gene expression-A3; NSCLC: non-small-cell lung cancer.

(A)

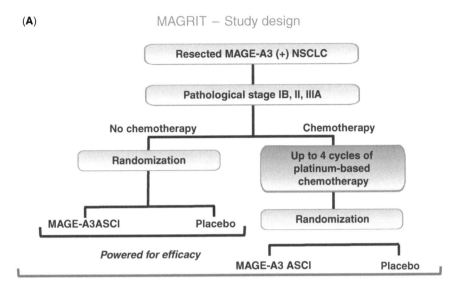

(B)

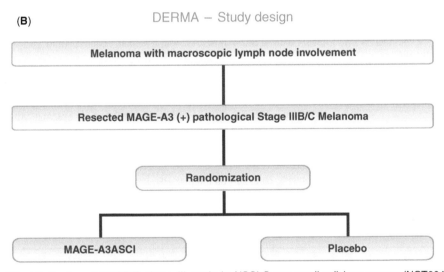

Figure 7.3 **(A)** Design of MAGRIT phase III study in NSCLC non-small-cell lung cancer (NCT00480025). **(B)** Design of DERMA phase III study in melanoma (NCT00796445).

immunotherapy when compared with placebo arm after a median followup of 44 months and the MAGE-A3 plus AS02$_B$ was well tolerated (64) (Table 7.1).

Concurrently with the PoC study, an open, parallel-group, randomized phase II study in MAGE-A3-positive unresected melanoma was performed to evaluate the two Adjuvant Systems (AS02$_B$ and AS15), with the aim of selecting the best one for further development. Seventy-five patients were enrolled. The vaccines were well tolerated by the patients. The main outcome of this study was the selection of AS15—based on increased immunological responses of the vaccinated patients and an increased overall survival—as the best immunostimulant for the phase III trials (65,66) (Table 7.2).

Consequently, two large randomized, double-blind, placebo-controlled phase III clinical trials have been designed—MAGRIT (MAGE-A3 as adjuvant non-small cell lung cancer Immunotherapy) in NSCLC and DERMA (Adjuvant Immunotherapy with MAGE-A3 in melanoma) in melanoma (Fig. 7.3A and 7.3B for study design respectively). In both trials, recMAGE-A3 combined with AS15 was administered to patients expressing MAGE-A3 in the adjuvant setting, with the aim of evaluating the efficacy and safety of the vaccine.

The MAGRIT study is the biggest phase III cancer clinical trial in the history of immunotherapeutics, aiming to enroll about 2300 NSCLC patients with MAGE-A3-positive stage IB, II, and IIIA cancers after resection. It is designed to demonstrate the efficacy of MAGE-A3 ASCI with or without standard-care adjuvant chemotherapy in this clinical setting. Treatment is being administered as 13 intramuscular injections over 27 months. Patients will be followed up every 6 months for 5 years and then annually until 10 years from the start of treatment. The primary endpoint will be disease-free survival and the secondary endpoint will be prospective validation of the gene signature (GS) predictive of benefit from MAGE-A3 ASCI therapy (discussed below). This multicentered (400), worldwide (33 countries from Europe, North and South America, Asia, and Australia), clinical trial was started in October 2007. DERMA is a phase III clinical trial aiming to enroll 1300 patients who have MAGE-A3-positive resected melanoma in stage III with a lymph-node involvement. Treatment is being administered as 13 intramuscular injections over 27 months. The primary endpoint will be disease-free survival and as for MAGRIT, one of the secondary endpoints will be the prospective validation of the GS predictive of benefit from the MAGE-A3 ASCI therapy (discussed below).

Table 7.1 Final Results from Phase II Clinical Study in NSCLC with a Median Followup Time of 44 Months (64)

Phase II NSCLC (NCT 00290355) ($N_{total}=182$)		recMAGE-A3 + AS02$_B$ (N = 122)
Primary endpoint	DFI	HR: 0.75 (95% CI: 0.46–1.23) recMAGE-A3 + AS02B vs. placebo $p=0.127$ in favor of MAGE-A3 ASCI
Secondary endpoints	Safety	Well tolerated
	Humoral immune response	CD4+ T-cell responses induced in >98% patients
	Cellular immune response	Response induced in 41% patients

Abbreviations: CI, confidence interval; DFI, disease-free interval; HR, hazard ratio; MAGE-A3, microarray and gene expression-A3; NSCLC, non-small-cell lung cancer.

Table 7.2 Results from Phase II Study in Cutaneous Metastatic Melanoma (65)

Phase II melanoma (NCT 00086866) $N_{total}=72$		recMAGE-A3 + AS02$_B$ N = 36	recMAGE-A3 + AS15 N = 36
Primary endpoint	Clinical objective responses	1 PR (7-mo) 5 SD (>16 wks)	3 CR (11, 32+, 23+) 1 PR (5 mo) 5 SD (>16 wks)
Secondary endpoints	Safety	Well tolerated	Well tolerated
	Overall survival	19.9 mo (95% CI: 15.4; 25.6)	31.1 mo (95% CI: 20.0; NR)
	Cellular immune response	CD4+ T-cell responses induced in 21% of patients	CD4+ T-cell responses induced in 76% of patients. 1 patient presented a detectable CD8+ T-cell response

Abbreviations: CR, complete response; CI, confidence interval; MAGE-A3, microarray and gene expression-A3; NR, not reached; PR, partial response; SD, stable disease.

PREDICTIVE BIOMARKERS ASSOCIATED WITH ASCI

The phase II clinical study on unresected metastatic melanoma was developed to evaluate the immunostimulants $AS02_B$ and AS15 (the Adjuvant Systems described earlier) was also used for the identification, by gene microarray analysis, of biomarkers linked to the clinical response. This analysis took place in biopsies obtained before immunotherapy and led to the identification of a short list of genes that predict the clinical benefit of recMAGE-A3 ASCI. The predictive GS was associated with significant improvement in median overall survival, from 16.2 months (GS negative) to 28 months (GS positive), and identified a subset of patients more likely to respond to the melanoma vaccine (67) (Table 7.3). The predictive GS was, as for the studies reported by Gajewski *et al.* (68), composed of genes related to immune infiltration, T-cell markers, and imprints of IFN signaling. These markers were confirmed by quantitative reverse polymerase chain reaction (67).

The results obtained in melanoma opened the road for the implementation of gene-expression analysis for the prospective evaluation of patients involved in active immunotherapy. The first assay was performed in the above-mentioned PoC phase II study in NSCLC (64). By taking advantage of the tissue samples available from this study, a gene-expression profiling was performed. The results obtained confirmed the hypothesis found in the phase II melanoma study. The predictive GS identified in melanoma could also be applied to the gene expression profile found in the NSCLC study (69). A calculation based on disease-free interval showed that the application of the predictive GS corresponded to an increase of about two folds in the relative risk of recurrence among MAGE-A3-vaccinated patients compared with the overall study population. Furthermore, among the GS-negative patients, no difference in disease-free interval was observed between the actively treated and placebo groups, thus supporting the hypothesis that the identified GS has little or no prognostic value (69).

Thus, the results obtained in melanoma and NSCLC cases by gene-expression profiling suggest a common predictive GS, indicative of the presence of an active in situ immune reaction to cancer cells and allowing the identification of patients with a likelihood, but not certainty, of responding to the active cancer immunotherapy. The GS will be validated in the MAGRIT and DERMA phase III studies.

IMPROVING ASCI EFFICACY

Unfortunately, for a majority of patients receiving active immunotherapies, the chances of tumor regression remain very small, regardless of the therapy applied (7). Nevertheless, administration of a high-dose IL-2 could show 20% objective responses in renal cell carcinoma (70). The current best success rate remains the ones achieved by the adoptive T-cell therapies developed by Steven Rosenberg's group, which reports objective responses for up to 70% of the patients treated (71). These adoptive therapies are based on individual success in isolating tumor- or antigen-specific T cells from lesions or peripheral blood. After a massive expansion

Table 7.3 Gene Signature Associated with the Clinical Benefit of MAGE-A3 ASCI: Identification in Phase II Study in Melanoma Patients and Confirmation in NSCLC Patients (67)

Phase II Studies Evaluating the MAGE-A3 ASCI	
Phase II NSCLC (NCT 00290355) 25% relative improvement in DFI in overall population 53% relative improvement in DFI in GS⁺ population	Phase II melanoma (NCT 00086866) OS of 16.2 mo in GS⁻ population OS of 28.0 mo in GS⁺ population

GS⁺: population for which a specific gene signature has been defined; GS⁻: population in which the gene signature was not found.
Abbreviations: ASCI, antigen-specific cancer immunotherapeutics; DFI, disease-free interval; GS, gene signature; MAGE-A3, microarray and gene expression-A3; NSCLC, non-small-cell lung cancer; OS, overall survival.

ex vivo, such cells are reinfused into the patients preconditioned with immunosuppressive agents that are thought to eliminate resource competition and immunosuppressive immune cells (71). Experimental models demonstrate that adoptive transferred T cells localize in the neoplastic lesions for which they express the antigen they are specific for (72), and these evidences reinforce the concept that tumor regression may be mediated by the local presence of antigen-specific T cells. Clinical observations also support this concept. The presence of activated CD8 T cells in the tumor microenvironment has been associated with positive clinical outcome in cancer (73). Why these findings only apply to certain tumors remains an intriguing question. A partial answer is suggested by the observation that some melanoma metastasis and tumor cells do produce chemokines supporting the infiltration and chemotaxis of CD8 T cells (74). Importantly, active immunotherapeutic intervention can also modify the cancer microenvironment and improve the outcome. An analysis of patients treated with peptide vaccines and high-dose IL-12 has shown that patients who responded clinically were the ones who presented evidence of immune tumor-infiltrated microenvironment characterized by the presence of chemokines and T-cell markers in pre-treatment biopsies (68). These clinical and experimental observations suggest strongly that immunotherapeutic interventions should aim not only at mobilizing the effector immune anti-tumor response but also at conditioning the tumor microenvironment.

The mobilization of the widest and most effective possible effector response, in particular of CD8 T cells, depends on the way antigens are presented by dendritic cells, upon co-stimulatory conditions, and upon the cytokine microenvironment (75). The anti-tumor immune response is linked to the efficiency of the delivery of antigens to antigen-presenting cells. Improving the way in which antigen-presenting cells capture and process the antigens included in the cancer vaccines is therefore a potential path to follow (76). Options such as linking a target antigen to antibodies specific for particular dendritic cell receptors, such as mannose receptor and DEC205, have been exploited successfully in vitro and in vivo (77–79), and are currently under development for delivering NY-ESO-1 to dendritic cells in cancer patients (80). Co-stimulation is another alternative for improving T-cell response, through enhancement of co-stimulatory molecules via triggering of CD154 (CD40L) (81) via CD40-activating antibodies, or by interfering with negative co-stimulatory signals such as PD1/PD-L1 (82) or CTLA-4 (83). Anti-CTLA-4 has also been suggested to interfere with the immunomodulatory activity of "T_{REGS}" and maximize anti-tumor activity effector function (84). Such approaches have provided interesting results associated with anti-tumor activity in melanoma patients (85,5), and in particular for anti-CTLA-4 (Ipilimumab and Tremelimumab), significant clinical responses have been reported in melanoma, either alone or in combination with IL-2 or peptide vaccination (86–89). Finally, the cytokine microenvironment of the antigen-presenting cells can be modified by providing cytokines along with vaccines such as IL-12, IFN-alpha and TNF-alpha or by stimulating antigen-presenting cells with Toll-like receptor ligands (TLRL), such as TLR7/8 agonists, that through triggering of TLRs can induce cytokines that are known to be beneficial for the establishment of adaptive responses (90–92). These lines of evidence suggest that some patients, but not all, might be potentially predisposed to respond clinically to active vaccination, because they present an "inflamed" tumor microenvironment characterized by the presence of chemokines and activated effector cells. Other lesions, in contrast, may require the induction of an "inflamed" microenvironment that can be prone to immune-mediated tumor regression. The current quest is aimed at the identification and validation of immunotherapeutic study designs that can attain such a goal. In an alternative approach, the identification of the biomarkers that characterize such an inflamed tumor-infiltrated environment can be of major interest for the identification of surrogate predictive markers of therapy, as well as for the potential selection of patients more likely to respond to therapy, thus improving the overall clinical efficacy of the immunotherapeutic approach (68).

NEW TRANSLATIONAL RESEARCH HURDLES

The identification and validation of therapy-predictive biomarkers in cancer is possibly one of the most exciting findings in recent years in cancer research, potentially boosting the clinical efficacy of safe, well-tolerated immunotherapies and, consequently, revolutionizing the care of cancer patients.

The data and information presented above are encouraging and support further development to pave the way to strike an approach of personalized medical treatment, where patients would be assessed for the presence of particular biomarkers, such as tumor antigens (37), mutated genes (93), and immune gene- and protein-associated patterns (68) to identify a suitable therapeutic avenue that is most likely to produce positive clinical results.

However, from the practical point of view, the application of predictive biomarkers is challenging, with significant hurdles for successful implementation (Table 7.4). These hurdles apply to research and development, clinical and regulatory activities, patients, and health-care providers (68).

From the standpoint of research and development, gene arrays commonly used to evaluate gene-expression patterns are difficult to validate. Classifiers generated from a complex bioinformatic analysis require significant collections of relevant data sets as well as a consensus regarding the appropriate mathematical and statistical analysis (94). Finally, the diversity of sample-preservation techniques used in clinical routine creates difficult issues for comparison of studies.

Clinically, access to samples is the cornerstone for the success of biomarker development and implementation. The patient's informed consent, careful sample-management logistics, and the quantity and quality of tissue are fundamental for the success of biomarker analysis. Restrictions or major difficulties in one or more of these elements might impair the clinical applicability or reduce the relevance of the biomarkers identified.

Table 7.4 Hurdles Identified from the Implementation of Predictive Biomarkers in the MAGE-A3 Clinical Development Program

The New Translational Research Hurdles	
Research & development (R&D)	Analytical validation of the gene array assay
	Development of performance classifier (GS)
	Adaptation from microarrays to quantitative reverse transcription polymerase chain reaction and from fresh/frozen tissue to formalin-fixed paraffin-embedded material
Clinical R&D	Consent, logistics, and availability/quantity of material
	Statistical adjustment of significance value
	Screening efficiency is a layer of complexity for accrual (in NSCLC study, 4053 tested; 1375 (+), 688 patients included)
Regulatory issues	Class III IVD-PMA required (assay used to make the decision regarding therapy)
	All instruments used in the assay need to be approved as part of the device
	Sample size consideration (not all patients have biomarkers, not 100% samples available)
Access to patients	No good analogs (suggestive of a lower/delayed uptake of a drug)
	Screening may discourage health-care providers/patients
	How will predictive biomarkers be integrated with other biomarkers (e.g., epidermal growth factor receptor by immunohistochemistry and fluorescence in situ hybridization, B-Raf mutations, etc.) in current practice?

Abbreviations: GS, gene signature; MAGE-A3, microarray and gene expression-A3; NSCLC, non-small-cell lung cancer; PMA, Pre-Market Approval. *Source:* Ref. 68.

From the regulatory standpoint, many global regulatory authorities apply stringent requirements to the development, approval, and commercialization of the diagnostic tool that measures the biomarker. The U.S. FDA, for instance, requires the submission and approval of a Class III IVD-PMA (Pre-Market Approval application) for predictive biomarkers as these assays are used to help make decisions regarding therapy. These applications contain not only the details of the assay development and validation from a technical perspective but also the clinical utility data from the clinical development studies for the companion therapy. The development and approval of the biomarker in conjunction with the immunotherapy fall under the umbrella of co-development, a relatively unprecedented regulatory pathway that brings additional challenges and complexities to the development and regulatory approval of the immunotherapy.

Practical challenges are also associated with the uptake and use of biomarkers in therapeutic decision making. Patients and health-care providers might not welcome complex, and sometimes lengthy, screening procedures that delay the standard or proposed therapeutic care, and thus the information and mobilization of both partners are fundamental for biomarker-based or -driven therapies, especially considering the wide number of predictive makers that have already been described in several clinical settings (95).

Thus, the consideration of predictive biomarkers in clinics and in cancer therapy brings government authorities, health-care providers, researchers, and the biotechnological and pharmaceutical industries to an unprecedented level of discussion and dialogue for the benefit of the patients. It is to be hoped that this collaborative effort will allow the adoption of tailored, patient-specific therapies that will make possible the identification of patient populations more likely to benefit from specific therapies and will, consequently, improve the efficacy of such therapeutic interventions in the control and elimination of cancer.

ACKNOWLEDGMENTS

The authors thank Amy Scott, David Rea, Paul Woolley, Ginny Campen, Damien O'Farrel, Slavka Baronikova, and Alberta Di Pasquale for their valuable input and critical review of this chapter. The authors are also grateful to Julie Vandekerchove and Helene Servais for their editorial assistance.

REFERENCES

1. Boon T, Coulie PG, Eynde BJ, et al. Human T Cell Responses Against Melanoma. Annu Rev Immunol 2006; 24: 175–208.
2. Gajewski TF, Meng Y, Blank C, et al. Immune resistance orchestrated by the tumor microenvironment. Immunol Rev 2006; 213: 131–45.
3. Zitvogel L, Tesniere A, Kroemer G. Cancer despite immunosurveillance: immunoselection and immunosubversion. Nat Rev Immunol 2006; 6: 715–27.
4. Hodi FS, O'Day SJ, McDermott DF, et al. Improved survival with ipilimumab in patients with metastatic melanoma. N Engl J Med 2010; 363: 711–23.
5. Brahmer JR, Drake CG, Wollner I, et al. Phase I study of single-agent anti-programmed death-1 (MDX-1106) in refractory solid tumors: safety, clinical activity, pharmacodynamics, and immunologic correlates. J Clin Oncol 2010; 28: 3167–75.
6. Smyth MJ, Dunn GP, Schreiber RD. Cancer immunosurveillance and immunoediting: the roles of immunity in suppressing tumor development and shaping tumor immunogenicity. Adv Immunol 2006; 90: 1–50.
7. Srivastava PK. Therapeutic cancer vaccines. Curr Opin Immunol 2006; 18: 201–5.
8. Eggermont AM. Therapeutic vaccines in solid tumours: can they be harmful? Eur J Cancer 2009; 45: 2087–90.
9. Schreiber TH, Raez L, Rosenblatt JD, et al. Tumor immunogenicity and responsiveness to cancer vaccine therapy: the state of the art. Semin Immunol 2010; 22: 105–12.
10. Longo DL. New therapies for castration-resistant prostate cancer. N Engl J Med 2010; 363: 479–81.

11. Kantoff PW, Higano CS, Shore ND, et al. Sipuleucel-T immunotherapy for castration-resistant prostate cancer. N Engl J Med 2010; 363: 411–22.

12. Baxevanis CN, Voutsas IF, Tsitsilonis OE, et al. Tumor-specific CD4+ T lymphocytes from cancer patients are required for optimal induction of cytotoxic T cells against the autologous tumor. J Immunol 2000; 164: 3902–12.

13. Sun JC, Bevan MJ. Defective CD8 T cell memory following acute infection without CD4 T cell help. Science 2003; 300: 339–42.

14. Vyas JM, Van d V, Ploegh HL. The known unknowns of antigen processing and presentation. Nat Rev Immunol 2008; 8: 607–18.

15. Jungbluth AA, Chen YT, Stockert E, et al. Immunohistochemical analysis of NY-ESO-1 antigen expression in normal and malignant human tissues. Int J Cancer 2001; 92: 856–60.

16. Juretic A, Spagnoli GC, Schultz-Thater E, et al. Cancer/testis tumour-associated antigens: immunohistochemical detection with monoclonal antibodies. Lancet Oncol 2003; 4: 104–9.

17. Jager E, Chen YT, Drijfhout JW, et al. Simultaneous humoral and cellular immune response against cancer-testis antigen NY-ESO-1: definition of human histocompatibility leukocyte antigen (HLA)-A2-binding peptide epitopes. J Exp Med 1998; 187: 265–70.

18. Jackson H, Dimopoulos N, Mifsud NA, et al. Striking immunodominance hierarchy of naturally occurring CD8+ and CD4+ T cell responses to tumor antigen NY-ESO-1. J Immunol 2006; 176: 5908–17.

19. Valmori D, Souleimanian NE, Tosello V, et al. Vaccination with NY-ESO-1 protein and CpG in Montanide induces integrated antibody/Th1 responses and CD8 T cells through cross-priming. Proc Natl Acad Sci USA 2007; 104: 8947–52.

20. Davis ID, Chen W, Jackson H, et al. Recombinant NY-ESO-1 protein with ISCOMATRIX adjuvant induces broad integrated antibody and CD4(+) and CD8(+) T cell responses in humans. Proc Natl Acad Sci USA 2004; 101: 10697–702.

21. Wada H, Sato E, Uenaka A, et al. Analysis of peripheral and local anti-tumor immune response in esophageal cancer patients after NY-ESO-1 protein vaccination. Int J Cancer 2008; 123: 2362–9.

22. Uenaka A, Wada H, Isobe M, et al. T cell immunomonitoring[V5] and tumor responses in patients immunized with a complex of cholesterol-bearing hydrophobized pullulan (CHP) and NY-ESO-1 protein. Cancer Immun 2007; 7.

23. Oesterling JE. Prostate specific antigen: a critical assessment of the most useful tumor marker for adenocarcinoma of the prostate. J Urol 1991; 145: 907–23.

24. Kiessling A, Fussel S, Wehner R, et al. Advances in specific immunotherapy for prostate cancer. Eur Urol 2008; 53: 694–708.

25. Harris DT, Matyas GR, Gomella LG, et al. Immunologic approaches to the treatment of prostate cancer. Semin Oncol 1999; 26: 439–47.

26. Meidenbauer N, Harris DT, Spitler LE, et al. Generation of PSA-reactive effector cells after vaccination with a PSA-based vaccine in patients with prostate cancer. Prostate 2000; 43: 88–100.

27. van der Bruggen P, Stroobant V, Vigneron N, Van den Eynde B. T-cell defined tumor antigens. [Available from: http://www.cancerimmunity.org/peptidedatabase/Tcellepitopes.htm].

28. Campbell PJ, Stephens PJ, Pleasance ED, et al. Identification of somatically acquired rearrangements in cancer using genome-wide massively parallel paired-end sequencing. Nat Genet 2008; 40: 722–9.

29. Greenman C, Stephens P, Smith R, et al. Patterns of somatic mutation in human cancer genomes. Nature 2007; 446: 153–8.

30. Wood LD, Parsons DW, Jones S, et al. The genomic landscapes of human breast and colorectal cancers. Science 2007; 318: 1108–13.

31. Wolfel T, Hauer M, Schneider J, et al. A p16INK4a-insensitive CDK4 mutant targeted by cytolytic T lymphocytes in a human melanoma. Science 1995; 269: 1281–4.

32. Mandruzzato S, Stroobant V, Demotte N, et al. A human CTL recognizes a caspase-8-derived peptide on autologous HLA-B*3503 molecules and two unrelated peptides on allogeneic HLA-B*3501 molecules. J Immunol 2000; 164: 4130–4.

33. Ikeda H, Ohta N, Furukawa K, et al. Mutated mitogen-activated protein kinase: a tumor rejection antigen of mouse sarcoma. Proc Natl Acad Sci USA 1997; 94: 6375–9.

34. Dubey P, Hendrickson RC, Meredith SC, et al. The immunodominant antigen of an ultraviolet-induced regressor tumor is generated by a somatic point mutation in the DEAD box helicase p68. J Exp Med 1997; 185: 695–705.

35. Matsutake T, Srivastava PK. The immunoprotective MHC II epitope of a chemically induced tumor harbors a unique mutation in a ribosomal protein. Proc Natl Acad Sci USA 2001; 98: 3992–7.

36. Lennerz V, Fatho M, Gentilini C, et al. The response of autologous T cells to a human melanoma is dominated by mutated neoantigens. Proc Natl Acad Sci USA 2005; 102: 16013–18.

37. Lucas S, Coulie PG. About human tumor antigens to be used in immunotherapy. Semin Immunol 2008; 20: 301–7.

38. Gure AO, Chua R, Williamson B, et al. Cancer-testis genes are coordinately expressed and are markers of poor outcome in non-small cell lung cancer. Clin Cancer Res 2005; 11: 8055–62.

39. Andrade VC, Vettore AL, Felix RS, et al. Prognostic impact of cancer/testis antigen expression in advanced stage multiple myeloma patients. Cancer Immun 2008; 8.

40. Simpson AJ, Caballero OL, Jungbluth A, et al. Cancer/testis antigens, gametogenesis and cancer. Nat Rev Cancer 2005; 5: 615–25.

41. Brasseur F, Rimoldi D, Lienard D, et al. Expression of MAGE genes in primary and metastatic cutaneous melanoma. Int J Cancer 1995; 63: 375–80.

42. Van Den Eynde BJ, van der Bruggen P. T cell defined tumor antigens. Curr Opin Immunol 1997; 9: 684–93.

43. De Plaen E, Arden K, Traversari C, et al. Structure, chromosomal localization, and expression of 12 genes of the MAGE family. Immunogenetics 1994; 40: 360–9.

44. Marchand M, Weynants P, Rankin E, et al. Tumor regression responses in melanoma patients treated with a peptide encoded by gene MAGE-3. Int J Cancer 1995; 63: 883–5.

45. Marchand M, Brasseur F, van der BP, et al. Perspectives for immunization of HLA-A1 patients carrying a malignant melanoma expressing gene MAGE-1. Dermatology 1993; 186: 278–80.

46. Chaux P, Vantomme V, Coulie P, et al. Estimation of the frequencies of anti-MAGE-3 cytolytic T-lymphocyte precursors in blood from individuals without cancer. Int J Cancer 1998; 77: 538–42.

47. Carrasco J, Van PA, Neyns B, et al. Vaccination of a melanoma patient with mature dendritic cells pulsed with MAGE-3 peptides triggers the activity of nonvaccine anti-tumor cells. J Immunol 2008; 180: 3585–93.

48. Marchand M, van Baren N, Weynants P, et al. Tumor regressions observed in patients with metastatic melanoma treated with an antigenic peptide encoded by gene MAGE-3 and presented by HLA-A1. Int J Cancer 1999; 80: 219–30.

49. Weber JS, Hua FL, Spears L, et al. A phase I trial of an HLA-A1 restricted MAGE-3 epitope peptide with incomplete Freund's adjuvant in patients with resected high-risk melanoma. J Immunother 1999; 22: 431–40.

50. Marchand M, Punt CJ, Aamdal S, et al. Immunisation of metastatic cancer patients with MAGE-3 protein combined with adjuvant SBAS-2: a clinical report. Eur J Cancer 2003; 39: 70–7.

51. Vantomme V, Dantinne C, Amrani N, et al. Immunologic analysis of a phase I/II study of vaccination with MAGE-3 protein combined with the AS02B adjuvant in patients with MAGE-3-positive tumors. J Immunother 2004; 27: 124–35.

52. Kruit WH, van Ojik HH, Brichard VG, et al. Phase 1/2 study of subcutaneous and intradermal immunization with a recombinant MAGE-3 protein in patients with detectable metastatic melanoma. Int J Cancer 2005; 117: 596–604.

53. Atanackovic D, Altorki NK, Stockert E, et al. Vaccine-induced CD4+ T cell responses to MAGE-3 protein in lung cancer patients. J Immunol 2004; 172: 3289–96.

54. Atanackovic D, Altorki NK, Cao Y, et al. Booster vaccination of non-small cell lung cancer (NSCLC) patients with MAGEA3 protein and AS02B adjuvant. Proc Natl Acad Sci U S A 2008; 105: 1065–5.

55. Pichyangkul S, Gettayacamin M, Miller RS, et al. Pre-clinical evaluation of the malaria vaccine candidate P. falciparum MSP1(42) formulated with novel adjuvants or with alum. Vaccine 2004; 22: 3831–40.

56. Garcon N, Chomez P, Van MM. GlaxoSmithKline Adjuvant Systems in vaccines: concepts, achievements and perspectives. Expert Rev Vaccines 2007; 6: 723–39.

57. Baldridge JR, McGowan P, Evans JT, et al. Taking a Toll on human disease: Toll-like receptor 4 agonists as vaccine adjuvants and monotherapeutic agents. Expert Opin Biol Ther 2004; 4: 1129–38.

58. Kensil CR, Kammer R. QS-21: a water-soluble triterpene glycoside adjuvant. Expert Opin Investig Drugs 1998; 7: 1475–82.

59. Hemmi H, Takeuchi O, Kawai T, et al. A Toll-like receptor recognizes bacterial DNA. Nature 2000; 408: 740–5.

60. Brichard VG, Lejeune D. Cancer immunotherapy targeting tumour-specific antigens: towards a new therapy for minimal residual disease. Expert Opin Biol Ther 2008; 8: 951–68.

61. Waldmann TA. Effective cancer therapy through immunomodulation. Annu Rev Med 2006; 57: 65–81.

62. Hoos A, Parmiani G, Hege K, et al. A clinical development paradigm for cancer vaccines and related biologics. J Immunother 2007; 30: 1–15.

63. Garcia M, Jemal A, Ward EM, et al. Global cancer facts & figures. Atlanta: GA: American Cancer Society, 2007.
64. Vansteenkiste J, Zielinski M, Linder A, et al. Phase II randomized study of MAGE-A3 immunotherapeutic as adjuvant therapy in stage IB/II Non-Small Cell Lung Cancer (NSCLC): 44 month follow-up, humoral and cellular immune response data. 2008; Abstract No. 148O–.
65. Kruit WH, Suciu S, Dreno B, et al. Immunization with the recombinant MAGE-A3 protein combined with Adjuvant Systems AS02B or AS15 in patients with metastatic melanoma: final results of a Phase II study of the EORTC Melanoma Group. Perspectives in Melanoma, 2009. 2009;
66. Spatz A, Dreno B, Chiarion-Sileni V, et al. MAGE-A3 Antigen-Specific Cancer Immunotherapy (ASCI) clinical activity in metastatic melanoma is associated with predictive biomarkers present in the tumor prior to immunization. Canadian Melanoma Conference. Conference document: 2010-FinalProgram. 2010; [Available from: http://www.buksa.com/melanoma/docs/2010-FinalProgram.pdf: p13].
67. Louahed J, Lehmann F, Ulloa-Montoya F, et al. Identification of a gene expression signature predictive of clinical activity following MAGE-A3 ASCI. AACR-NCI-EORTC_International Conference: Molecular Targets and Cancer Therapeutics-Mol Cencer Ther. 2009;8:abstract n° A37-.
68. Gajewski TF, Louahed J, Brichard VG. Gene signature in melanoma associated with clinical activity: a potential clue to unlock cancer immunotherapy. Cancer J 2010; 16: 399–403.
69. Vansteenkiste J, Zielinski M, Dahabreh J, et al. Gene expression signature is strongly associated with clinical efficacy of MAGE-A3 Antigen-Specific Cancer Immunotherapeutic (ASCI) as adjuvant therapy in resected stage IB/II Non-Small Cell Lung Cancer (NSCLC[V6]). J Clin Oncol 2008; 26 [15S (May 20 Supplement)]: 7501.
70. Klapper JA, Downey SG, Smith FO, et al. High-dose interleukin-2 for the treatment of metastatic renal cell carcinoma : a retrospective analysis of response and survival in patients treated in the surgery branch at the National Cancer Institute between 1986 and 2006. Cancer 2008; 113: 293–301.
71. Yee C. Adoptive therapy using antigen-specific T-cell clones. Cancer J 2010; 16: 367–73.
72. Koya RC, Mok S, Comin-Anduix B, et al. Kinetic phases of distribution and tumor targeting by T cell receptor engineered lymphocytes inducing robust antitumor responses. Proc Natl Acad Sci USA 2010; 107: 14286–91.
73. Pages F, Galon J, eu-Nosjean MC, et al. Immune infiltration in human tumors: a prognostic factor that should not be ignored. Oncogene 2010; 29: 1093–102.
74. Harlin H, Meng Y, Peterson AC, et al. Chemokine expression in melanoma metastases associated with CD8+ T-cell recruitment. Cancer Res 2009; 69: 3077–85.
75. Mescher MF, Curtsinger JM, Agarwal P, et al. Signals required for programming effector and memory development by CD8+ T cells. Immunol Rev 2006; 211: 81–92.
76. Keler T, He L, Ramakrishna V, et al. Antibody-targeted vaccines. Oncogene 2007; 26: 3758–67.
77. He LZ, Crocker A, Lee J, et al. Antigenic targeting of the human mannose receptor induces tumor immunity. J Immunol 2007; 178: 6259–67.
78. Idoyaga J, Cheong C, Suda K, et al. Cutting edge: langerin/CD207 receptor on dendritic cells mediates efficient antigen presentation on MHC I and II products in vivo. J Immunol 2008; 180: 3647–50.
79. Bozzacco L, Trumpfheller C, Huang Y, et al. HIV gag protein is efficiently cross-presented when targeted with an antibody towards the DEC-205 receptor in Flt3 ligand-mobilized murine DC. Eur J Immunol 2010; 40: 36–46.
80. Dhodapkar MV, Osman K, Teruya-Feldstein J, et al. Expression of cancer/testis (CT) antigens MAGE-A1, MAGE-A3, MAGE-A4, CT-7, and NY-ESO-1 in malignant gammopathies is heterogeneous and correlates with site, stage and risk status of disease. Cancer Immun 2003; 3: 9–.
81. O'Sullivan B, Thomas R. CD40 and dendritic cell function. Crit Rev Immunol 2003; 23: 83–107.
82. Ohigashi Y, Sho M, Yamada Y, et al. Clinical significance of programmed death-1 ligand-1 and programmed death-1 ligand-2 expression in human esophageal cancer. Clin Cancer Res 2005; 11: 2947–53.
83. van EA, Hurwitz AA, Allison JP. Combination immunotherapy of B16 melanoma using anti-cytotoxic T lymphocyte-associated antigen 4 (CTLA-4) and granulocyte/macrophage colony-stimulating factor (GM-CSF)-producing vaccines induces rejection of subcutaneous and metastatic tumors accompanied by autoimmune depigmentation. J Exp Med 1999; 190: 355–66.
84. Peggs KS, Quezada SA, Chambers CA, et al. Blockade of CTLA-4 on both effector and regulatory T cell compartments contributes to the antitumor activity of anti-CTLA-4 antibodies. J Exp Med 2009; 206: 1717–25.
85. Vonderheide RH, Flaherty KT, Khalil M, et al. Clinical activity and immune modulation in cancer patients treated with CP-870,893, a novel CD40 agonist monoclonal antibody. J Clin Oncol 2007; 25: 876–83.

86. Downey SG, Klapper JA, Smith FO, et al. Prognostic factors related to clinical response in patients with metastatic melanoma treated by CTL-associated antigen-4 blockade. Clin Cancer Res 2007; 13: 6681–8.

87. Phan GQ, Yang JC, Sherry RM, et al. Cancer regression and autoimmunity induced by cytotoxic T lymphocyte-associated antigen 4 blockade in patients with metastatic melanoma. Proc Natl Acad Sci USA 2003; 100: 8372–7.

88. Maker AV, Phan GQ, Attia P, et al. Tumor regression and autoimmunity in patients treated with cytotoxic T lymphocyte-associated antigen 4 blockade and interleukin 2: a phase I/II study. Ann Surg Oncol 2005; 12: 1005–16.

89. Ribas A. Overcoming immunologic tolerance to melanoma: targeting CTLA-4 with tremelimumab (CP-675,206). Oncologist 2008; 13(Suppl 4): 10–15.

90. Stary G, Bangert C, Tauber M, et al. Tumoricidal activity of TLR7/8-activated inflammatory dendritic cells. J Exp Med 2007; 204: 1441–51.

91. Ramakrishna V, Vasilakos JP, Tario JD Jr, et al. Toll-like receptor activation enhances cell-mediated immunity induced by an antibody vaccine targeting human dendritic cells. J Transl Med 2007; 5: 5–.

92. Poulin LF, Salio M, Griessinger E, et al. Characterization of human DNGR-1+ BDCA3+ leukocytes as putative equivalents of mouse CD8alpha+ dendritic cells. J Exp Med 2010; 207: 1261–71.

93. Davies H, Bignell GR, Cox C, et al. Mutations of the BRAF gene in human cancer. Nature 2002; 417: 949–54.

94. Aliferis CF, Statnikov A, Tsamardinos I, et al. Factors influencing the statistical power of complex data analysis protocols for molecular signature development from microarray data. PLoS One 2009; 4.

95. Oldenhuis CN, Oosting SF, Gietema JA, et al. Prognostic versus predictive value of biomarkers in oncology. Eur J Cancer 2008; 44: 946–53.

8 | Antigen-targeted, synthetic vaccines for metastatic cancer

Zhiyong Qiu, David C. Diamond, Kent A. Smith, Dar Rosario, Sabrina Miles, Mihail Obrocea, Thomas M. Kundig, and Adrian Bot

INTRODUCTION AND THE RATIONALE

An Integrated Model of Immune Responsiveness

Secondary lymphoid organs, including lymph nodes, spleen, and mucosa-associated lymphoid tissue, are highly organized anatomical structures encompassing a wide variety of bone marrow–derived cell types in close proximity. Regulation of immunity in the periphery is largely confined to the secondary lymphoid organs and includes the following functions: maintenance of tolerance in a steady-state fashion, homeostatic proliferation, induction and expansion of immune responses, differentiation of effector and memory cells, and retraction of immune responses through tolerance, anergy, or exhaustion. Furthermore, the proximity of complementary immune cell phenotypes is developmentally programmed (1,2) and key to the successful immunoregulatory function of secondary lymphoid organs described earlier.

During the 1990s, several models emerged aimed at explaining immune regulation and self–non-self discrimination. The geographical concept of immune induction (3,4) explains immunity as a function of where the antigen exposure occurs. If an antigen—presented in context of a relatively innocuous, noninfectious process—remains confined to non-lymphoid organs and is dealt with by natural barriers of protection or innate defense mechanisms, then no substantial adaptive immune response should emerge. However, if the antigen penetrates these defenses and reaches the secondary lymphoid organs, irrespective of its infectious potential, a strong immune response emerges, presumably due to an appropriate immunostimulatory environment within such anatomical structures. The observation that intrasplenic administration of transfected fibroblasts resulted in effective immunity (4) provided a compelling argument in support of this paradigm, since it eliminated the infectious nature of the antigen from the equation. On the other hand, this "one-signal" model is challenged by data which indicate that a number of cells resident to lymphoid organs are involved in maintaining peripheral tolerance and, thus, participate in self–non-self discrimination (5–7). We now know that a specific immunity type is regulated in a multifaceted fashion via three categories of signals. The immune response is initiated through antigen receptors (signal 1, recognition), complemented by co-stimulatory and co-inhibitory receptors (signal 2, verification), and regulated by soluble mediators such as cytokines and chemokines (signal 3) (8). Signals 2 and 3 are key for determining the magnitude and profile of immune responses and are orchestrated by the recognition of immune cues via germ-line receptors for exogenous pathogen-associated molecular patterns, pattern recognition receptors (9), and endogenous "danger signals" released during tissue damage (10) or cellular stress (11,12). In addition, this model calls for potent signal 2 and 3 signaling to induce substantial immunity, a key component of the self– non-self discrimination process that complements the immune repertoire formation. Mere exposure to antigen (even within secondary lymphoid organs) in the absence of appropriate co-stimulation will therefore result in a lack of immune response or even immune tolerance, responsible for immune homeostasis in a noninfective steady-state situation (13).

How can one reconcile the two seemingly contradictory perspectives from above? In fact, the two models seem to be complementary facets of an integrated overarching mechanism. First, it is quite clear that antigen exposure within lymphoid organs occurs as a natural consequence of almost any antigen exposure outside the lymphoid system, due to trafficking of antigen-presenting cells (APCs) such as certain dendritic cells like Langerhans cells which monitor the mucosal and skin areas, along with other mechanisms such as direct lymphatic circulation (14). Furthermore, this process is significantly enhanced by infection-associated signals (15). It is expected that limiting antigen influx into lymph nodes by blocking the incoming APCs and lymphatic fluid will severely restrict the magnitude of immune responses (16) even in the context of strong signals 2 and 3. Conversely, while more recent studies showed that the antigen exposure within lymph nodes, using noninvasive approaches, actually resulted in immune tolerance (17), it is not very surprising that a direct intrasplenic injection of transfected cells (4) would provoke an array of "danger signals" that could switch on immunity. Thus, key elements of both models seem to be required to explain how and when an immune response versus immune tolerance occurs (Fig. 8.1). Under this integrated model, induction of immune response requires both antigen presentation within lymphoid organs and the presence of robust signals 2 and 3 within the same microenvironment, in addition to the default co-stimulatory environment within lymphoid organs in the steady state. In all other circumstances, a suboptimal (deviated/ dwarfed) immune response or tolerance will ensue, depending on the nature of the antigen and the presence or lack of low-level co-stimulation.

Based on this integrated model, we expect that direct administration of antigens and biological response modifiers into lymph nodes represents a unique and effective approach to achieve induction or modulation of immune responses for the following three reasons. (*i*) Bioavailability ceases to be a critical parameter. When delivered through other routes of administration, several categories of reagents and vectors such as polypeptides, small molecules, and noninfectious, nonreplicating vectors in general will have limited immunogenic potential due to limited exposure in the secondary lymphoid tissues. Thus, a direct lymph node administration broadens up the range of viable options for vaccines and immune modulating agents. (*ii*) Signals 1, 2, and 3 can be modulated independently and more easily by utilizing appropriately timed and dosed antigens, and biological response modifiers. (*iii*) A broader, more effective dose range is achievable for both antigens and immune modulators thereby minimizing the importance of DC trafficking and lymphatic drainage. In all, the direct lymph node administration will enhance the range of useful antigens and immune modulators, and amplify their biological effect. The only limiting parameter will be the inherent production of "danger signals" as a natural consequence of injection.

Geographical model[1]	Co-stimulation model[2]
• Focuses on antigen compartmentalization and distribution as major determinant of immunity *(one-signal model)* • Antigen reaching secondary lymphoid organs is necessary and sufficient for induction of immunity, provided a competent immune repertoire • Less emphasis on the profile of immune response and immune regulation per se	• Emphasis on the importance of co-stimulatory signals through non-antigen specific receptors as a prerequisite to immunity *(multiple signal model)* • The magnitude and nature of signals 2 (co-receptors) and 3 (cytokines) determine the nature, magnitude and profile of response • Assumes antigen availability within lymphoid organs
An integrated model	
• Prerequisites for induction of an immune response are both optimal antigen availability within secondary lymphoid organs, as well as additional co-stimulation beyond the default state. • The primary immune repertoire is comprehensive and includes self and non-self specific clonotypes. Primary repertoire selection is inherently imperfect. Self / non-self discrimination relies on multiple mechanisms (central and peripheral, antigen and non-antigen specific). • The relative strength and nature of signals 1 (antigen specific) vs signals 2 and 3 within secondary lymphoid organs, control the immune response magnitude and profile, from tolerance to immunity.	

Figure 8.1 Models of immune responsiveness. [1]Key elements of this model were advanced by Zinkernagel and Hengartner as a one-signal model essentially (18). [2]This integrates aspects of two models: Cohn's time-based two-signal model and a development–context model that assumes distinct central and peripheral tolerance mechanisms as responsible for self–non-self discrimination as discussed by Anderson C.C. (19).

Several preclinical studies during the last decade illustrate these aspects and also reinforce the integrated model depicted in Figure 8.1. For example, a direct intra-lymph node or intrasplenic administration of diverse molecules and vectors including peptides (20), proteins (21), recombinant DNA (22), and whole cells (4,23) were more immunogenic than other routes of delivery, presumably due to a much higher antigen exposure. In addition, a direct intra-lymph node administration of biological response modifiers, such as Toll-like receptor (TLR) 9 ligand (unmethylated CpG), afforded an increased therapeutic index measured as the ratio of doses inducing immune modulation and side effects due to a systemic exposure to this potent adjuvant (24). Further, independently varying signals 1 and 2 through intra-lymph node co-administration of peptide and TLR ligand in different proportions resulted in a wide range of immune responses from a magnitude and quality standpoint. While intermediate peptide doses accompanied by a robust TLR ligation resulted in a robust expansion of specific CD8+ T cells, excessive peptide doses without adjuvants resulted in a greatly reduced T cell expansion with an anergy-prone phenotype (25). Similarly, a high peptide exposure within lymph nodes, even in the context of TLR ligand provision, resulted in diminished immunity accompanied by an anergic phenotype (25). Interestingly, a very limited exposure to antigen, coupled with an optimal co-stimulation, generated a robust CD8+ T-cell immunity with low levels of programmed cell death-1 (PD-1) expression, thus, resulting in T cells with increased functional competence and proliferative capacity (25,26). Together with a concordant lack of acquisition of other co-inhibitory molecules such as cytotoxic T-lymphocyte antigen 4 (CTLA-4) and lymphocyte activation gene-3 (LAG-3), these results suggest that the programming of T cells to be more refractory to negative regulatory mechanisms is achievable through vaccination (27). In addition, this finding is not merely a reflection of a lack of differentiation since the expression of CD62L (a marker distinguishing the central memory vs. peripheral memory effector cells) on these cells did not correlate with PD-1 expression. Furthermore, an exponential increase of exogenous antigen within lymph nodes over the course of immunization resulted in an exponentially higher T cell immunity (23). Finally, intra-lymph node immunization with peptide and TLR ligand was also more effective in vivo than other routes of administration in inducing an immune response protective against an immunogenic tumor described in a murine cancer model (28,29). Altogether, these preclinical studies (Table 8.1) while supporting the model described in Figure 8.1, suggest that direct intra-lymph node delivery offers an exquisitely potent approach to induce and modulate immunity over a wide range of magnitudes and profiles as compared to conventional immunization. The aspect of whether immune tolerance could be effectively achieved by means of this strategy remains to be elucidated as certain unavoidable "danger signals" accompanying direct injection procedures may impede this end.

Immunizing Vectors

Immunization utilizing replicating or nonreplicating vectors carries a remarkable potential because of the feasibility of co-delivering substantial co-stimulatory signals and thereby generating a range of immune responses encompassing innate, B cell, T-helper, and CTL immunity. Among the possible vectors with practical applicability, nonreplicating vectors such as naked plasmids pose little, if any, safety concerns and are quite easy to manufacture and formulate. Upon delivery through a wide range of means (from intramuscular injection to dermal particle bombardment), plasmids are taken up by somatic and bone marrow derived cells with differential roles in initiating immunity, depending primarily on the route and means of administration (32–34). Typically, only a few hundred or thousand cells are transfected in situ and capable of producing modest levels of antigen for several days to a few weeks, with plasmids persisting transiently in an episomal state rather than integrating within the genome (35,36). Extensive preclinical evaluation of the mechanism of action afforded by plasmid immunization showed that the number of antigen-expressing APCs is clearly a limiting factor for the magnitude of immunity (34). Despite some initial excitement based on preclinical modeling, many subsequent clinical trials with plasmids essentially confirmed that this category of vectors results in

Table 8.1 Preclinical Evaluation of Immunization by Antigen Administration to Secondary Lymphoid Organs

Category	References	Summary
Comparison of intra-lymph node/ splenic administration with other routes	Kündig et al., 1995 (4)	Immune response against viral proteins was achieved more effectively by intrasplenic immunization with fibroblasts, than other routes (s.c., i.p.)
	Maloy et al., 2001 (22)	DNA immunization by intra-lymph node or splenic injection was more effective than other routes (s.c., i.d., i.m., i.v.) at inducing CTL immunity against a virus
	Johansen et al., 2005 (20)	Peptide + CpG immunization by intra-lymph node injection was more effective than other routes (s.c., i.d., i.m., i.v.) at inducing CTL immunity against a virus and a transplantable tumor
	Von Beust et al., 2005 (24)	Intra-lymph node administration of peptide with CpG was superior in generating a CTL response against a tumor antigen. Similarly, this approach was superior in generating an antibody response
	Johansen et al., 2005 (21)	Intra-lymph node administration of protein (denatured allergen) was more effective than other parenteral routes at inducing antibody responses
	Smith et al., 2009 (26)	Intra-lymph node administration of plasmid followed by peptides was more effective than other parenteral routes at inducing CTL immunity against human tumor antigens
	Smith et al., 2009 (28)	Intra-lymph node administration of peptide + TLR ligand was more effective than other routes, in inducing an immune response leading to prevention or regression of transplantable tumors
Modulation of immunity by intra-lymph node immunization	Johansen et al., 2005 (30)	Intra-lymph node administration of a range of TLR ligands plus allergenic protein resulted in T2/T1 immune modulation and induction of neutralizing antibodies
	Johansen et al., 2008 (23)	Intra-lymph node immunization with exponentially increasing doses of antigen achieved elevated CTL immunity over shorter intervals
	Wong et al., 2009 (25)	Modulation of acquisition of PD-1 and other co-inhibitory molecules by T cells, by intra-lymph node immunization with peptide and CpG
	Smith et al., 2010 (31)	Immunization by gene transfer (plasmid) into lymph nodes elicits low PD-1 expressing T cells that expand more effectively upon peptide boosting and uncovers a distinct T cell activation program linked to differential co-expression of inhibitory molecules

Abbreviations: CTL, cytotoxic T-lymphocyte antigen; PD-1, programmed cell death-1; TLR, Toll-like receptor.

modest immune responses at best (37). Attempts to improve on plasmid vector efficacy by in vivo electroporation (38) or direct intra-lymph node administration (39,40) have resulted in some promising preliminary results that require confirmation through additional clinical studies. As we will outline below, plasmid immunization may offer a platform to build more potent immunotherapy strategies.

An important potential advantage of plasmid immunization that could be utilized to build safe and potent immunization regimens is the quality, or the profile, of the immune response generated by this approach. In a preclinical setting, a direct intra-lymph node administration of a plasmid shifted the dose–effect curve toward minimal amounts of vector (22).

Strikingly, plasmid immunization elicited a population of CD8$^+$ T cells with special characteristics (26,31) including low expression levels of the co-inhibitory receptors PD-1 and CTLA-4. There were also substantial differences at the transcriptome level of these molecules compared to T cells resulting from intranodal peptide immunization without an adjuvant (25,31). In addition, a similar PD-1^{low} CD8$^+$ T cell phenotype could be recapitulated by a repeat low-dose peptide intranodal immunization in the context of TLR9 ligation (25). In contrast, a high-dose peptide elicited PD-1^{high} / CD8$^+$ T cells that were unable to proliferate upon subsequent antigen stimulation. The restoration of T cell proliferation and function by the PD-1 blocking antibody demonstrated the pivotal role of PD-1 in this process (25). Interestingly, the dichotomy between high and low PD-1-expressing T cells was independent of CD62L co-expression distinguishing essentially between CD62L$^+$ central memory (CM) and CD62L$^-$ peripheral memory/effector cells. This suggests that the programming of CD8$^+$ T cells that retain low expression levels of co-inhibitory receptors is, to some degree, imprinted during priming and carried through key steps of differentiation, thus defining a special lineage that could be less prone to major immune inhibitory mechanisms within lymphoid organs, sanctuary tissues, or tumors (Fig. 8.2). Possibly, a key prerequisite for generating this PD-1^{low} CD8$^+$ lineage consists in exposure to low levels of antigen for a prolonged interval, yet in the presence of an optimal level of innate immune activation through pathogen-associated molecular patterns or danger signals. This could be an important mechanism to accelerate the generation of immune memory and ensure a timely immune readiness in a manner dependent on the nature of the threat should it persist or reoccur. Therefore, it provides a veritable "standby immune status" anticipating imminent, massive penetration of virulent pathogens through first barriers of defense. In addition, this could explain why certain heterologous prime–boost approaches encompassing plasmid priming are so effective in eliciting highly elevated immune responses, as shown 15 years ago, for example that neonatal DNA vaccination of mice followed by virus boosting during adulthood resulted in an unparalleled CTL immune response (41). Importantly, however, it remains to be established whether entraining of CD8$^+$T cells to have a PD-1/CTLA-4/LAG-3 low phenotype ("fit T cells"; Fig. 8.2) renders these effector T cells more functional within the immune-hostile tumor microenvironment and can result in more clinically efficacious therapeutic vaccines for cancer. This paradigm is quite different from those utilized to design and optimize such investigational agents in the past, which have been based primarily on elevating the absolute numbers of vaccine-specific T cells.

Based on these considerations, plasmid immunization could be utilized to build, through prime–boost strategies, safe and more effective immune interventions for cancer immunotherapy. In addition, this may prove to be more practical and efficacious than blocking inhibitory receptors, one at a time, via antibody therapy (42,43). As expected, based on the localization of APCs and their proximity to T cells, direct intra-lymph node delivery of plasmid was found to be a more effective priming approach compared to subcutaneous or intra-muscular delivery (22,26). Furthermore, based on preclinical evaluation, plasmid priming elicited long-lasting CM-T cells with an exceptionally high proliferative potential following antigen re-exposure (26). In addition, using a single-epitope system, heterologous plasmid priming followed by peptide boost, both delivered intranodally, achieved very high frequencies of epitope-specific T cells in the order of 1/10-1/2 CD8$^+$ T cells (26). Furthermore, the antigen exposure derived from the plasmid was essential since co-expression by the same plasmid vector of an shRNA specific to the antigen effectively turned off the vaccine antigen expression and obliterated the priming effect of the plasmid (26). Moreover, reversing the sequence of the heterologous prime boost by priming with the peptide and boosting with plasmid, failed to reproduce the magnitude of T cell expansion or PD-1^{low} phenotype resulting from the heterologous plasmid priming followed by peptide boost (26). While plasmid priming resulted in long lasting CD62L$^+$ CM-T cells with significant expansion capability, peptide boosting induced their rapid expansion and differentiation to CD62L$^-$ peripheral memory effector T cells that displayed elevated PD-1 expression levels and thus were more susceptible to immune exhaustion (44). Based on these findings, we designed a novel intranodal immunization regimen using iterative cycles of plasmid prime and

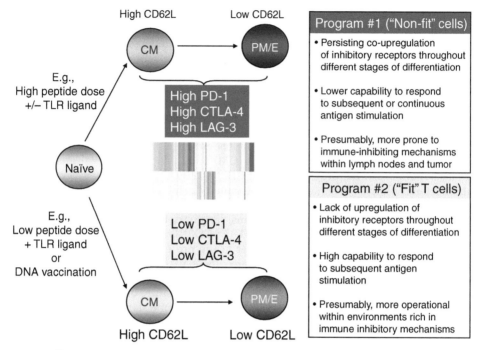

Figure 8.2 Differential programming of T cells based on the expression of inhibitory molecules. *Abbreviations*: CM, central memory; CTLA-4, cytotoxic T-lymphocyte antigen 4; LAG-3, lymphocyte activation gene-3; PD-1, programmed cell death-1; PM, peripheral memory; TLR, Toll-like receptor.

peptide boost to repeatedly elicit and replenish the pool of antigen-specific CM-T cells and effector cells (26,31). In preclinical murine tumor models, this approach resulted in effector cells that migrated to established tumors or emerging metastatic lesions and were able to eradicate tumors in prophylactic and therapeutic settings (26,31). Furthermore, intra-lymph node plasmid priming offers the potential to build multitargeted immunization regimens by utilizing a variety of boosting vectors including peptides, recombinant proteins, and viruses. A peptide-boosting approach will be "epitope centric", carrying the potential of generating a robust yet ultra-focused response. On the other hand, larger vectors encompassing antigen fragments or whole antigens could potentially trigger a more diversified response across many epitopes though with an expected lower magnitude of response for any given epitope. While the former approach carries the promise of being more potent in select patient populations and practical vis-à-vis several categories of vectors, the latter could have a much wider applicability although currently there is very little, if any, clinical information comparing these two strategies. Finally, in regard to heterologous prime–boost approaches that utilize plasmid priming, there are some initial promising data from clinical trials (45–50) but more studies are needed in the areas of infectious disease and oncology.

Target Antigens

The process of immune self–non-self discrimination does not rely entirely on the central tolerance established in the thymus for T cells and in bone marrow for B cells. In other words, the process of negative repertoire selection against a range of self antigens is leaky (51,52). This explains the inherent existence of self-reactive or cross-reactive T- and B-cell clonotypes in the periphery (51–53). In addition, this creates an exciting opportunity to harness this self-reactive

T-cell repertoire against a broader range of tumor antigens, beyond those generated by mutational events (neo-antigens), encompassing unmutated sequences which are immunogenic and antigenic and expressed differentially on cancer cells. The most interesting category of antigens is that which plays a significant biological role in tumor progression or involved in the metastatic process. Such antigens do not necessarily have an expression pattern restricted to tumors though exceptions do exist, such as developmentally regulated (oncofetal) or cancer testes antigens (expressed only by germinal cells during adult stage) that may assume cellular functions upon re-expression or ectopic expression. It is of course a well accepted paradigm that effective immune-targeting of molecules that play a role in tumorigenesis can have a profound and deleterious impact on the tumor process by interfering with the tumor's viability and also decreasing the chances for immune escape of the tumor through a range of mechanisms (54). The pros and cons for various categories of tumor antigens have been described already (55). In summary, antigens that have a very limited expression pattern, such as tissue specific antigens, may be more immunogenic, yet frequently lack key biological roles in cancer progression since they tend to be associated with ancillary tissue-specific functions. On the other hand, antigens with pivotal roles in cancer cell viability and progression usually have housekeeping roles in normal cells, thus potentially leading to autoimmune side effects. A particular case, at the junction between these two categories, involves neoantigens resulting from mutational events which are only rarely conserved within certain patient populations. While some may be appealing from a biological point of view, their translatability to safe, effective, synthetic ("off the shelf") vaccines with broader applicability is questionable. Finally, a quite special category of target antigens are in fact not expressed by cancerous cells but are expressed by stromal cells (56) and have the advantage that they may be less susceptible to clonal immune-escape mechanisms.

With the goal of developing effective immunotherapy regimens for the treatment of various cancers, we selected our target antigens based on the following major considerations (Table 8.2):

1. A demonstrated expression within metastatic lesions
2. Expression across various tumor types
3. A documented role in tumor biology

Two of the target antigens selected were the tissue-specific and differentiation antigens, Melan A/MART-1 (melanoma antigen recognized by T cells-1) and Tyrosinase (60,61) expressed on malignant melanoma, each of which had known immunogenic major histocompatibility complex (MHC) class I restricted epitopes (62–65). In the case of Melan A/MART-1, an objective tumor regression upon adoptive T cell transfer of antigen-specific T cells in man has demonstrated its target value (66). This was quite a unique circumstance in the current state of affairs of vaccine target development. Tyrosinase, on the other hand, was validated as a cancer-antigen target as the first approved veterinary cancer vaccine for melanoma (67). Since the function of these antigens is merely related to melanin synthesis rather than being required for tumor growth or metastasis one might expect immune evasion to occur rapidly through a variety of processes (54) although this remains to be tested in ongoing and future clinical studies (Ref). Nevertheless, the hope is that this type of immunization method will result in rapid and effective epitope spreading, involving an increasing number of antigens and effector mechanisms, (68) and will ultimately lead to a lasting clinical effect.

Prostate-specific membrane antigen (PSMA) is a tissue-specific antigen selected by our laboratory for clinical development with distinct characteristics from Melan A/MART-1 and Tyrosinase. PSMA is expressed by prostate carcinoma tumor cells in a manner proportional with the degree of cancer aggressiveness (69) and is also expressed by endothelial cells of the tumor neovasculature (70), playing a key role in angiogenesis (71). Nevertheless, PSMA is also expressed by other nontransformed cells such as prostate epithelial cells. Interestingly, PSMA is not a typical tissue-specific antigen and has multiple roles. It is a transmembrane enzyme (dihydrofolate reductase) (72) and presumably a vitamin transporter. In addition, upon

Table 8.2 Target Antigens: Main Features

Antigen	Melan A/MART-1	Tyrosinase	PRAME	PSMA	NY-ESO-1	SSX2
Category	Tissue differentiation antigen	Tissue differentiation antigen	Cancer testis antigen[a]	Tissue-specific antigen[b]	Cancer testis antigen	Cancer testis antigen
Expression in normal tissues	Melanocytes (neural crest)	Melanocytes (neural crest)	Germinal cells; Some expression in a variety of somatic and bone marrow derived cells	High expression in prostate epithelial cells; Low expression in brain, salivary gland, kidneys, blood vessels	Germinal cells	Germinal cells
Biological function in normal tissues	Melanin synthesis	Melanin synthesis	Regulation of cellular Differentiation, proliferation and death	Glutaminergic neurotransmission; Folate transport; Angiogenesis	Cellular motility (?)	Unknown
Expression in cancer	Melanoma	Melanoma	Diverse solid tumors and hematological malignancies	In localized and metastatic PC (higher in latter); In blood vessels of diverse solid tumors	Diverse solid tumors and hematological malignancies	Diverse solid tumors and hematological malignancies
Biological consequences in cancer	Unknown	Unknown	Block of cellular differentiation; Cell proliferation; Increased resistance to apoptosis	Angiogenesis; Genetic instability	Cellular motility (?)	Transcription inhibition
Evidence of immunogenicity and antigenicity	(60–67)		(74,78)	(57–59)	(81)	(82)
Previous clinical experience[c]	Peptides; DNA vaccines; Adoptive cell transfer; Viral vectors	Peptides; DNA vaccines	Peptides; Protein; DNA vaccines	Peptides; Protein; DNA vaccine; Adoptive cell transfer; Antibodies	Peptide; Protein; DNA vaccine; Adoptive cell transfer; Viral vectors	None

[a]PRAME is not a typical cancer testis antigen since it is expressed at low levels on other normal cells (somatic or bone marrow derived).
[b]PSMA is not a typical tissue specific antigen since it is expressed at various levels on other normal cells.
[c]http://clinicaltrials.gov/
Abbreviations: PRAME, preferential expressed antigen of melanoma; PC, prostate cancer; PSMA, prostate-specific membrane antigen.

overexpression, it interacts and interferes with the cell division machinery resulting in genomic instability (73). This could be a feature that favors the selection of cancer clonotypes with an increased invasiveness thereby facilitating the tumor progression. In addition, PSMA expression by the neovasculature will potentially enable the co-targeting of a PSMA expressing tumor and its vasculature simultaneously, along with the added advantage that immune escape mechanisms may be less operational in the noncancerous endothelial cells. It can also be used to target the neovasculature of tumors in which the neoplastic cells do not express PSMA, particularly in bivalent vaccines, also targeting an antigen expressed in the cancer cells themselves.

A fourth target antigen selected for development by our group was preferential expressed antigen of melanoma (PRAME) that has an expression profile reminiscent of a cancer testes antigen. In fact, PRAME, which is a retinoic acid receptor inhibitor (74), is expressed at low physiological levels by a range of nontransformed cells and is a member of a large family of related molecules (75). Most interestingly, PRAME seems to be involved in blocking pro-differentiation and anti-proliferation signals (76). This may explain why PRAME expression is substantially upregulated in both hematological and solid malignancies (77). PRAME is also an immunogenic antigen encompassing defined antigenic epitopes restricted to MHC class I molecules (78). However, compared to Melan A/MART-1, Tyrosinase, and PSMA, PRAME has been evaluated, to a much lesser extent, as a possible therapeutic target, although some late breaking clinical information is imminent (79,80).

NY-ESO-1 and SSX2 (synovial sarcoma X gene family) are two "cancer testis" antigens we selected for our pipeline (Table 8.2). As they were widely described before (81,82) and not part of our clinical stage portfolio at this time, we will not cover them in this chapter.

In summary, we initially employed an epitope-centric strategy to select our target antigens. By doing so we designed a series of investigational agents (Fig. 8.3) to favor the immunogenicity of select epitopes in the hope of generating robust immune responses against epitopes that could be targeted in tumor cells. This is in contrast to whole antigen strategies

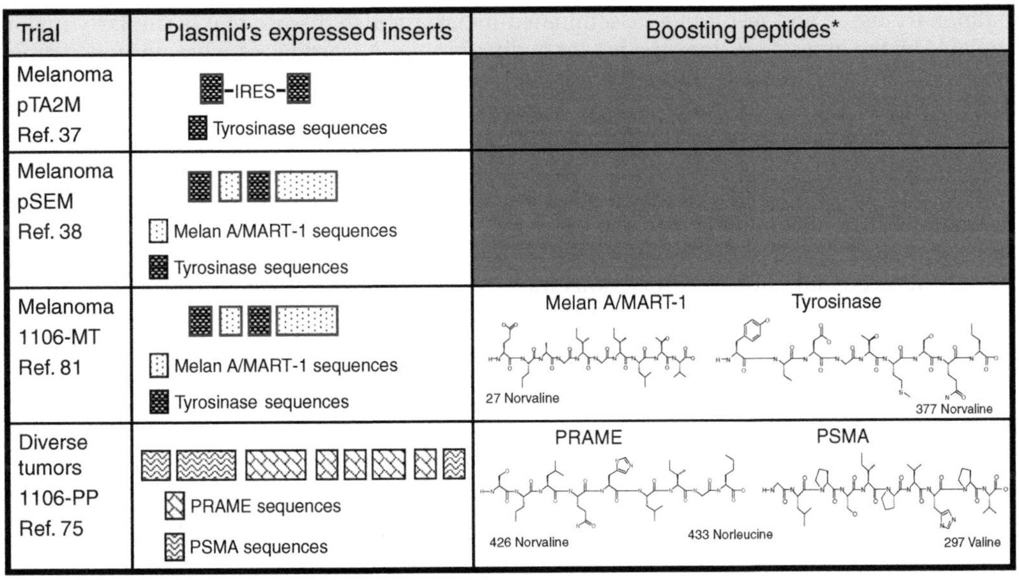

Trial	Plasmid's expressed inserts	Boosting peptides*
Melanoma pTA2M Ref. 37	▦–IRES–▦ ▦ Tyrosinase sequences	
Melanoma pSEM Ref. 38	▦ ▦ ▦ ▦ ▦ Melan A/MART-1 sequences ▦ Tyrosinase sequences	
Melanoma 1106-MT Ref. 81	▦ ▦ ▦ ▦ ▦ Melan A/MART-1 sequences ▦ Tyrosinase sequences	Melan A/MART-1 Tyrosinase 27 Norvaline 377 Norvaline
Diverse tumors 1106-PP Ref. 75	▦ ▦ ▦ ▦ ▦ ▦ ▦ PRAME sequences ▦ PSMA sequences	PRAME PSMA 426 Norvaline 433 Norleucine 297 Valine

Figure 8.3 A schematic representation of investigational agents. The peptides are analogous with substitutions at second or last position to increase MHC–peptide complex half-life, of Melan A/MART-1 26–35, Tyrosinase 369–377, PRAME 425–433 and PSMA 288–297 epitopes while maintain the cross-reactivity of induced T cells to native epitopes (*). *Abbreviations*: IRES, internal ribosome entry site; MART-1, melanoma antigen recognized by T cells-1; MHC, major histocompatibility complex; PRAME, preferential expressed antigen of melanoma; PSMA, prostate-specific membrane antigen.

that may elicit modest responses per a given epitope, yet may have a broader applicability. Nevertheless, we acknowledge that a head-to-head comparison between an "epitope-focused" and "whole-antigen approach," burdened as it will be with technical difficulties and issues with interpretability, has not been done yet.

Disease Indications

In order to more optimally position our novel investigational agents in early clinical development, we executed a series of in vivo preclinical studies designed to generate relevant and reliable immune correlates of clinical response and to help guide optimization of our platform technology and clinical trial design. The literature suggests that active immunotherapy is most suited for treatment in a minimal residual disease or adjuvant setting, presumably to keep the patients in remission once the standard therapy has achieved a significant reduction or debulking of their cancer (83). Under this paradigm, cancer vaccine researchers sought to evaluate vaccine regimens in patients free of clinical disease and mostly based on putative immune correlates of clinical activity. We will discuss the risks related to this approach at the end of the chapter. Conversely, evaluation of active immunotherapy in a measurable disease or a rapidly progressing disease setting, provided a reasonable likelihood of therapeutic success exists, will improve on drug evaluation considerably since clinical signals of efficacy are now part of the equation.

Utilizing an intra-lymph node immunization regimen comprised of peptides derived from tumor-associated antigens in combination with a potent TLR ligand as an adjuvant, we used a mouse model of transplantable, immunogenic tumor to evaluate the potentials and limitations of vaccination in various stages of cancer (28). The tumor cells are murine epithelioid cells transformed with the human papilloma virus (HPV) genome and expressing a dominant E7 epitope (84). Following subcutaneous injection, these cancerous cells from solid tumors that progress rapidly and eventually overwhelm the animal's immune system and ability to cope with this challenge. In the case of intravenous infusion, these cells lodge within the pulmonary tissue and result in a disseminated metastatic-like disease that is similarly uncontrollable by the immune system and is eventually terminal. Nevertheless, a lymph-node administration of HPV E7 peptide plus adjuvant led to a considerable expansion of E7-specific CD8$^+$ T cells (reaching a proportion of 1/10–1/2 specific cells per total CD8$^+$ T cells) and resulted in complete tumor protection, irrespective of the route of tumor challenge (28). Once the prophylactic benefit of the vaccine was established we wanted to test our active immunotherapy regimen in a more "physiological" or relevant therapeutic tumor setting to evaluate the disease indication where this regimen had the greatest likelihood of success and, equally valuable, to determine the limitations of this approach. To that aim, mice were first inoculated with tumors by subcutaneous injection or intravenous infusion and after various intervals of time, immunized against E7 antigen by intranodal injection using an ultra-potent regimen similar to the one described earlier (28). Not surprisingly, while the regimen was quite effective in inducing a similar level of immunity irrespective of the tumor stage at the start of immunization, the impact of the immune response on tumor progression was widely different. In the early, minimal residual disease or limited tumor size stage, immunotherapy significantly slowed the tumor progression and induced tumor regression in most of the animals. In the late disease stage, when tumors reached beyond 0.25% of the mouse's weight, immunization alone ceased to be effective in controlling tumor progression. Interestingly, while T cells could still massively infiltrate the tumor tissue, they were quite unable to exert an effect upon target cells within the tumor microenvironment (28). Isolation of these tumor-infiltrating T cells (TILs) followed by in vitro manipulation, at least partially restored their functional capabilities, indicating that the TILs were effectively silenced within the tumor microenvironment, even in the context of a robust systemic immune response. Utilization of low, immune modulating doses of cyclophosphamide (at sub-cytotoxic doses, affecting T regulatory (T$_{REG}$) cells but not the tumor progression) (85) partially restored the functional capability of the TILs in vivo and enabled immune-mediated tumor control in later stage disease (28). In addition, a key observation was made when immunized mice with large tumors were infused with E7 peptide-pulsed lymphocyte target cells. In this situation, E7-immunized mice were perfectly capable of eliminating the target cells systemically or within lymphoid organs but were unable to exert cytotoxicity against peptide-pulsed target cells within their tumor unless a T_{REG} cell depletion was performed (28), thus, highlighting the immunosuppressive microenvironment within large established tumors. This supports the view that therapeutic vaccination could be a very potent approach to interfere with cancer in minimal residual disease (localized or disseminated) or at the stage when tumor cells have spread throughout the lymphatic system. In essence, this could be due to the fact that as tumors progress from primary, to localized lymphatic, to lymphatic metastatic, and finally to visceral involvement, there is a gradual accumulation of immune evasion and inhibiting mechanisms that curb the activity of tumor-specific T cells. Therefore, it may be possible that the lymphatic localization of tumor cells may be associated with a narrower range of immune inhibiting mechanisms and thus more amenable to active immunotherapy compared with the treatment of well-established, vascularized tumors although this hypothesis needs to be further tested.

In light of these considerations, for malignant melanoma we explored a range of disease stages spanning visceral metastasis, generalized systemic lymphatic metastatic disease, to an earlier "in transit" disease or a localized, yet rapidly progressing lymph node disease.

To clinically test our PRAME and PSMA immunotherapy regimen, and due to the wide applicability of the target antigens in cancer, we enrolled patients with several tumor types that met the antigen expression profile, with the goal of pursuing the most responsive tumor types and indications for future clinical studies.

In summary, the strategy of evaluating active immunotherapy in rapidly progressing metastatic disease offers the opportunity of generating clinical efficacy signals earlier in the course of development and in a more reliable fashion, at two levels:

1. Assessing whether there is tumor regression or a cytostatic effect in progressing lesions, measurable at the start of therapy.
2. Evaluating whether there is an inhibition in the onset of new metastatic lesions.

Effectively, this allows a concurrent evaluation of a therapeutic effect in two biologically different circumstances (measurable tumors within internal organs, lymph nodes, soft tissue, or skin; and a more indirect evaluation of microlesions). The risk associated with assessing and deciding upon new cancer vaccines in a measurable disease setting is to inadvertently discard approaches that, while not potent enough to afford clinical signals of efficacy in an advanced disease stage, may still be useful in much earlier stages. This is a price that perhaps we need to pay until we realize breakthroughs at several levels including, but not limited to, defining reliable immune response correlates of clinical efficacy.

CLINICAL EVALUATION OF EARLY AND CURRENT CANDIDATES
Overall Clinical Trial Strategy and Rationale

The main objectives of the four trials completed to date were to characterize the overall safety and immune response, as well as to evaluate and document any evidence of clinical benefit afforded by intranodal plasmid immunization (39,40) or intranodal plasmid prime and peptide boost (80,86), respectively. In the most recently completed phase 1 trials we evaluated our active immunotherapy regimen in patients with measurable, metastatic disease with a goal of generating safety data, immune response results, and quantifiable early clinical signals. To maximize the trials' output and improve on the likelihood of clinical and technical success we optimized the investigational agents, selected the patient population based on tumor antigen expression, and set endpoints that were supported through comprehensive clinical and laboratory evaluation. The immune monitoring strategy was to employ commonly used, clinically applicable real-time analysis to confirm the biological effect of the vaccine along with preserving samples for ulterior in-depth immunological analysis pertaining to the quality and profile of the immune response.

First, to enhance the immune activity we designed plasmids that yield preferentially immunodominant HLA-A2-restricted epitopes from well-characterized target antigens, MART-1/Melan A and Tyrosinase for melanoma and PRAME and PSMA applicable to a variety of solid tumors [Fig. 8.3 and (26,39,40,80,86)]. As boosting agents, we utilized peptides that had substitutions at key MHC anchor residues (26,80,86) to increase the half-life of the MHC–peptide complex, a crucial parameter leading to the stabilization of the immune synapse (87). Such substitutions, while abrogating immune reactivity of the native epitope, maintained reactivity of the induced T cells with the native epitope. Based on limited immune response data and owing to a scarcity of efficacy data from clinical trials with plasmid alone (39,40), we utilized a recently tested heterologous prime–boost approach (80,86); (Fig. 8.4) that has been complemented by preclinical studies using strategies to build on the advantages of plasmid priming through heterologous prime–boost immunization (26). This strategy afforded an increased immune response rate and most importantly, signals of clinical benefit. Nevertheless, the information derived from these early clinical trials pointed to some key challenges as well as opportunities to redirect development of cancer vaccines and immune monitoring as discussed below.

Secondly, we enrolled HLA-A*0201 patients who co-expressed the target antigens within their tumors. Further, acknowledging the likelihood of cytostatic rather than cytoreductive effects and, the delayed clinical benefit, a hallmark of several immune interventions (88), the trials were designed to allow patients who did not show signs of disease progression to remain on study and receive multiple cycles of treatment. In addition, a key eligibility criterion was the presence of measurable disease and clear progression on prior therapies which was documented at the time of enrollment either clinically, radiologically, or through biomarkers, as applicable by tumor types.

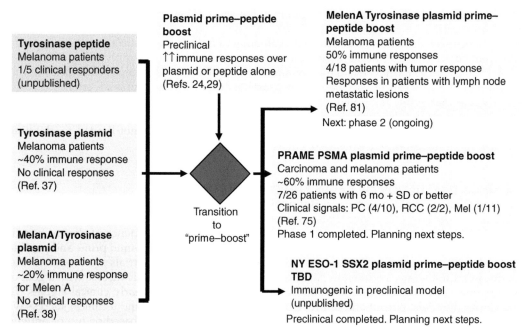

Figure 8.4 Evolution of investigational agents for intra-nodal immunization. *Abbreviations*: PC, programmed cell death-1; Me, melanoma; RCC, renal cell carcinoma; SD, stable disease.

Feasibility and Safety of Intra-Lymph Node Immunization

Our four trials (39,40,80,86) (Table 8.3) along with independent studies executed with cell-based vaccines (89,90) in cancer, or antigens for allergy desensitization (91,92), showed that intra-lymph node immunization, either by infusion or bolus injection, is a relatively simple and feasible procedure. The administration of the vaccine was accomplished by ultrasound-guided injection, either via an infusion set and portable pump (39,40) or by bolus injections using a unibody syringe having fixed echogenic needles (80,86,91,92), into the superficial inguinal or axillary lymph nodes. These nodes were selected for their relatively long major axes (1–2 cm) and their easy accessibility. The infusion or injection did not require anesthesia and while the portable infusion pump was connected for up to 96 hours, the bolus injection was administrated within a few minutes. During earlier trials with intra-lymph node infusion of plasmids the most common treatment-related adverse events (AEs) reported were local pain, lymph node swelling, redness at the infusion site, and systemic flu-like syndrome that occurred only in a few patients. Overall, toxicity from intra-lymph node infusion of plasmids was minimal with no dose-limiting toxicities. Out of dozens of patients treated with plasmid alone there was only one documented grade 3 drug-related toxicity which was a deep venous thrombosis reported at the highest plasmid dose level (1500 µg) (40). In addition, data from the two recently completed phase 1 trials utilizing a plasmid prime–peptide boost regimen (80,86) also indicated that a repeat bolus injection into inguinal lymph nodes of the three-component regimens was well tolerated and associated with over 90% compliance. The longest treatment duration was in a melanoma trial [Table 8.3, (86)] where a patient received 9 treatment cycles spanning over a year with 54 bilateral intra-lymph node immunization procedures and without any serious adverse events (AEs) reported. In these latter prime–boost trials the safety profile was similar to that in earlier plasmid trials with generally mild or grade 1 or 2 drug-related AEs reported. In addition to some mild or moderate pain at the site of administration, the most common AEs reported were flu-like symptoms such as fever and fatigue along with diarrhea, vomiting, pyrexia, decreased appetite, and hyperglycemia. No dose-limiting toxicities were reported and no grade 3–4 AEs were related to the study regimen. Taken together, our clinical experience demonstrated feasibility and safety of repeat intranodal immunization by infusion or bolus injection in patients with advanced cancer (malignant melanoma or carcinomas).

Intra-Lymph Node Immunization Induces Antigen-Specific T-Cell Immunity in Cancer Patients

We commonly utilized two immunological assays to assess the antigen-specific immune response in vaccinated patients: enumeration of antigen (epitope) specific CD8$^+$ T cells by tetramer analysis using flow cytometry and complemented, in three out of four trials, by enzyme-linked immunosorbent spot analysis. In all cases we prospectively defined immune responders as having a two-fold post-treatment increase in tetramer value and/or a three-fold increase in the enzyme-linked immunosorbent spot value over the screening value, provided that these values were significantly different from background. The immune analysis was done on peripheral blood mononuclear cells utilizing qualified and validated assays and executed in independent academic laboratories (39,40) or contract research organizations (80,86). Nevertheless, we acknowledge two serious pitfalls of these assays that are commonly used to evaluate the immune efficacy of vaccines. First, they cannot provide any insight regarding the immune response within tumors; and secondly, they do not capture key functional parameters such as polyfunctionality, affinity to the target antigen, avidity of the target antigen, and expression of co-inhibitory receptors that could trump the quantitative aspect represented by the frequency of vaccine antigen-specific T cells.

While previous trials executed with plasmid alone demonstrated an immune response to a single antigen in about one-third of the treated patients (39,40), two recently completed phase I trials utilizing a plasmid-prime and peptide-boost approach showed an immune response against two antigens in a simple majority (>50%) of patients [Table 8.3 and (80,86)]. While the

Table 8.3 Early Stage Clinical Trials with Intra-Lymph Node Administration of Plasmids and Peptides

Trial/Investigational Agents	Plasmid (pTA2M)	Plasmid (pSEM)	Plasmid & Peptides (pSEM Plasmid + Melan A/MART-1 and Tyrosinase Peptides)	Plasmid & Peptides (pPRA-PSM Plasmid + PRAME and PSMA Peptides)
Target antigens	Tyrosinase	Melan A/MART-1 Tyrosinase	Melan A/MART-1 Tyrosinase	PRAME PSMA
Method	Continuous infusion	Continuous infusion	Bolus injection	Bolus injection
Tumor type (number of patients)	Advanced melanoma (26 pts)	Advanced melanoma (19 pts)	Advanced melanoma (18 pts)	• Diverse tumors (carcinoma, melanoma), advanced stage (26 pts) • Prostate carcinoma: 10 pts • Melanoma: 10 pts • Renal cell carcinoma: 2 pts • Mesothelioma: 2 pts • Basal cell carcinoma: 1 pt • Esophageal carcinoma: 1 pt
Disease stage	Stage IV IV M1a: 4 pts IV M1b: 12 pts IV M1c: 10 pts	Stage IV IV M1a: 6 pts IV M1b: 6 pts IV M1c: 7 pts	Stages III B/C and IV IIIC: 1 pt IV M1a: 6 pts IV M1b: 2 pts IV M1c: 9 pts	
Dosing regimen	Plasmid dose escalation (200, 400 or 800 ug over 96 hours x 4 times, every 2 weeks)	Plasmid dose escalation (500, 1000 or 1500 ug over 96 hours x 4 times, every 2 weeks)	Multiple cycles of DNA-priming, peptide-boosting (1200 ug DNA on cycle days 1, 4, 15 and 18; 100 or 300 ug of each peptide on cycle days 29 and 32)	Multiple cycles of DNA-priming, peptide-boosting (1200 ug DNA on cycle days 1, 4, 15 and 18; 22.5 or 150 ug of PRAME peptide and 30 or 300 ug of PSMA peptide on cycle days 29 and 32)
Immune response rate[a]	42% to Tyrosinase	21% to Melan A/MART-1	50% overall 39% to Melan A/MART-1 33% to Tyrosinase	58% overall 42% to PRAME 53% to PSMA
Objective tumor regression	None	None	4/18 (4/7 with stage III/IV M1a)	1 prostate cancer patient with transient lymph node regression
Stable disease # patients Median (Range)	6 pts 2 (2–4 months)	6 pts 2 (2–4.5 months)	6 pts 12 (3–12 months)	10 pts 6 (3–11 months)
References	Tagawa et al., 2003 (39)	Weber et al., 2008 (40)	Ribas et al., 2011 (86)	Weber et al., In press (80)

[a]Criteria were defined prospectively.

Abbreviations: MART-1, melanoma antigen recognized by T cells-1; PSMA, prostate-specific membrane antigen; PRAME, preferential expressed antigen of melanoma.

immune response rate was higher in these latter trials, it is not clear whether peptide boost was solely responsible for this result since there were other differences including the dosing regimen, drug formulation, and administration by bolus injection in the recent studies (80,86), compared with a slow intranodal infusion in the previous trials (39,40). In addition, there was no apparent difference in immune response between the low- and high-peptide boost cohorts (80,86) except for a higher tendency to respond to the subdominant peptide in the high-peptide dose group (86). Several patients apparently showed a reduction in the frequency of antigen-specific T cells in blood upon peptide boost; however, we cannot rule out differentiation and emigration of T cells from the circulation to lymph nodes or tumor sites following the boost as we know repeat antigen exposure can result in further T-cell differentiation.

In general, enumeration of antigen-specific T cells in blood showed three patterns: (*i*) induction of persisting levels of specific T cells over the duration of treatment; (*ii*) transient induction or enhancement of specific T cells followed by decline upon continuing immunization; and (*iii*) no elevation compared to pre-treatment values. Intriguingly, a number of patients with malignant melanoma and various carcinomas showed a specific measurable immunity prior to vaccination confirming that these tumor antigens are endogenously presented and yield target epitopes recognized by the unmanipulated immune system (83,86). The significance of this pre-existing immunity could be complex.

While these data confirm the immunogenicity of the investigational agents in man, there is discordance with earlier preclinical results employing similar prime boosting in murine models (26,28,31), especially in regard to the relatively modest magnitude of the immune response seen in the clinic. This is perhaps not surprising considering the differences in immune status between previously treated heterogeneous cancer patients, and the inbred and fully immune competent transgenic rodents. While these results suggest that there is an additional opportunity to improve the potency of vaccines in man, this conclusion is somewhat tempered by a lack of understanding of what the appropriate immune correlates of clinical efficacy are and whether the immune environment or repertoire in cancer patients is inherently limitative.

Preliminary Evidence of Disease Control by Intra-Lymph Node Immunization with Plasmid–Prime and Peptide–Boost Regimens

Earlier trials with plasmids expressing Melan A/MART-1 and Tyrosinase antigens, in stage IV malignant melanoma patients with visceral or lymphatic metastatic disease, showed no evidence of tumor regression or change of disease progression (Table 8.3) (39,40). However, there was a correlation between immunity against Melan A/MART-1 and time-to-progression in one trial (40) while the other showed a slightly increased survival rate compared with historical references (39).

Of note, in one of the recently concluded trials in patients with advanced melanoma (MKC1106-MT) encompassing a peptide boost subsequent to plasmid immunization, there was a significant slowdown in disease progression associated with a durable tumor regression in four patients with measurable, metastatic disease localized to the lymphatic system [Table 8.3, (86)]. These patients remained on treatment for at least eight cycles, or one year from treatment initiation. Two out of these four patients remained free of disease progression for two years after the first dose, while the others progressed after one year of treatment. The rest of the patients in this melanoma trial—mostly with metastatic disease already affecting viscera—progressed within the first three months (two cycles) of therapy or immediately afterwards (about eight weeks), in fitting with the expected natural progression of disease in patients with advanced metastatic melanoma.

In the PRAME/PSMA prime-boost trial (MKC1106-PP) involving 26 patients with various tumor types [Table 8.3; (80)], seven patients showed some evidence of disease control which was defined as having stable disease for at least six months, or in patients with advanced prostate cancer, a favorable Prostate-specific antigen response. Of these responders four were prostate carcinoma patients (out of 10 patients with this tumor type) showed stable disease for

>6 months, a decline in Prostate-specific antigen levels, or in one case reduction of tumor volume in the pelvic lymph nodes. Two other patients with advanced renal cell carcinoma showed also evidence of disease control; one patient with rapidly advancing subcutaneous metastases lesions of which stabilized upon administration of four cycles of treatment and then successfully surgically resected with no evidence of disease at 1.5 years post vaccination. The other patient with advanced kidney cancer completed full course of treatment and remained stable on therapy for over nine months. The remaining patient who showed evidence of clinical benefit presented with advanced melanoma metastatic to lungs and liver (one out of 10 patients with melanoma) and experienced long-term stable disease lasting for at least 18 months.

Correlation Between Immune and Clinical Response

Based on the putative mechanism of action of immunotherapy which involves the generation, expansion, and/or activation of tumor antigen-specific T cells, one could expect a relationship between the clinical outcome and immune response. It is important to mention that immune monitoring in this trial was limited to only to enumerate specific T cells in peripheral blood mononuclear cell. As mentioned above, there was no evidence of clinical response in the earlier trials with plasmid alone in metastatic melanoma (39,40), although there was an association between immunity against Melan A/MART-1 and time to progression in one of the studies (40). Instead, in the prime–boost trial employing PRAME and PSMA as target antigens (80), six out of seven patients with evidence of disease control defined as stable disease for six months or better, had low or no detectable antigen-specific T cells at baseline, yet mounted an immune response against both antigens. In contrast, less than half of the remaining patients with a rapidly progressing disease showed an elevation of T cells against either epitope upon immunization, with most of them having pre-existing antigen-specific T cells. This finding suggests that de novo induction of specific T cells against the select target epitopes resulted in a beneficial clinical effect, with the caveat that we cannot exclude at this stage in development that the induced immunity was an epiphenomenon. Furthermore, the data suggest that a pre-existing immunity against these two antigens, presumably elicited through exposure of the immune system to the tumor, is somewhat linked to an impairment of these peripheral T cells, leading to lack of expansion, or activation of T cells subsequent to immunization.

Surprisingly, although the number of patients was smaller, a similar trend comparing the induction or elevation of antigen-specific T cells and clinical response was not apparent in the MKC1106-MT prime–boost trial involving metastatic melanoma patients (86). Strikingly, however, all four patients who showed durable tumor regression with no evidence of additional lesions, displayed a pre-existing Melan A/MART-1-specific T cells response prior to immunization, which generally persisted throughout the immunization protocol (86). In contrast, the other 14 patients who showed no clinical response displayed a minimal or nonpersisting Melan A/MART-1-specific T cell response. Notably, there was a triple association between pre-existing T cells against Melan A/MART-1, the disease stage (lesions generally confined to the lymph nodes), and disease control (86) defined as durable stable disease or better. The best evidence to date that this investigational agent afforded disease control and provided clinical benefit consisted in the independent confirmation of durable tumor regression; although quantitatively, these patients failed short of the PR criteria for a RECIST (Response Evaluation Criteria in Solid Tumors) response (86). Interestingly, the results are somewhat reminiscent of previous data from a trial carried out with the identical plasmid but devoid of any peptide boost component. In this study an association between ongoing T-cell immunity against Melan A/MART-1, pre-existing or induced, and time to progression was found but no evidence of tumor regression was reported even though some of the patients had disease confined to the lymph nodes (40). In the absence of detailed mechanistic information from the ongoing phase II clinical trial, and prior to completing a comprehensive analysis of stored samples from the phase I trials, we could only speculate that the prime–boost vaccination effectively converted the pre-existing but potentially functional, rather than anergic Melan A/MART-1 specific T cells, to highly effective anti-tumoral T cells. In addition, it is quite possible that this pre-existing Melan

A/MART-1-specific repertoire emerges (and is potentially functional) upon tumor progression from in situ to lymphatic involvement, but degenerates later on into anergic cells, or disappears altogether in more advanced disease stages. In any case, a preliminary and limited evaluation of TILs in regressing lesions showed that only a fraction of functionally active, resident T cells are specific against the vaccine target antigens, compatible with an "epitope-spreading" process quite common in autoimmune diseases (93).

Altogether, these results warrant further evaluation of the prime–boost regimens (MKC1106-MT and MKC1106-PP) in select clinical indications—such as disease mostly confined to lymph nodes in melanoma—and with a purpose of evaluating both the clinical and immune response in a comprehensive fashion (Fig. 8.4).

CONCLUSIONS, MECHANISTIC CONSIDERATIONS, AND OUTSTANDING QUESTIONS

Our preclinical and early clinical evaluation of intra-lymph node vaccines, to date, yielded some surprising conclusions, with dual theoretical and practical impact (Fig. 8.5).

A key observation was that immunization against the tissue-specific antigens (Melan A/MART-1 and Tyrosinase) could indeed elicit durable tumor regression in patients with metastatic melanoma depending on the disease localization. Lesions localized within the lymph nodes seemed to be more susceptible to control by this active immunotherapy as opposed to visceral metastases. These early stage results need to be confirmed in larger trials; however, the clinical responses to date seem to be durable and encompassing not only regression but also nonoccurrence of new metastatic lesions indicating at least a temporarily slowdown effect in disease progression. Preliminary data on the mechanism of action of this vaccine revealed that in regressing lesions approximately 1% of the TILs with an effector phenotype were antigen specific and suggestive of intramolecular epitope spreading after immunization (86). Furthermore, the presence of both antigen-positive tumor cells and TILs within regressing or stable lesions provides a strong evidence for a "stand-off" mechanism in which the tumor is contained by the surrounding immune cells and which is reminiscent of what occurs in several autoimmune diseases (94). Overall, these results are similar to our earlier preclinical findings that

	Major findings in phase 1	Next steps
1106-MT Melan A Tyrosinase prime–boost (Melanoma)	• Safe, feasible • Immunogenic in ~50% patients • Tumor regression in most lymphatic metastatic patients • No regression in visceral metastatic patients • Disease control correlated with pre-existing immunity; lack of correlation with immune response in blood • Preliminary evidence of active tumor infiltrating T cells	• Phase II proof of concept clinical trial in malignant melanoma (ongoing) • Lymphatic localized or metastatic disease (stage III B/C, IV) • Objectives: clinical response, comprehensive evaluation of immunity (including in situ) • Future: expansion to adjuvant setting and adjunctive to targeted therapies
1106-PP PRAME PSMA prime–boost (Various solid tumors)	• Safe, feasible • Immunogenic in ~60% patients • Evidence of disease control (SD for 6 months or better, or PSA drop) in prostate carcinoma, kidney cancer and melanoma • Clinical signals were associated with induction and persistence of immunity against both antigens	• Phase II proof of concept clinical trials in planning • Option 1: prostate carcinoma, rising PSA; or metastatic, pre-chemotherapy • Option 2: kidney cancer, adjunctive therapy to small molecules; or relapsing after standard of care, or in neo-adjuvant setting

Figure 8.5 Summarized next steps with prime-boost investigational agents 1106-MT and 1106-PP. *Abbreviations*: PSA, prostate-specific antigen; SD, stable disease.

suggest effector T cells within lymphoid organs do not face as stringent an immune inhibiting environment as found in established, vascularized tumors (28). This premise provides a foundation for testing novel immunotherapies more reliably, in measureable lymphatic metastatic disease for example, as opposed to minimal residual disease that requires lengthier, less informative trials (unless randomized) or in later stages associated with visceral metastases. In addition, it emphasizes a possible key indication for active immunotherapy in cancer with the potential to suppress disease progression via the lymphatic system, to prevent long-term metastatic disease. Both aspects have practical importance since they may expedite the progress and decision-making processes involved in cancer drug development programs within smaller biotech companies that are pursuing highly innovative yet riskier technologies. It indeed seems that the clinical response profile afforded by this class of immune interventions differs significantly from that of small molecules such as tyrosine kinase inhibitors showing a rapid debulking, yet a transient effect, while the former show a prolonged clinical effect with a quite moderate impact on the tumor burden, yet a significant slowdown of disease progression. Conversely, these data also reinforce the need for more elaborate, combinatorial approaches for the management of visceral metastatic disease which are needed to co-target a diverse array of immune inhibiting mechanisms.

Somewhat related to the critical goal of eliciting immune responses refractory to immune-inhibiting mechanisms within the tumor microenvironment, is the exciting prospect of programming specific T cells through immunization to retain optimal effector capabilities and yet express minimal levels of co-inhibitory receptors such as PD-1 and CTLA-4 (27). While preclinical results point to the existence of a separate lineage of differentiated specific T cells that fail to acquire PD-1 expression and have enhanced proliferative capabilities (31), more research needs to be done to validate this model in man and establish its translational value. It appears though that immunization mediated by plasmid administration can elicit this CD8$^+$ PD-1^{low} T cell phenotype emphasizing this methodology as a viable priming approach. This of course is linked to the ever-lasting mechanistic debate: What is more crucial, the magnitude or quality of the immune response, or both? In addition, what are the appropriate immune correlates of clinical efficacy? Despite some evidence suggesting that the magnitude of the immune response is absolutely critical for its efficacy, even in the context of early disease (95), so far clinical results do not support this paradigm (96–98). In addition, surprisingly, even in preclinical models suggestive of T-cell expansion as being a key immune correlate of anti-tumor efficacy, a closer look shows that only about 1% or less of the vaccine-specific T cells reacted against tumor cells; this indicates that most of the vaccine-induced cells have uncertain or no relevance vis-à-vis tumor control (26). Furthermore, different dosing approaches showed that a substantial expansion of T cells was not required for a tumor response (28) suggesting that *quality* of immune response could very well trump the overall magnitude of immunity, or at least has similar importance. This is an absolutely key aspect that complements a general lack of correlation between the frequency of vaccine-specific T cells and the clinical outcome in man and points to the importance of functional avidity, polyspecificity, and the migratory capability of tumor reactive T cells (99–103) as alternate or multiparametric immune correlates. A more comprehensive systems biology approach (104) defining the immune gene signature of response within tumor (105,106), prior and after immunization for example, needs to be employed to gather a more accurate picture of the mechanism of action of immune interventions that afford clinical benefit in a subset of treated patients. It is our conviction that a breakthrough in this regard must rely on a systematic, comprehensive, and nonbiased hypothesis generating assessment of immunity at baseline, after therapy, within target tumor lesions as well as systemically in patients who respond clinically to a given immune intervention versus nonresponders.

While the field will undoubtedly witness a tremendous progress in the development of potent next-generation immune interventions that will complement small-molecule and molecular diagnostics in the quest of achieving long-term management of cancer, there are a few immediate challenges that we face: (*i*) how to optimize and expedite proof of concept studies in man and achieve regulatory approval of novel active immune therapies that are mostly

Preclinical findings	Clinical findings	Inferences
• Vaccine's effect is severely limited in established tumors; mostly active in minimal residual disease or initially, in disseminated disease	• A plasmid-priming, peptide-boost regimen elicited tumor regression in lymph node but not visceral metastatic disease • Disease stabilization observed as well	• Active immunotherapy (vaccination) may be effective alone in measurable disease setting, in addition to minimal residual disease, in select indications such lymph node metastatic disease
• Strong correlation between immune response and tumor regression or tumor control in models • Only a minute fraction of T cells seem to respond to tumor	• Modest correlation between immune response in blood and clinical signals or outcome • Association between pre-existing immunity and disease control was antigen- and disease dependent	• Measurement of global magnitude of immunity in blood may not be a reliable immune correlate for clinical response • A comprehensive immune evaluation, including intratumoralimmunity, may be needed to define and optimize immune correlates
• Very robust induction of immunity by plasmid-priming, peptide-boost in immune competent, inbred mice	• Relatively limited expansion of T cells upon prime–boost • No apparent peptide boosting effect measured in blood	• Limited translational value of animal models to immune compromised cancer patients • Dosing regimen could be further optimized through addition of biological response modifiers or vector and regimen changes

Outstanding questions

• Does immunization based on gene transfer or other methods "program" T cells with low inhibitory receptor expression, more operational within tumor environment?

• Could active immunotherapy be harnessed to elicit tumor regression or disease stabilization in measurable disease setting? How do we enable active immunotherapy in visceral metastatic disease?

• What are more reliable immune correlates of clinical response ?

• Are "epitope-centric/focused" approaches inherently more or less potent than whole antigen vaccination?

• How do we design broadly applicable—across HLAs—yet potent, therapeutic vaccines?

• How do we design next-generation immune interventions that rely to a lesser extent on patient's immune status?

Figure 8.6 Key learning and outstanding questions.

applicable to minimal residual disease; (*ii*) how to fully leverage the lessons learned from other immune interventions to create practical, more potent, and widely applicable synthetic vaccines to minimal and measurable disease alike; (*iii*) how to more reliably monitor the performance of such therapeutic vaccines in the clinic in light of the complex mechanism of action and the heterogeneous nature of the target population; and (*iv*) how to exactly integrate immune interventions with standard-of-care and other evolving targeted therapies to achieve durable control of cancer.

Above all, our results based on a novel platform technology encompassing synthetic molecules, carry the promise that active immunotherapy can be safely and effectively applied for long-term management of metastatic cancer by blocking the disease's spread from the lymphatic system to viscera.

REFERENCES

1. Mebius RE. Organogenesis of lymphoid tissues. Nat Rev Immunol 2003; 3: 292–303.
2. Müller G, Lipp M. Concerted action of the chemokine and lymphotoxin system in secondary lymphoid-organ development. Curr Opin Immunol 2003; 15: 217–24.
3. Zinkernagel RM, Ehl S, Aichele P, et al. Antigen localisation regulates immune responses in a dose- and time-dependent fashion: a geographical view of immune reactivity. Immunol Rev 1997; 156: 199–209.

4. Kündig TM, Bachmann MF, DiPaolo C, et al. Fibroblasts as efficient antigen-presenting cells in lymphoid organs. Science 1995; 268: 1343–7.
5. Hawiger D, Inaba K, Dorsett Y, et al. Dendritic cells induce peripheral T cell unresponsiveness under steady state conditions in vivo. J Exp Med 2001; 194: 769–79.
6. Steinman RM, Hawiger D, Liu K, et al. Dendritic cell function in vivo during the steady state: a role in peripheral tolerance. Ann NY Acad Sci 2003; 987: 15–25.
7. Fletcher AL, Malhotra D, Turley SJ, et al. Lymph node stroma broaden the peripheral tolerance paradigm. Trends Immunol 2011; 32: 12–18.
8. Medzhitov R, Janeway CA Jr. How does the immune system distinguish self from nonself? Semin Immunol 2000; 12: 185–8.
9. Medzhitov R, Janeway CA Jr. Decoding the patterns of self and nonself by the innate immune system. Science 2002; 296: 298–300.
10. Matzinger P. Tolerance, danger, and the extended family. Annu Rev Immunol 1994; 12: 991–1045.
11. Zhang K, Shen X, Wu J, et al. Endoplasmic reticulum stress activates cleavage of CREBH to induce a systemic inflammatory response. Cell 2006; 124: 587–99.
12. Bot A, Patterson J. Sensing Immune Danger through Unfolded Protein Response plus Pathogen Recognition Receptors; and Immune Modulation for Cancer and HIV-1 Disease. Int Rev Immunol 2011; in press.
13. Hernandez J, Aung S, Redmond WL, et al. Phenotypic and functional analysis of CD8(+) T cells undergoing peripheral deletion in response to cross-presentation of self-antigen. J Exp Med 2001; 194: 707–17.
14. Kaplan DH. In vivo function of Langerhans cells and dermal dendritic cells. Trends Immunol 2010; 31: 446–51.
15. López-Bravo M, Ardavín C. In vivo induction of immune responses to pathogens by conventional dendritic cells. Immunity 2008; 29: 343–51.
16. Barker CF, Billingham RE. The role of regional lymphatics in the skin homograft response. Transplantation 1967; 5(Suppl): 962–6.
17. Fletcher AL, Lukacs-Kornek V, Reynoso ED, et al. Lymph node fibroblastic reticular cells directly present peripheral tissue antigen under steady-state and inflammatory conditions. J Exp Med 2010; 207: 689–97.
18. Zinkernagel RM, Hengartner H. On immunity against infections and vaccines: credo 2004. Scand J Immunol 2004; 60: 9–13.
19. Anderson CC. Time, space and contextual models of the immunity tolerance decision: bridging the geographical divide of Zinkernagel and Hengartner's 'Credo 2004'. Scand J Immunol 2006; 63: 249–56.
20. Johansen P, Häffner AC, Koch F, et al. Direct intralymphatic injection of peptide vaccines enhances immunogenicity. Eur J Immunol 2005; 35: 568–74.
21. Johansen P, Senti G, Martínez Gómez JM, et al. Heat denaturation, a simple method to improve the immunotherapeutic potential of allergens. Eur J Immunol 2005; 35: 3591–8.
22. Maloy KJ, Erdmann I, Basch V, et al. Intralymphatic immunization enhances DNA vaccination. Proc Natl Acad Sci USA 2001; 98: 3299–303.
23. Johansen P, Storni T, Rettig L, et al. Antigen kinetics determines immune reactivity. Proc Natl Acad Sci USA 2008; 105: 5189–94.
24. von Beust BR, Johansen P, Smith KA, et al. Improving the therapeutic index of CpG oligodeoxynucleotides by intralymphatic administration. Eur J Immunol 2005; 35: 1869–76.
25. Wong RM, Smith KA, Tam VL, et al. TLR-9 signaling and TCR stimulation co-regulate CD8(+) T cell-associated PD-1 expression. Immunol Lett 2009; 127: 60–7.
26. Smith KA, Tam VL, Wong RM, et al. Enhancing DNA vaccination by sequential injection of lymph nodes with plasmid vectors and peptides. Vaccine 2009; 27: 2603–15.
27. Bot A, Qiu Z, Wong R, et al. Programmed cell death-1 (PD-1) at the heart of heterologous prime-boost vaccines and regulation of CD8+ T cell immunity. J Transl Med 2011; in press.
28. Smith KA, Meisenburg BL, Tam VL, et al. Lymph node-targeted immunotherapy mediates potent immunity resulting in regression of isolated or metastatic human papillomavirus-transformed tumors. Clin Cancer Res 2009; 15: 6167–76.
29. Bot A, Smith KA, Liu X, et al. In situ targeting of antigen presenting cells within secondary lymphoid organs as a means to control immune responses. J Immunother 2005; 28: 653.
30. Johansen P, Senti G, Martinez Gomez JM, et al. Toll-like receptor ligands as adjuvants in allergen-specific immunotherapy. Clin Exp Allergy 2005; 35: 1591–8.

31. Smith KA, Qiu Z, Wong R, et al. Multivalent immunity targeting tumor-associated antigens by intra-lymph node DNA-prime, peptide-boost vaccination. Cancer Gene Ther 2011; 18: 63–76.

32. Fu TM, Ulmer JB, Caulfield MJ, et al. Priming of cytotoxic T lymphocytes by DNA vaccines: requirement for professional antigen presenting cells and evidence for antigen transfer from myocytes. Mol Med 1997; 3: 362–71.

33. Corr M, Lee DJ, Carson DA, et al. Gene vaccination with naked plasmid DNA: mechanism of CTL priming. J Exp Med 1996; 184: 1555–60.

34. Bot A, Stan AC, Inaba K, et al. Dendritic cells at a DNA vaccination site express the encoded influenza nucleoprotein and prime MHC class I-restricted cytolytic lymphocytes upon adoptive transfer. Int Immunol 2000; 12: 825–32.

35. Manthorpe M, Cornefert-Jensen F, Hartikka J, et al. Gene therapy by intramuscular injection of plasmid DNA: studies on firefly luciferase gene expression in mice. Hum Gene Ther 1993; 4: 419–31.

36. Chastain M, Simon AJ, Soper KA, et al. Antigen levels and antibody titers after DNA vaccination. J Pharm Sci 2001; 90: 474–84.

37. Lu S, Wang S, Grimes-Serrano JM, et al. Current progress of DNA vaccine studies in humans. Expert Rev Vaccines 2008; 7: 175–91.

38. Low L, Mander A, McCann K, et al. DNA vaccination with electroporation induces increased antibody responses in patients with prostate cancer. Hum Gene Ther 2009; 20: 1269–78.

39. Tagawa ST, Lee P, Snively J, et al. Phase I study of intranodal delivery of a plasmid DNA vaccine for patients with Stage IV melanoma. Cancer 2003; 98: 144–54.

40. Weber J, Boswell W, Smith J, et al. Phase 1 trial of intranodal injection of a Melan-A/MART-1 DNA plasmid vaccine in patients with stage IV melanoma. J Immunother 2008; 31: 215–23.

41. Bot A, Bot S, Garcia-Sastre A, et al. DNA immunization of newborn mice with a plasmid-expressing nucleoprotein of influenza virus. Viral Immunol 1996; 9: 207–10.

42. Korman AJ, Peggs KS, Allison JP. Checkpoint blockade in cancer immunotherapy. Adv Immunol 2006; 90: 297–339.

43. Wolchok JD, Yang AS, Weber JS. Immune regulatory antibodies: are they the next advance? Cancer J 2010; 16: 311–17.

44. Blank C, Mackensen A. Contribution of the PD-L1/PD-1 pathway to T-cell exhaustion: an update on implications for chronic infections and tumor evasion. Cancer Immunol Immunother 2007; 56: 739–45.

45. Wang S, Kennedy JS, West K, et al. Crosssubtype antibody and cellular immune responses induced by a polyvalent DNA prime-protein boost HIV-1 vaccine in healthy humanvolunteers. Vaccine 2008; 26: 3947–57.

46. Bansal A, Jackson B, West K, et al. Multifunctional T-cell characteristics induced by a polyvalent DNA prime/protein boost human immunodeficiency virus type 1 vaccine regimen given to healthy adults are dependent on the route and dose of administration. J Virol 2008; 82: 6458–69.

47. Harari A, Bart PA, Stöhr W, et al. An HIV-1 clade C DNA prime, NYVAC boost vaccine regimen induces reliable, polyfunctional, and long-lasting T cell responses. J Exp Med 2008; 205: 63–77.

48. Todorova K, Ignatova I, Tchakarov S, et al. Humoral immune response in prostate cancer patients after immunization with gene-based vaccines that encode for a protein that is proteasomally degraded. Cancer Immunol 2005; 5: 1.

49. Dangoor A, Lorigan P, Keilholz U, et al. Clinical and immunological responses in metastatic melanoma patients vaccinated with a high-dose poly-epitope vaccine. Cancer Immunol Immunother 2010; 59: 863–73.

50. McConkey SJ, Reece WH, Moorthy VS, et al. Enhanced T-cell immunogenicity ofplasmid DNA vaccines boosted by recombinant modified vaccinia virus Ankara in humans. Nat Med 2003; 9: 729–35.

51. Guerau-de-Arellano M, Martinic M, Benoist C. Neonatal tolerance revisited: a perinatal window for Aire control of autoimmunity. J Exp Med 2009; 206: 1245–52.

52. Meffre E, Wardemann H. B-cell tolerance checkpoints in health and autoimmunity. Curr Opin Immunol 2008; 20: 632–8.

53. Schoenberger SP, Sercarz EE. Harnessing self-reactivity in cancer immunotherapy. Semin Immunol 1996; 8: 303–9.

54. Gajewski TF, Meng Y, Blank C, et al. Immune resistance orchestrated by the tumor microenvironment. Immunol Rev 2006; 213: 131–45.

55. Cheever MA, Allison JP, Ferris AS, et al. The prioritization of cancer antigens: a national cancer institute pilot project for the acceleration of translational research. Clin Cancer Res 2009; 15: 5323–37.

56. Zhou H, Luo Y, Mizutani M, et al. T cell-mediated suppression of angiogenesis results in tumor protective immunity. Blood 2005; 106: 2026–32.

57. Slovin SF. Targeting novel antigens for prostate cancer treatment: focus on prostate-specific membrane antigen. Expert Opin Ther Targets 2005; 9: 561–70.
58. Lu J, Celis E. Recognition of prostate tumor cells by cytotoxic T lymphocytes specific for prostate-specific membrane antigen. Cancer Res 2002; 62: 5807–12.
59. Harada M, Matsueda S, Yao A, et al. Prostate-related antigen-derived new peptides having the capacity of inducing prostate cancer-reactive CTLs in HLA-A2+ prostate cancer patients. Oncol Rep 2004; 12: 601–7.
60. Coulie PG, Brichard V, Van Pel A, et al. A new gene coding for a differentiation antigen recognized by autologous cytolytic T lymphocytes on HLA-A2 melanomas. J Exp Med 1994; 180: 35–42.
61. Brichard V, Van Pel A, Wölfel T, et al. The tyrosinase gene codes for an antigen recognized by autologous cytolytic T lymphocytes on HLA-A2 melanomas. J Exp Med 1993; 178: 489–95.
62. Cormier JN, Salgaller ML, Prevette T, et al. Enhancement of cellular immunity in melanoma patients immunized with a peptide from MART-1/Melan A. Cancer J Sci Am 1997; 3: 37–44.
63. Slingluff CL Jr, Chianese-Bullock KA, Bullock TN, et al. Immunity to melanoma antigens: from self-tolerance to immunotherapy. Adv Immunol 2006; 90: 243–95.
64. Kawakami Y, Eliyahu S, Sakaguchi K, et al. Identification of the immunodominant peptides of the MART-1 human melanoma antigen recognized by the majority of HLA-A2-restricted tumor infiltrating lymphocytes. J Exp Med 1994; 180: 347–52.
65. Kang X, Kawakami Y, el-Gamil M, et al. Identification of a tyrosinase epitope recognized by HLA-A24-restricted, tumor-infiltrating lymphocytes. J Immunol 1995; 155: 1343–8.
66. Morgan RA, Dudley ME, Wunderlich JR, et al. Cancer regression in patients after transfer of genetically engineered lymphocytes. Science 2006; 314: 126–9.
67. Bergman PJ, McKnight J, Novosad A. Long-term survival of dogs with advanced malignant melanoma after DNA vaccination with xenogeneic human tyrosinase: a phase I trial. Clin Cancer Res 2003; 9: 1284–90.
68. Ribas A, Timmerman JM, Butterfield LH. Determinant spreading and tumor responses after peptide-based cancer immunotherapy. Trends Immunol 2003; 24: 58–61.
69. Murphy GP, Elgamal AA, Su SL, et al. Current evaluation of the tissue localization and diagnostic utility of prostate specific membrane antigen. Cancer 1998; 83: 2259–69.
70. Chang SS, O'Keefe DS, Bacich DJ, et al. Prostate-specific membrane antigen is produced in tumor-associated neovasculature. Clin Cancer Res 1999; 5: 2674–81.
71. Conway RE, Petrovic N, Li Z, et al. Prostate-specific membrane antigen regulates angiogenesis by modulating integrin signal transduction. Mol Cell Biol 2006; 26: 5310–24.
72. Rajasekaran AK, Anilkumar G, Christiansen JJ. Is prostate-specific membrane antigen a multifunctional protein? Am J Physiol Cell Physiol 2005; 288: C975–81.
73. Rajasekaran SA, Christiansen JJ, Schmid I, et al. Prostate-specific membrane antigen associates with anaphase-promoting complex and induces chromosomal instability. Mol Cancer Ther 2008; 7: 2142–51.
74. Epping MT, Wang L, Edel MJ, et al. The human tumor antigen PRAME is a dominant repressor of retinoic acid receptor signaling. Cell 2005; 122: 835–47.
75. Birtle Z, Goodstadt L, Ponting C. Duplication and positive selection among hominin-specific PRAME genes. BMC Genomics 2005; 6: 120.
76. Paydas S. Is everything known in all faces of iceberg in PRAME? Leuk Res 2008; 32: 1356–7.
77. Matsushita M, Yamazaki R, Ikeda H, et al. Preferentially expressed antigen of melanoma (PRAME) in the development of diagnostic and therapeutic methods for hematological malignancies. Leuk Lymphoma 2003; 44: 439–44.
78. Griffioen M, Kessler JH, Borghi M, et al. Detection and functional analysis of CD8+ T cells specific for PRAME: a target for T-cell therapy. Clin Cancer Res 2006; 12: 3130–6.
79. Krymskaya L, Do L, Hong S, et al. Ex vivo immunogenicity of PRAME native epitopes and MHC anchor modified analogues: implications on active immunotherapeutic approaches. J Immunother 2006; 29: 674.
80. Weber JS, Vogelzang NJ, Ernstoff MS, et al. A Phase 1 Study of a Vaccine Targeting Preferentially Expressed Antigen in Melanoma (PRAME) and Prostate Specific Membrane Antigen (PSMA) in Patients with Advanced Solid Tumors. J Immunoth; In press.
81. Old LJ. Cancer vaccines: an overview. Cancer Immun 2008; 8(Suppl 1): 1.
82. Ayyoub M, Stevanovic S, Sahin U, et al. Proteasome-assisted identification of a SSX-2-derived epitope recognized by tumor-reactive CTL infiltrating. J Immunol 2002; 168: 1717–22.
83. Klebanoff CA, Acquavella N, Yu Z, et al. Therapeutic cancer vaccines: are we there yet? Immunol Rev 2011; 239: 27–44.

84. Feltkamp MC, Smits HL, Vierboom MP, et al. Vaccination with cytotoxic T lymphocyte epitope-containing peptide protects against a tumor induced by human papillomavirus type 16-transformed cells. Eur J Immunol 1993; 23: 2242–9.

85. Machiels JP, Reilly RT, Emens LA, et al. Cyclophosphamide, doxorubicin, and paclitaxel enhance the antitumor immune response of granulocyte/macrophage-colony stimulating factor-secreting whole-cell vaccines in HER-2/neu tolerized mice. Cancer Res 2001; 61: 3689–97.

86. Ribas A, Weber JS, Chmielowski B, et al. Intra-Lymph Node Prime-Boost Vaccination Against Melan A and Tyrosinase for the Treatment of Metastatic Melanoma: Results of a Phase 1 Clinical Trial. Clin Cancer Res 2011; 17: 2987–96.

87. Micheletti F, Bazzaro M, Canella A, et al. The lifespan of major histocompatibility complex class I/peptide complexes determines the efficiency of cytotoxic T-lymphocyte responses. Immunology 1999; 96: 411–15.

88. Hoos A, Eggermont AM, Janetzki S, et al. Improved endpoints for cancer immunotherapy trials. J Natl Cancer Inst 2010; 102: 1388–97.

89. Lesimple T, Neidhard EM, Vignard V, et al. Immunologic and clinical effects of injecting mature peptide-loaded dendritic cells by intralymphatic and intra-nodal routes in metastatic melanoma patients. Clin Cancer Res 2006; 12: 7380–8.

90. Gilliet M, Kleinhans M, Lantelme E, et al. Intranodal injection of semimature monocyte-derived dendritic cells induces T helper type 1 responses to protein neoantigen. Blood 2003; 102: 36–42.

91. Senti G, Johansen P, Kündig TM. Intralymphatic immunotherapy. Curr Opin Allergy Clin Immunol 2009; 9: 537–43.

92. Senti G, Prinz Vavricka BM, Erdmann I, et al. Intralymphatic allergen administration renders specific immunotherapy faster and safer: a randomized controlled trial. Proc Natl Acad Sci USA 2008; 105: 17908–12.

93. Fujinami RS, von Herrath MG, Christen U, et al. Molecular mimicry, bystander activation, or viral persistence: infections and autoimmune disease. Clin Microbiol Rev 2006; 19: 80–94.

94. Waid DM, Vaitaitis GM, Pennock ND, et al. Disruption of the homeostatic balance between autoaggressive (CD4+CD40+) and regulatory (CD4+CD25+FoxP3+) T cells promotes diabetes. J Leukoc Biol 2008; 84: 431–9.

95. Sioud M. Does our current understanding of immune tolerance, autoimmunity, and immunosuppressive mechanisms facilitate the design of efficient cancer vaccines? Scand J Immunol 2009; 70: 516–25.

96. Nielsen MB, Marincola FM. Melanoma vaccines: the paradox of T cell activation without clinical response. Cancer Chemother Pharmacol 2000; 46(Suppl): S62–6.

97. Lee KH, Wang E, Nielsen MB, et al. Increased vaccine-specific T cell frequency after peptide-based vaccination correlates with increased susceptibility to in vitro stimulation but does not lead to tumor regression. J Immunol 1999; 163: 6292–300.

98. Monsurrò V, Nagorsen D, Wang E, et al. Functional heterogeneity of vaccine-induced CD8(+) T cells. J Immunol 2002; 168: 5933–42.

99. Wieckowski S, Baumgaertner P, Corthesy P, et al. Fine structural variations of alphabetaTCRs selected by vaccination with natural versus altered self-antigen in melanoma patients. J Immunol 2009; 183: 5397–406.

100. Lin Y, Gallardo HF, Ku GY, et al. Optimization and validation of a robust human T-cell culture method for monitoring phenotypic and polyfunctional antigen-specific CD4 and CD8 T-cell responses. Cytotherapy 2009; 11: 912–22.

101. Jackson HM, Dimopoulos N, Chen Q, et al. A robust human T-cell culture method suitable for monitoring CD8+ and CD4+ T-cell responses from cancer clinical trial samples. J Immunol Methods 2004; 291: 51–62.

102. Krug LM, Dao T, Brown AB, et al. WT1 peptide vaccinations induce CD4 and CD8 T cell immune responses in patients with mesothelioma and non-small cell lung cancer. Cancer Immunol Immunother 2010; 59: 1467–79.

103. Domchek SM, Recio A, Mick R, et al. Telomerase-specific T-cell immunity in breast cancer: effect of vaccination on tumor immunosurveillance. Cancer Res 2007; 67: 10546–55.

104. Buonaguro L, Pulendran B. Immunogenomics and systems biology of vaccines. Immunol Rev 2011; 239: 197–208.

105. Bedognetti D, Wang E, Sertoli MR, et al. Gene-expression profiling in vaccine therapy and immunotherapy for cancer. Expert Rev Vaccines 2010; 9: 555–65.

106. Mandruzzato S, Callegaro A, Turcatel G, et al. A gene expression signature associated with survival in metastatic melanoma. J Transl Med 2006; 4: 50.

9 | Clinical perspectives in cancer vaccines for hematological diseases

Maurizio Chiriva-Internati, Leonardo Mirandola, Marjorie Jenkins, Martin Cannon, Everardo Cobos, and W. Martin Kast

PERSPECTIVES IN CANCER VACCINES

The idea that suffering from an infectious disease affords protection against it in the future originated before the birth of modern medicine. The first documentation, dated 429 BC, observed that the survivors of the plague of Athens could not catch the disease a second time. Nonetheless, it is only in the 19th century AD that the first scientific proof of principle of vaccination was reported. In 1800, E.A. Jenner published his book "An Inquiry into the Causes and Effects of the Variolae Vaccinae," where he described his experiments conducted on 23 subjects that were protected from smallpox virus after inoculation with material from cowpox-infected animals. Since then, vaccinology has realized dramatic successes: vaccination is the most relevant public health measure of the past century. Despite striking advances, the idea that not only microbes but also tumor cells could be the target of vaccination strategies is more recent, and initiated with R. Virchow's studies in 1863, who described the presence of abundant immune cells in the stroma of different tumor lesions. Now it has been universally accepted that the immune system plays a critical role in cancer progression (1). The incidence of hepatocellular carcinoma has been significantly decreased thanks to the introduction of the hepatitis-B vaccine, while human papillomavirus (HPV) vaccines significantly prevent HPV-associated cervical malignancies by protecting against HPV infection. However, human cancers with a clear infective etiology account for less than 20% of all tumor cases worldwide. Therefore, cancer vaccinology has been exploiting tumor targets different from cancer-inducing microbes, that is, tumor antigens. Intriguing tumor antigens as vaccine targets were firstly identified in melanoma, belonging to the class of tumor-specific antigens and cancer testis antigens (CTAs). Many clinical trials showed that cancer vaccines frequently induced the generation of cytotoxic T lymphocytes (CTLs), or more generally elicited immune responses activation, but they inexorably fail to afford a clinically significant advantage in phase III clinical trials. The reason for this unsuccessful outcome is to be found in the suboptimal trial design. Most of the cancer vaccine trials carried out so far have been on end-stage patients. This is a limitation to unravel the potential of cancer vaccines, because advanced-stage patients have undergone previous treatments that are potentially harmful for the immune system's response to vaccination, and a chronic exposure to tumor antigens can lead to dysfunctional T-cell responses. In contrast, vaccination at early tumor stages affords excellent responses and significantly improves survival in preclinical studies. These observations point out the urgent need of evaluating cancer vaccine strategies in early-stage patients to fully exploit their potential.

ADOPTIVE AND INNATE STRATEGIES

Adoptive vaccination strategies consist of transferring immunity through the administration of specific antibodies or immune cells such as T-cells or dendritic cells (DCs). DCs represent a critical bridge between innate and adaptive responses (2). They are initially activated by invariant receptors that belong to innate immunity and recognize the molecular patterns associated with microbes or tumors, but subsequently they prime and direct adaptive T- and B-cell responses. Recently, a new subset of DC-termed IFNγ-producing killer dendritic cells (IKDCs) has been discovered. These express some NK markers, produce interferon-gamma (IFNγ), and have cytotoxic activities (3), and therefore represent a clear link between adaptive and innate immunity.

Innate Strategies

Microbial DNA can be taken up in DC endosomes and it is recognized by Toll-like receptor 9 (TLR9), one of the major drivers of innate immunity. In turn, TLR9 triggers the secretion of inflammatory signals, such as IFNα, that activates the cascade of differentiation and recruits different immune cells. TLRs belong to the set of germ-line encoded receptors that function as "sensors" of conserved molecular structures expressed by pathogens. At present, TLRs are promising targets of innate immunotherapy in cancer vaccinology. In murine models, TLR9 agonists have been shown to significantly protect from tumor development alone or in combination with monoclonal antibodies (4), cytokines (5), epidermal growth factor receptor (EGFR), and angiogenesis inhibitors (6). Another promising target for cancer immunotherapy is TLR7 as it recognizes single-stranded RNA and is physiologically critical to mount efficient antiviral responses. Several low-molecular-weight compounds are available that can selectively activate TLR7, such as imiquimod that exerts its anti-tumor activity by inducing inflammatory cytokines such as IFNγ and IL-12 (7). In 2004, a topical formulation of imiquimod has received FDA approval for the treatment of external genital warts and basal cell carcinoma.

Adoptive Strategies

Adoptive strategies are based on the administration of DC or T-cells modified to recognize and specifically target cancer cells. The rationale is that growing tumor-specific immune cells outside the host allow their expansion in large numbers, overcoming the immune suppressive mechanisms.

Adoptive immunotherapy originated from the pioneer work of S.A. Rosenberg on unselected T-cells in vitro activated with IL-2 in melanoma (8). Recent advances in molecular biology have provided the tools to genetically modify T-cells to redirect normal peripheral blood T-cells against tumor antigens. One option is to transfer specific, natural TCR receptor genes into T-cells. As an alternative, it is possible to transfer chimeric TCR comprised of an antibody fragment fused with the TCR signal transduction domain. Both the approaches revealed not only exceptional efficacy but also high levels of risk due to toxic T-cell mediated reactions. Toxicity seems to be a common issue in both natural TCR- and chimeric TCR-transduced T-cell adoptive therapies owing to the difficulty in predicting the pharmacodynamics of engineered T-cells. T-cell adoptive transfer strategies have been evaluated in hematological malignancies also. In a recent trial (9), patients with recurrent leukemia after MHC-matched allogeneic hematopoietic stem cell transplantation received donor-derived CTL expanded ex vivo and selected for tissue-restricted minor histocompatibility antigens (mHAg) expressed by the recipients. Adoptively transferred CTLs were detected in the blood for over 21 days after infusion; 71% of patients achieved complete remission. However, 42% of patients displayed potentially life-threatening pulmonary toxicity. Another recent clinical trial investigated adoptive transfer of genetically modified T-cells in advanced follicular lymphoma (10). Autologous T-cells genetically modified to express a chimeric antigen receptor binding the B-cell antigen CD19, produced a significant reduction of B-cell precursors in the bone marrow. A log-lasting selective eradication of B-lineage cells was observed, together with a normalization of circulating immunoglobulin levels. This effect was associated with cytopenia and fever, consistent with acute toxicities. T-cell adoptive transfer has been the object of a recent clinical trial on multiple myeloma (MM) (11). Fifty-four MM patients received auto-transplantation followed by infusion of anti-CD3/anti-CD28 stimulated autologous T-cells expanded ex vivo and were selected for the ability to recognize the tumor-associated antigens (TAA) survivin or hTERT (11). The therapy produced an evident increase in T-cell counts, above the physiologic levels, associated with a reduction in regulatory T-cells. Noteworthy, adoptive transfer of survivin tumor antigen vaccine-primed and co-stimulated T cells improved and accelerated immune reconstitution, and improved antitumor immunity, after autologous stem cell transplantation. Major toxic effects were grade I–III GvHD (13% of subjects) and indurations caused by a DTH response. DCs have been the target of a large number of adoptive vaccination strategies against infectious diseases, autoimmunity, and cancer (12). Their potentials and superior safety compared with T-cells have been reported in both preclinical and clinical settings. DC manipulation techniques include pulsing DC with tumor antigens or tumor fragments, or antigen transfer by viral vectors. Recombinant adeno-associated viral vectors (rAAV) have been successfully used to transfer HPV E6 in DC in a model of cervical cancer (13). An rAAV infection resulted in efficient priming of tumor-specific CTL in vitro (13). Pre-clinical rAAV-based manipulation of DCs are promising in the context of ovarian cancer (OC), targeting the tumor antigen, Her-2/Neu (14). Efficacy of rAAV in manipulating DC was reported also in MM (15). The self antigen HM1.24, expressed by MM cells, was used as the target. CTLs were generated with only one stimulation from patient PBMCs after co-culturing with autologous rAAV-HM1.24 transduced DC.

These studies provided the pre-clinical proof of principle for the use of adenoviral vectors in the DC manipulation preceding adoptive transfer strategies. In MM, the generation of clinically significant immune response following DC transfer has been shown to be a challenging procedure (16). While in other malignancies, such as prostate cancer (17), DC administration was proved to prolong survival, no improvement was shown in MM, compared with standard chemotherapy (18). In a pre-clinical murine study (19), DC pulsed in vitro with idiotype proteins induced therapeutic immunity in tumor-bearing animals. Adoptive DC transfer protected from tumor growth and eradicated plasma cells in 60% of mice. A novel strategy with intranodal adoptive transfer of reprogrammed DC has been developed, and a recent clinical trial showed the potential of this approach in human MM (20). Intranodal injection of idiotype and keyhole limpet hemocyanin-pulsed, in vitro matured DC with CD40L induced idiotype-specific immune responses (20). This protocol was proved to be safe, with no major side effects and six out of nine patients had stable disease at the five-year followup. Very recently, a more holistic approach has been evaluated, consisting of a vaccination with the adoptive transfer of DC fused with whole tumor cells in vitro (21). In a phase I clinical trial, DC fused with bone marrow-derived MM cells expressed co-stimulatory and maturation markers and the tumor-associated antigens CD38 and CD138. The absence of relevant side effects and the observation that disease stabilization was achieved in most of the patients indicated the feasibility of this approach (21).

In summary, adoptive transfer of in vitro manipulated DC with different methods is likely to be one of the most promising therapeutic options for MM patients in the near future. However, there is no general accordance concerning the strategies for DC preparation. At present, clinical trials are underway to identify the optimal conditions for DC manipulation. Ideally, two main goals have to be achieved: maximizing the efficiency of tumor antigen transfer in DC and optimizing the manipulation techniques in order to obtain DCs capable of overcoming immune tolerance (22).

SMALL MOLECULES

The concept that monotherapy strategies will most likely prove ineffective is gaining growing consensus in the field of cancer vaccines. The use of adjuvants and other drug-based therapies to boost immunological responses is currently explored. The final goal is to exploit the synergism between chemotherapy and immunotherapy to generate long-lasting memory immunity, overcoming tolerance and immune suppressive mechanisms (23). Most of the drugs developed for this purpose belong to the class of small molecules (heterogeneous compounds, generally with a low molecular weight).

Synthetic Compounds

Immune suppression inhibitors are promising candidates as adjuvants of vaccines against cancer. Relevant examples are indoleamine 2, 3-dioxygenase-1 (IDO) inhibitors. IDO converts the amino acid tryptophan to N-formylkynurenine. It has been shown that IDO is a key regulator of immunosuppressive mechanisms in tumor escape (24). Two recent studies provided a pre-clinical evaluation for the use of the synthetic hydroxyamidine IDO inhibitor INCB024360 in vivo (25,26). INCB024360 reactivated host DC and increased the frequency of IFNγ-secreting T-cells and reduced T regulatory cells (T_{REGS}).

A major issue with DC vaccine in MM arises from DC dysfunction, a deficiency associated with this disease (27,28). Studies to unravel the molecular mechanisms of DC dysfunction in MM reported the central role played by the mitogen-activated protein kinase 14 (p38α). Accordingly, the use of p38α inhibitor, SB203580, is a promising strategy to improve the efficacy of DC-based MM immunotherapy (29). The p38 inhibition could be instrumental also for OC vaccines: p38 is required for IL-10 production by DC (30), which is responsible for T_{REGS} differentiation, and accordingly, p38 inhibition results in the complete loss of T_{REG} function in preclinical studies (31).

Nucleic Acids

Short nucleic acid sequences can improve the efficacy of tumor vaccinations through multiple pathways. Unmethylated CpG-rich microbial DNA is recognized by the pathogen recognition receptor, TLRs that act as "danger sensors" of microbial infections and initiate potent immune responses. A phase I–II clinical trial (NCI no. NCT00185965) to evaluate the use of agatolimod in combination with local radiation in recurrent low-grade lymphomas was recently completed, but official results are not available. CpG treatment was reportedly effective in melanoma in a randomized phase II clinical trial. A hundred and eighty-four patients with metastatic melanoma received agatolimod alone or in combination with dacarbazine, and a significant treatment improvement was observed with agatolimod (32). Very recently, the effectiveness of CpG as a cancer vaccine adjuvant was shown in a murine model of OC (33). A CpG-adjuvanted peptide vaccine against the tumor-associated antigen Sperm Protein 17 (SP17) displayed its ability to overcome tumor-induced tolerance and afforded long-term protection from the development of tumors in a therapeutic way.

In conclusion, TLR agonists have generated great interest in tumor immunology in the past 10 years. Despite initial enthusiasm, they have obtained limited success so far, mainly because of inhibitory mechanisms that hamper TLR agonists' efficacy in vivo. For instance, it was reported that systemic CpG administration induces a decrement in spleen CTL activity, most likely due to IDO activation and T_{REG} upregulation (34). Therefore, more extensive studies are warranted to completely understand the still unrevealed mechanisms of action of TLR agonists and their potential benefits and risks for cancer patients.

RNAs are mainly exploited to regulate gene expression by tumor or immune system cells, with the final goal to break immune tolerance. An attractive alternative was recently developed with an aim of triggering the expression of specific novel antigens by tumor cells by inhibiting the nonsense-mediated messenger RNA decay (35). Small interfering RNA (siRNA)-mediated inhibition of nonsense-mediated messenger RNA decay in cancer cells resulted in the expression of antigenic proteins that in turn, potentiated immune responses and significantly inhibited the tumor growth.

Novel alternatives are DNA-siRNA fusion molecules (36). An siRNA targeting the transcription factor STAT3 is particularly an attractive strategy because activation of STAT3 is a key promoter of oncogenesis mediated by tumor-infiltrating myeloid and B-cells (37). Unfortunately, in vivo delivery of siRNA is challenging because of their high instability and reduced half-life (38). Linking anti-STAT3 siRNA to the TLR9 agonist CpG1668 has been shown to enable siRNA delivery to myeloid and B-cells and induction of a potent anti-tumor immune response in the B16 murine model of melanoma (36).

DC-BASED CANCER VACCINES AND PERSONALIZED IMMUNOTHERAPIES

As previously explained, DCs are the most powerful APC and are able to activate and regulate both innate and acquired immune mechanisms and they play a key role in balancing immunity and tolerance. Is has been extensively proved that tumor antigens can be loaded on DCs to initiate immune responses in vitro and in vivo. Accordingly, a number of clinical trials have explored the effect of antigen-pulsed DC vaccination in different types of tumors, including breast, prostate, colorectal and non-small-cell lung cancer, renal cell carcinoma, melanoma, and MM. The general outcome of these studies show that DC-based vaccines are safe, but the advantage that they are expected to offer in the clinical practice is still to be elucidated. In general, DC vaccines induce potent tumor-specific T-cell responses and occasionally tumor regression, but the average therapeutic significance is limited. At present, about 200 clinical trials have evaluated DC-based cancer vaccines, a majority of which focused on monocyte-derived DC (MoDC), obtained by culturing patients' monocytes with GM-CSF and IL-4 in vitro (Fig. 9.1). Some studies evaluated DCs generated from CD34⁺ hematopoietic stem cells or directly circulating DCs (Fig. 9.1). Depending on the study, the administration route varied from intradermal, to subcutaneous and intranodal. Although a large number of manipulation strategies were attempted, a typical trend of clinical trials was an initial optimal response in phase I–II followed by a general failure in phase III studies. At present, there is no accordance concerning the optimal DC-based strategy with regard to the source of the antigens, the optimal loading procedure (Fig. 9.1), the route, and the timing for vaccination.

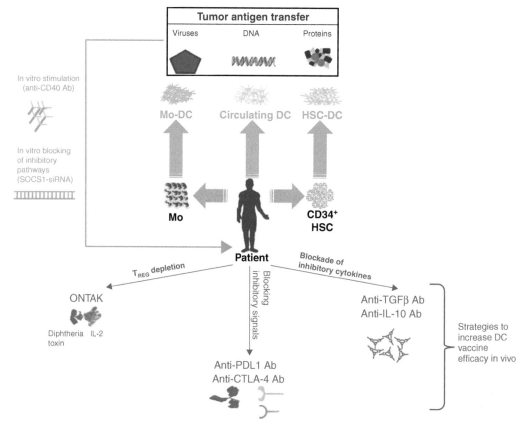

Figure 9.1 Dendritic cell (DC) vaccine techniques for cancer patients. The source of DCs can be monocytes (Mo's), hematopoietic stem cells (HSCs), or circulating DCs. Tumor antigen transfer can be performed through virus infection, vector DNA transduction, or direct protein loading. DCs are then transferred back to the patient after in vitro stimulation with different methods, such as CD40 activation, or after inhibition of regulatory pathways, such as SOCS1 silencing. DC transfer can be followed by adjuvant therapies aimed to deplete T_REGS, or block inhibitory signals (see text for details). *Abbreviations*: IL, interleukin; SOCS, suppressor of cytokine signaling; TGF-β, transforming growth factor beta.

New strategies point to overcome the multiple mechanisms of immune tolerance against tumor cells that account for the general disappointing clinical outcomes of DC-based vaccines. These include the hampering of co-stimulation, expression of inhibitory molecules, induction of T_{REG} cells, increased IDO activity, and secretion of immune suppressive cytokines (39).

Antibodies designed to block the T-cell inhibitory ligand PDL-1 frequently expressed by tumor and DC have been shown to enhance tumor-specific T-cell responses in vitro; accordingly, the humanized anti-PDL1 antibody CA-011 has been reported to increase the number of circulating $CD4^+$ T-cells in a phase I clinical trial for advanced hematological malignancies (40) (Fig. 9.1). An alternative strategy attempts to block the activation of T_{REG} subtypes. This result was obtained with an anti-CTLA antibody therapy (41): anti-CTLA-4 treatment with ipilimumab and tremelimumab yielded promising results in melanoma (42) and non-Hodgkin's lymphoma (43) (Fig. 9.1). A completely different approach consists of interfering with intracellular pathways that block DC functions in vivo, like the suppressor of cytokine signaling (SOCS) protein family. SOCS1 inhibition obtained through specific siRNA (Fig. 9.1) resulted in an improved antigen presentation by DC and enhanced IL-12 production (44).

A promising strategy to enhance the DC vaccine efficiency is the inhibition of T_{REGS}. Because T_{REGS} express high levels of IL-2 high affinity receptor CD25, an IL-2-diphteria toxin fusion protein denileukin diftitox (ONTAK) has been designed to preferentially target and kill this lymphocyte subset (45) (Fig. 9.1). Because TGF-β and IL-10 are potent DC-derived T_{REG} inducers, blocking agents to target these two key cytokines have been researched (Fig. 9.1). Combined CpG-IL10 receptor blocking antibodies resulted in an increased IL-12 production, while anti-TGF-β treatment increased the number of tumor-specific T-cells and decreased the proliferation of T_{REGS} (46).

In conclusion, the lack of significant clinical responses in most DC vaccine trials highlights the need for optimizing of DC vaccine protocols. New strategies in combination with DC vaccines to break tumor-induced immune tolerance are expected to enhance their efficacy in vivo and are required to achieve durable anti-tumor immune responses.

VACCINES AGAINST HEMATOLOGICAL MALIGNANCIES

It should be noted that hematopoietic stem cell transplantation (HSCT), frequently included in therapies against various hematological malignancies, is a form of a cancer vaccine itself (47) (Fig. 9.2), because it generates a graft versus tumor (GvT) response that plays a critical role in the eradication of the disease or the control of disease relapse.

It is extremely complex to control the balance between GvT and graft-versus-host disease (GvHD), a form of autoimmunity reaction against non-tumor tissues. Chronic GvHD has been correlated with a reduced risk of relapse, while a reduced frequency of GvHD is accompanied by a higher frequency of relapse, particularly in chronic myelogenous leukemias (CMLs) (48). The donor lymphocyte infusion procedure was developed to boost GvT effect in transplanted patients after malignant relapse (49). Based on the idea that allogeneic HSCT could act as a sort of immune therapy, many studies evaluated innovative strategies to avoid full myeloablative regimens before HSC administration. Results indicate that preconditioning regimens with reduced intensity are less efficient in killing the tumor, but afford a reduced treatment-related mortality and more efficient GvT responses. Non-myeloablative conditioning is indicated for aged patients who can benefit from the GvT mechanisms and can undergo a milder and less toxic chemotherapy. Introduction of non-myeloablative regimens also increased the median age of patients undergoing allogeneic HSCT by 11 years. This has made HSCT available for age-associated hematological malignancies.

In addition to the context of allogeneic or autologous HSCT, peptide-, cellular- and DNA-based vaccination strategies have been explored in hematological tumors such as acute myelogenous leukemia (AML), CML, B-cell lymphoma, and MM (50).

Clinical trials evaluating the efficacy and safety of peptide-based vaccines for AML have been initiated only recently. A recent study analyzed the cellular and humoral mechanisms

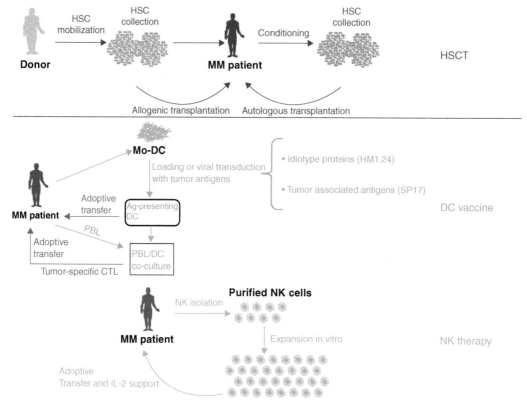

Figure 9.2 Immunotherapy approaches for multiple myeloma (MM). Hematopoietic stem cell transplantation (HSCT) can be considered a form of immunotherapy. Because dendritic cells (DCs) are dysfunctional in MM patients, autologous Mo-DC vaccinations have been attempted. DCs can be modified to express idiotypic proteins or tumor-associated antigens such as SP17. As an alternative, cytotoxic T lymphocytes (CTL) from patient's peripheral blood lymphocytes (PBL) can be obtained in vitro by co-culture with DCs. Recently, a natural killer (NK) based therapy has been tested using autologous NK expanded in vitro and adoptively transferred to MM patients with interleukin-2 (IL-2) support therapy.

associated with a complete remission achieved in an AML patient who received a Wilms Tumor Protein 1 (WT1) peptide vaccine (51). The study identified a WT1-sopecific T-cell predominant clone that was present both in the peripheral blood and bone marrow during clinical remission. After an initial decrease in the frequency of the predominant clone, a relapse phase occurred; that was associated with a rise of the WT1-specific clone cells in the peripheral blood, but not in the bone marrow. Interestingly, this secondary response was driven by a clone that is unable to produce IFN-γ. Overall, these results support the hypothesis that the compartmentalization of T-cell responses against peptide vaccines plays a critical role in the outcome of the vaccine therapy.

WT1 has also been tested as a target for DC-based vaccines in two AML patients displaying partial remission after receiving chemotherapy (52). Intradermal administration of full-length WT1 mRNA-electroporated dendritic cells led to a complete remission in both patients. In these and in other two subjects who were in complete remission after chemotherapy, the WT1-DC vaccine produced a decrease in the AML-associated tumor marker. The clinical response was accompanied by an expansion of WT1-specific CD8$^+$ T cells and activated NK cells. These data indicate the effectiveness of DC-based vaccines to prevent full relapse in remission phase AML.

CML is characterized by a chromosomal abnormality consisting of t(9;22) chromosomal translocation, which moves the c-abl oncogene 1 (ABL1) from chromosome 9 into the breakpoint cluster region (BCR) on chromosome 22. The resulting BCR–ABL1 fusion gene encodes a 210 kDa protein with constitutive tyrosine kinase activity (53). Therefore, the BCR-ABL1 protein is a specific tumor antigen that can be exploited in vaccine strategies. Two main alternative p210 proteins, p210–b2a2 and p210–b3a2 exist, depending on the exons of ABL1 and BCR that are combined by the translocation. The study by Bonecchia M. et al. (54) reports the outcome of an immunogenic 25-mer b2a2 breakpoint-derived peptide (CMLb2a2–25) in a 63-year-old woman with CML, who had received IFN-α treatment for six years. A significant b2a2–25 peptide-specific CD4[+] T-cell response and a decrease in the BCR–ABL1 transcript levels were detected after nine boosts of vaccine. No toxic effects were reported. The patient achieved a complete remission lasting more than 39 months, with a vaccine boost given every three months as the sole treatment.

Although immunotherapy has been primarily used as a treatment to consolidate remission after chemotherapy, the study by Navarrete M. A. et al. (55) showed that idiotype protein-based vaccination is efficacious as the primary intervention for treatment of indolent B-cell lymphoma. After six intradermal injections of adjuvanted recombinant idiotype Fab fragment (Fab[Id]), 76% of patients displayed anti-idiotype antibodies and/or cell-mediated responses. Induction of anti-idiotype antibodies correlated with progression-free survival. To increase vaccine effectiveness, a reengineering of the idiotypic lymphoma antigen has been evaluated. By genetically linking the *Escherichia coli* heat-labile enterotoxin (EtxB) to a single-chain Fv sequence of the idiotypic immunoglobulin antigen, Chen C. G. et al. (56) developed an effective vaccine against the mouse BCL1 B-cell lymphoma. The increased efficacy of the fusion protein over the native idiotypic protein stems from the EtxB's ability to bind the GM1ganglioside. In turn, the GM1 ganglioside acts as an endocytosis receptor in DC, facilitating the uptake of the idiotypic antigen.

MM (Fig. 9.2) can be considered a relatively weak immunogenic tumor. However, various TAA have been identified in MM that are potentially targetable by immune responses, including MUC1, HM1.24, PRAME, WT1, CYP1B1, GP96, and PTTG-1 (15,57). At present, a number of WT1-derived peptides have been shown to induce specific HLA-A*2402, HLA-A*0201, and HLA-A*0206 CTL responses and a durable disease stabilization (58). Originally, HM1.24 was discovered as a cell-surface protein aberrantly expressed by MM cells. It encodes for a HLA-A2-restricted T-cell epitope presented on MHC class-I complexes. DC transduced with HM1.24-derived peptide or transduced with HM1.24-expressing adenovirus (15) (Fig. 9.2) efficiently prime CD8[+] autologous cytotoxic T-cells.

Cell-based vaccinations for MM have been widely explored because of their superior ability to overcome immune dysfunction issues compared with peptide-based vaccines. Specifically, MM patients typically display quantitatively and qualitatively impaired DC functions. Serum from MM patients contains high levels of DC inhibitor factors, as IL-6 and TGF-β (59). The possibility to obtain large amounts of functionally active DC from MM patients in vitro supports the rationale for the use of DC-based vaccines in this malignancy. The safety and efficacy of DC infusion after transplantation have been clinically proved (Fig. 9.2). A study including 12 MM patients vaccinated with idiotype-pulsed DC, intravenously infused, showed no serious adverse effects and a cellular idiotype-specific response in two patients (16). Later, the feasibility of idiotype-loaded DC vaccination for MM was reported (60), and it was also validated in transplant settings. As alternative cellular immunotherapies for MM, natural killer (NK) cells were explored as well (Fig. 9.2). They play a fundamental role in innate immune responses and efficiently kill a variety of tumor cells without the assistance of MHC molecules. NK cells isolated from MM patients were shown to efficiently lyse autologous plasma cells in vitro, but not CD34[+] cells or allogeneic lymphocytes (61). NK cells were pre-clinically validated in vivo using murine models. Adoptive transfer of activated NK cells combined with IL-2 adjuvant therapy to myeloma-bearing mice prolonged the survival time compared with single treatments alone (62). Finally, MM patient-derived NK cells can be efficiently expanded ex vivo under GMP guidelines, and the obtained NK cells have high ability to kill autologous MM cells (63). In conclusion, recent advances in the field of MM immunotherapy hold the promise of successful future developments. Numerous antigens have been discovered to be expressed by malignant plasma cells and targetable by vaccination strategies. In a subset of patients, clinical responses were demonstrated, but strategies to improve immunotherapy for MM are still an urgent need. Of note, many clinical trials enroll patients with refractory and advanced disease, but these subjects' immune responses are dysfunctional; therefore, tumor immunotherapies will be more effective in patients with low tumor burden.

Furthermore, it is worthy of note that vaccination strategies against hematological tumors are more challenging compared with vaccines for solid cancers. Indeed, despite the fact that the expansion of antigen-specific T-cell responses is associated with anti-tumor effects, the clinical significance of such observation is disappointing in most cases. This is due to the limited number of tumor antigens identified in hematological malignancies compared with solid tumors and their low immunogenicity (64). Additionally, patients with hematological tumors frequently present functional deficiencies in the cellular and molecular antigen-presenting machinery (29,64–68). Among these, the low efficiency of hematological tumor antigens in binding to HLA class I molecules has been reported, and recent reports indicate that this is the major cause of immune escape in B-lymphomas (69). It has been hypothesized that this effect is due to the fact that hematological tumor cells tend to present TAA early in the natural history of the malignancy (70). This causes the selection of tumor variants which efficiently present TAA-HLA-I complexes, and the consequent outgrowth of tumor clones with impaired presentation abilities (69,70).

CTA TARGETING IN CANCER VACCINES FOR HEMATOLOGICAL MALIGNANCIES: THE CASE FOR MM

Studies evaluating the expression of CTAs in cancers have primarily focused on solid tumors. Only recently, more CTAs have been found to be expressed in hematological malignances (71-76), including SP17, MAGE-1, NY-ESO-1, SEMG-1, SPAN-Xb, SCP1, SSX, PASD1 and HAGE. In hematological malignancies, not only are CTAs expressed by tumor cells but they also induce frequent B-cell responses, as indicated by high levels of specific antibodies and CD4$^+$ T-cell clones in tumor-bearing patients (77,78). CTAs are also able to induce CTL responses with high efficiency. SP17-specific CTLs that are able to lyse tumor cells can be generated from the peripheral blood mononucleated cells of patients with hematological tumors and healthy donors (79). These results strongly support the feasibility of CTA-targeted vaccines for patients with hematological malignancies. Almost all studies evaluating CTA as targets for hematological tumor vaccines have focused on MM, probably because of the poor prognosis of the disease, the need for alternative therapies different from standard treatments, and the frequent CTA hyperexpression displayed by malignant plasma cells (73). Interestingly, there is a positive correlation between CTA expression and poor outcomes in MM patients (78).

A recent study analyzing the expression of 14 CTAs in 39 MM patients reported 77% positivity for MAGE-C1 (80) which was also associated with a more malignant phenotype and reduced survival time (81). A successful approach to identify CTAs that elicit CTL responses in MM patients and thereby representing good candidates for cancer vaccines exploited 12 peptide epitopes derived from a panel of CTAs to screen for a specific CTL in the blood of MM patients (82). In about 30% of subjects, a CTL response was identified against at least one of the tested CTA. NY-ESO-1-specific T-cells were identified and isolated from the peripheral blood of MM patients. These T-cells were shown to lyse autologous MM cells in vitro (78). Importantly, it was suggested that allogeneic effects of HSCT and GvT in MM should be boosted by CTA-targeted immunotherapy, since they were shown to induce systemic immunity and long-lasting protection after transplantation (83). As stated, a powerful technique to improve the outcome of peptidic lies in exploiting DCs to achieve a more potent and durable induction of T cell–mediated responses. To improve DC antigen presentation, Batchu R. B. et al. (84) reengineered

NY-ESO-1 protein by fusing it with the HIV-Tat protein transduction domain (PTD), which enabled the peptidic vaccine to freely cross cellular membranes. In vitro studies showed that the reengineered vaccine induced a higher frequency of CD8+ T-cells specific for NY-ESO-1, compared with NY-ESO-1 alone. NY-ESO-1-specific T-cells generated actively produced IFN-γ and type 1 cytokines. Thus, PTD-NY-ESO-1 accesses the cytoplasm by protein transduction, is processed by the proteosome, and the NY-ESO-1 peptides presented by HLA class I elicit NY-ESO-1-specific T lymphocytes.

Another CTA SPAN-Xb is targeted by specific CD8+ T-cells from MM patients, as indicated in a study using ELISPOT assays for IFN-γ (85).

So far, SP17 is the only CTA evaluated in a clinical trial for active immunotherapy in hematological tumors (86), using SP17-loaded autologous DCs in a patient with relapsed MM that underwent allogeneic HSCT (Fig. 9.3). SP17-specific immunity was achieved, as indicated by anti-SP17 circulating IgG following immunization. Immune response reduced serum paraptrotein to 10%. The GvT effect was accompanied by a GvHD reaction, probably exacerbated by the use of adjuvant IL-2 administration. This study, however, provided the proof of principle for the use of CTA-active immunization in hematological malignancies, and further evaluations in a broader cohort of subjects, possibly with early disease, are warranted.

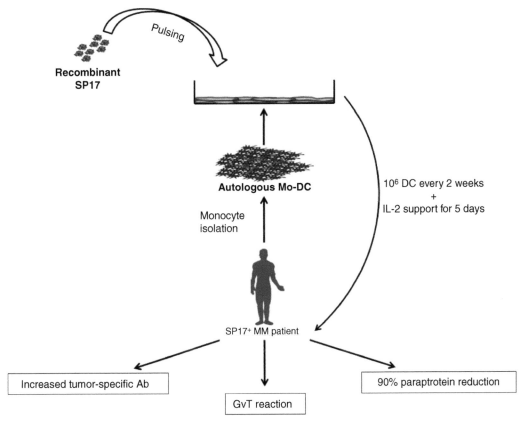

Figure 9.3 Vaccination with cancer testis antigen (CTA) in multiple myeloma (MM) patients. So far, the only clinical trial using CTA as MM vaccine targets has been performed using SP17 (see text for details). Autologous Mo-DCs were pulsed with recombinant SP17 protein, and then repetitively transferred to the patient with interleukin-2 (IL-2) support therapy. The advantages were increased anti-tumor antibody (Ab) response, graft versus tumor reaction, and a significant reduction in tumor burden (assessed as paraptrotein levels).

In conclusion, despite that CTAs are ideal targets for vaccine strategies in hematological malignancies, and specifically in MM, there is no effective CTA-based vaccine available. The lack of success could be partially explained by the heterogeneous nature of CTA expression between cells composing the same tumor mass. Therefore, if the immune system successfully deletes one tumor clone, the malignancy could be sustained by the emergence of a tumor variant with a different CTA expression pattern. Most importantly, however, the potential of vaccine interventions are likely to be masked by the heavy tumor burden characterizing the advanced-stage disease that has been tested so far. For these reasons, future studies should be performed to identify novel CTA antigens, to simultaneously target multiple CTAs and to include early-stage patients.

ACKNOWLEDGMENTS

W. Martin Kast holds the Walter A. Richter Cancer Research Chair.

REFERENCES

1. Hanahan D, Weinberg RA. The hallmarks of cancer. Cell 2000; 100: 57–70.
2. Novak N, Koch S, Allam JP, Bieber T. Dendritic cells: bridging innate and adaptive immunity in atopic dermatitis. J Allergy Clin Immunol 2010; 125: 50–9.
3. Chan CW, Crafton E, Fan HN, et al. Interferon-producing killer dendritic cells provide a link between innate and adaptive immunity. Nat Med 2006; 12: 207–13.
4. Wooldridge JE, Ballas Z, Krieg AM, Weiner GJ. Immunostimulatory oligodeoxynucleotides containing CpG motifs enhance the efficacy of monoclonal antibody therapy of lymphoma. Blood 1997; 89: 2994–8.
5. Chaudhry UI, Kingham TP, Plitas G, et al. Combined stimulation with interleukin-18 and CpG induces murine natural killer dendritic cells to produce IFN-gamma and inhibit tumor growth. Cancer Res 2006; 66: 10497–504.
6. Damiano V, Caputo R, Bianco R, et al. Novel toll-like receptor 9 agonist induces epidermal growth factor receptor (EGFR) inhibition and synergistic antitumor activity with EGFR inhibitors. Clin Cancer Res 2006; 12: 577–83.
7. Hemmi H, Kaisho T, Takeuchi O, et al. Small anti-viral compounds activate immune cells via the TLR7 MyD88-dependent signaling pathway. Nat Immunol 2002; 3: 196–200.
8. Rosenberg SA, Packard BS, Aebersold PM, et al. Use of tumor-infiltrating lymphocytes and interleukin-2 in the immunotherapy of patients with metastatic melanoma. A preliminary report. N Engl J Med 1988; 319: 1676–80.
9. Warren EH, Fujii N, Akatsuka Y, et al. Therapy of relapsed leukemia after allogeneic hematopoietic cell transplantation with T cells specific for minor histocompatibility antigens. Blood 2010; 115: 3869–78.
10. Kochenderfer JN, Wilson WH, Janik JE, et al. Eradication of B-lineage cells and regression of lymphoma in a patient treated with autologous T cells genetically engineered to recognize CD19. Blood 2010; 116: 4099–102.
11. Rapoport AP, Aqui NA, Stadtmauer EA, et al. Combination immunotherapy using adoptive T-cell transfer and tumor antigen vaccination on the basis of hTERT and survivin after ASCT for myeloma. Blood 2011; 117: 788–97.
12. Palucka K, Banchereau J, Mellman I. Designing vaccines based on biology of human dendritic cell subsets. Immunity 2010; 33: 464–78.
13. Chiriva-Internati M, Liu Y, Salati E, et al. Efficient generation of cytotoxic T lymphocytes against cervical cancer cells by adeno-associated virus/human papillomavirus type 16 E7 antigen gene transduction into dendritic cells. Eur J Immunol 2002; 32: 30–8.
14. Yu Y, Pilgrim P, Zhou W, et al. rAAV/Her-2/neu loading of dendritic cells for a potent cellular-mediated MHC class I restricted immune response against ovarian cancer. Viral Immunol 2008; 21: 435–42.
15. Chiriva-Internati M, Liu Y, Weidanz JA, et al. Testing recombinant adeno-associated virus-gene loading of dendritic cells for generating potent cytotoxic T lymphocytes against a prototype self-antigen, multiple myeloma HM1.24. Blood 2003; 102: 3100–7.
16. Reichardt VL, Okada CY, Liso A, et al. Idiotype vaccination using dendritic cells after autologous peripheral blood stem cell transplantation for multiple myeloma—a feasibility study. Blood 1999; 93: 2411–19.

17. Tanimoto T, Hori A, Kami M. Sipuleucel-T immunotherapy for castration-resistant prostate cancer. N Engl J Med 2010; 363: 1966; author reply 1967–8.

18. Eubel J, Enk AH. Dendritic cell vaccination as a treatment modality for melanoma. Expert Rev Anticancer Ther 2009; 9: 1631–42.

19. Wang S, Hong S, Wezeman M, et al. Dendritic cell vaccine but not idiotype-KLH protein vaccine primes therapeutic tumor-specific immunity against multiple myeloma. Front Biosci 2007; 12: 3566–75.

20. Yi Q, Szmania S, Freeman J, et al. Optimizing dendritic cell-based immunotherapy in multiple myeloma: intranodal injections of idiotype-pulsed CD40 ligand-matured vaccines led to induction of type-1 and cytotoxic T-cell immune responses in patients. Br J Haematol 2010; 150: 554–64.

21. Rosenblatt J, Vasir B, Uhl L, et al. Vaccination with DC/tumor fusion cells results in cellular and humoral anti-tumor immune responses in patients with multiple myeloma. Blood 2010; 28: 28.

22. Skalova K, Mollova K, Michalek J. Human myeloid dendritic cells for cancer therapy: does maturation matter? Vaccine 2010; 28: 28.

23. Copier J, Dalgleish AG, Britten CM, et al. Improving the efficacy of cancer immunotherapy. Eur J Cancer 2009; 45: 1424–31.

24. Muller AJ, DuHadaway JB, Donover PS, Sutanto-Ward E, Prendergast GC. Inhibition of indoleamine 2,3-dioxygenase, an immunoregulatory target of the cancer suppression gene Bin1, potentiates cancer chemotherapy. Nat Med 2005; 11: 312–19.

25. Liu X, Shin N, Koblish HK, et al. Selective inhibition of IDO1 effectively regulates mediators of antitumor immunity. Blood 2010; 115: 3520–30.

26. Koblish HK, Hansbury MJ, Bowman KJ, et al. Hydroxyamidine inhibitors of indoleamine-2,3-dioxygenase potently suppress systemic tryptophan catabolism and the growth of IDO-expressing tumors. Mol Cancer Ther 2010; 9: 489–98.

27. Ratta M, Fagnoni F, Curti A, et al. Dendritic cells are functionally defective in multiple myeloma: the role of interleukin-6. Blood 2002; 100: 230–7.

28. Brown RD, Pope B, Murray A, et al. Dendritic cells from patients with myeloma are numerically normal but functionally defective as they fail to up-regulate CD80 (B7-1) expression after huCD40LT stimulation because of inhibition by transforming growth factor-beta1 and interleukin-10. Blood 2001; 98: 2992–8.

29. Wang S, Hong S, Yang J, et al. Optimizing immunotherapy in multiple myeloma: Restoring the function of patients' monocyte-derived dendritic cells by inhibiting p38 or activating MEK/ERK MAPK and neutralizing interleukin-6 in progenitor cells. Blood 2006; 108: 4071–7.

30. Jarnicki AG, Conroy H, Brereton C, et al. Attenuating regulatory T cell induction by TLR agonists through inhibition of p38 MAPK signaling in dendritic cells enhances their efficacy as vaccine adjuvants and cancer immunotherapeutics. J Immunol 2008; 180: 3797–806.

31. Adler HS, Kubsch S, Graulich E, et al. Activation of MAP kinase p38 is critical for the cell-cycle-controlled suppressor function of regulatory T cells. Blood 2007; 109: 4351–9.

32. Wagner S, Weber J, Redman B, et al. CPG 7909, a TLR9 agonist immunomodulator in metastatic melanoma: a randomized phase II trial comparing two doses and in combination with DTIC. ASCO Meeting Abstracts 2005; 23(16 Suppl): 7526.

33. Chiriva-Internati M, Yu Y, Mirandola L, et al. Cancer testis antigen vaccination affords long-term protection in a murine model of ovarian cancer. PLoS One 2010; 5: e10471.

34. Wingender G, Garbi N, Schumak B, et al. Systemic application of CpG-rich DNA suppresses adaptive T cell immunity via induction of IDO. Eur J Immunol 2006; 36: 12–20.

35. Maquat LE. Nonsense-mediated mRNA decay: splicing, translation and mRNP dynamics. Nat Rev Mol Cell Biol 2004; 5: 89–99.

36. Kortylewski M, Swiderski P, Herrmann A, et al. In vivo delivery of siRNA to immune cells by conjugation to a TLR9 agonist enhances antitumor immune responses. Nat Biotechnol 2009; 27: 925–32.

37. Yu H, Kortylewski M, Pardoll D. Crosstalk between cancer and immune cells: role of STAT3 in the tumour microenvironment. Nat Rev Immunol 2007; 7: 41–51.

38. Ryther RC, Flynt AS, Phillips JA, 3rd, Patton JG. siRNA therapeutics: big potential from small RNAs. Gene Ther 2005; 12: 5–11.

39. Bronte V, Mocellin S. Suppressive influences in the immune response to cancer. J Immunother 2009; 32: 1–11.

40. Berger R, Rotem-Yehudar R, Slama G, et al. Phase I safety and pharmacokinetic study of CT-011, a humanized antibody interacting with PD-1, in patients with advanced hematologic malignancies. Clin Cancer Res 2008; 14: 3044–51.

41. Keilholz U. CTLA-4: negative regulator of the immune response and a target for cancer therapy. J Immunother 2008; 31: 431–9.
42. Yuan J, Gnjatic S, Li H, et al. CTLA-4 blockade enhances polyfunctional NY-ESO-1 specific T cell responses in metastatic melanoma patients with clinical benefit. Proc Natl Acad Sci USA 2008; 105: 20410–15.
43. O'Day SJ, Hamid O, Urba WJ. Targeting cytotoxic T-lymphocyte antigen-4 (CTLA-4): a novel strategy for the treatment of melanoma and other malignancies. Cancer 2007; 110: 2614–27.
44. Evel-Kabler K, Song XT, Aldrich M, Huang XF, Chen SY. SOCS1 restricts dendritic cells' ability to break self tolerance and induce antitumor immunity by regulating IL-12 production and signaling. J Clin Invest 2006; 116: 90–100.
45. Foss F. Clinical experience with denileukin diftitox (ONTAK). Semin Oncol 2006; 33: S11–16.
46. Fujita T, Teramoto K, Ozaki Y, et al. Inhibition of transforming growth factor-beta-mediated immuno-suppression in tumor-draining lymph nodes augments antitumor responses by various immunologic cell types. Cancer Res 2009; 69: 5142–50.
47. Jenq RR, van den Brink MR. Allogeneic haematopoietic stem cell transplantation: individualized stem cell and immune therapy of cancer. Nat Rev Cancer 2010; 10: 213–21.
48. Marmont AM, Horowitz MM, Gale RP, et al. T-cell depletion of HLA-identical transplants in leukemia. Blood 1991; 78: 2120–30.
49. Dodero A, Carniti C, Raganato A, et al. Haploidentical stem cell transplantation after a reduced-intensity conditioning regimen for the treatment of advanced hematologic malignancies: posttrans-plantation CD8-depleted donor lymphocyte infusions contribute to improve T-cell recovery. Blood 2009; 113: 4771–9.
50. Joseph-Pietras D, Gao Y, Zojer N, et al. DNA vaccines to target the cancer testis antigen PASD1 in human multiple myeloma. Leukemia 2010; 24: 1951–9.
51. Ochsenreither S, Fusi A, Busse A, et al. "Wilms Tumor Protein 1" (WT1) peptide vaccination-induced complete remission in a patient with acute myeloid leukemia is accompanied by the emergence of a predominant T-cell clone both in blood and bone marrow. J Immunother 2011; 34: 85–91.
52. Van Tendeloo VF, Van de Velde A, Van Driessche A, et al. Induction of complete and molecular remis-sions in acute myeloid leukemia by Wilms' tumor 1 antigen-targeted dendritic cell vaccination. Proc Natl Acad Sci USA 2010; 107: 13824–9.
53. Hehlmann R, Hochhaus A, Baccarani M. Chronic myeloid leukaemia. Lancet 2007; 370: 342–50.
54. Bocchia M, Defina M, Aprile L, et al. Complete molecular response in CML after p210 BCR-ABL1-derived peptide vaccination. Nat Rev Clin Oncol 2010; 7: 600–3.
55. Navarrete MA, Heining-Mikesch K, Schüler F, et al. Upfront immunization with autologous recombi-nant idiotype Fab fragment without prior cytoreduction in indolent B-cell lymphoma. Blood 2011; 117: 1483–91.
56. Chen CG, Lu Y-T, Lin M, et al. Amplification of immune responses against a DNA-delivered idiotypic lymphoma antigen by fusion to the B subunit of E. coli heat labile toxin. Vaccine 2009; 27: 4289–96.
57. Chiriva-Internati M, Ferrari R, Prabhakar M, et al. The pituitary tumor transforming gene 1 (PTTG-1): an immunological target for multiple myeloma. J Transl Med 2008; 6: 15.
58. Oka Y, Tsuboi A, Fujiki F, et al. WT1 peptide vaccine as a paradigm for "cancer antigen-derived peptide"-based immunotherapy for malignancies: successful induction of anti-cancer effect by vacci-nation with a single kind of WT1 peptide. Anticancer Agents Med Chem 2009; 9: 787–97.
59. Hayashi T, Hideshima T, Akiyama M, et al. Ex vivo induction of multiple myeloma-specific cytotoxic T lymphocytes. Blood 2003; 102: 1435–42.
60. Guardino AE, Rajapaksa R, Ong KH, Sheehan K, Levy R. Production of myeloid dendritic cells (DC) pulsed with tumor-specific idiotype protein for vaccination of patients with multiple myeloma. Cyto-therapy 2006; 8: 277–89.
61. Frohn C, Hoppner M, Schlenke P, et al. Anti-myeloma activity of natural killer lymphocytes. Br J Haematol 2002; 119: 660–4.
62. Alici E, Konstantinidis KV, Sutlu T, et al. Anti-myeloma activity of endogenous and adoptively trans-ferred activated natural killer cells in experimental multiple myeloma model. Exp Hematol 2007; 35: 1839–46.
63. Alici E, Sutlu T, Bjorkstrand B, et al. Autologous antitumor activity by NK cells expanded from myeloma patients using GMP-compliant components. Blood 2008; 111: 3155–62.
64. Avigan D, Tzachanis D. Cancer vaccines in hematologic malignancies: advances, challenges and therapeutic potential. Expert Rev Vaccin 2010; 9: 451–4.

65. van Luijn MM, van den Ancker W, Chamuleau ME, et al. Impaired antigen presentation in neoplasia: basic mechanisms and implications for acute myeloid leukemia. Immunotherapy 2010; 2: 85–97.
66. Amria S, Cameron C, Stuart R, Haque A. Defects in HLA class II antigen presentation in B-cell lymphomas: Leuk Lymphoma 2008; 49: 353–5.
67. Wetzler M, McElwain BK, Stewart CC, et al. HLA-DR antigen-negative acute myeloid leukemia. Leukemia 2003; 17: 707–15.
68. Wetzler M, Baer MR, Stewart SJ, et al. HLA class I antigen cell surface expression is preserved on acute myeloid leukemia blasts at diagnosis and at relapse. Leukemia 2001; 15: 128–33.
69. Strothmeyer AM, Papaioannou D, Duhren-von Minden M, et al. Comparative analysis of predicted HLA binding of immunoglobulin idiotype sequences indicates T cell-mediated immunosurveillance in follicular lymphoma. Blood 2010; 116: 1734–6.
70. Bogen B. Lymphoma invisibility–vaccination–attack? Blood 2011; 117: 1437–8.
71. Chiriva-Internati M, Wang Z, Salati E, et al. Sperm protein 17 (Sp17) is a suitable target for immunotherapy of multiple myeloma. Blood 2002; 100: 961–5.
72. Wang Z, Zhang Y, Liu H, et al. Gene expression and immunologic consequence of SPAN-Xb in myeloma and other hematologic malignances. Blood 2003; 101: 955–60.
73. van Baren N, Brasseur F, Godelaine D, et al. Genes encoding tumor-specific antigens are expressed in human myeloma cells. Blood 1999; 94: 1156–64.
74. Zhang Y, Wang Z, Liu H, Giles FJ, Lim SH. Pattern of gene expression and immune responses to Semenogelin 1 in chronic hematologic malignancies. J Immunother 2003; 26: 461–7.
75. Tarte K, De Vos J, Thykjaer T, et al. Generation of polyclonal plasmablasts from peripheral blood B cells: a normal counterpart of malignant plasmablasts. Blood 2002; 100: 1113–22.
76. Adams SP, Sahota SS, Mijovic A, et al. Frequent expression of HAGE in presentation chronic myeloid leukaemias. Leukemia 2002; 16: 2238–42.
77. Wang Z, Zhang Y, Ramsahoye B, Bowen D, Lim SH. Sp17 gene expression in myeloma cells is regulated by promoter methylation. Br J Cancer 2004; 91: 1597–603.
78. van Rhee F, Szmania SM, Zhan F, et al. NY-ESO-1 is highly expressed in poor-prognosis multiple myeloma and induces spontaneous humoral and cellular immune responses. Blood 2005; 105: 3939–44.
79. Chiriva-Internati M, Wang Z, Salati E, Wroblewski D, Lim SH. Successful generation of sperm protein 17 (Sp17)-specific cytotoxic T lymphocytes from normal donors: implication for tumour-specific adoptive immunotherapy following allogeneic stem cell transplantation for Sp17-positive multiple myeloma. Scand J Immunol 2002; 56: 429–33.
80. Andrade VC, Vettore AL, Felix RS, et al. Prognostic impact of cancer/testis antigen expression in advanced stage multiple myeloma patients. Cancer Immun 2008; 8: 2.
81. Atanackovic D, Luetkens T, Hildebrandt Y, et al. Longitudinal analysis and prognostic effect of cancer-testis antigen expression in multiple myeloma. Clin Cancer Res 2009; 15: 1343–52.
82. Goodyear O, Piper K, Khan N, et al. CD8+ T cells specific for cancer germline gene antigens are found in many patients with multiple myeloma, and their frequency correlates with disease burden. Blood 2005; 106: 4217–24.
83. Atanackovic D, Arfsten J, Cao Y, et al. Cancer-testis antigens are commonly expressed in multiple myeloma and induce systemic immunity following allogeneic stem cell transplantation. Blood 2007; 109: 1103–12.
84. Batchu RB, Moreno AM, Szmania SM, et al. Protein transduction of dendritic cells for NY-ESO-1-based immunotherapy of myeloma. Cancer Res 2005; 65: 10041–9.
85. Frank C, Hundemer M, Ho AD, Goldschmidt H, Witzens-Harig M. Cellular immune responses against the cancer-testis antigen SPAN-XB in healthy donors and patients with multiple myeloma. Leuk Lymphoma 2008; 49: 779–85.
86. Dadabayev AR, Wang Z, Zhang Y, et al. Cancer immunotherapy targeting Sp17: when should the laboratory findings be translated to the clinics? Am J Hematol 2005; 80: 6–11.

10 | Epitope-based vaccines for cancer

Vy Phan-Lai, Denise L. Cecil, Gregory E. Holt, Daniel R. Herendeen, Forrest Kievit, Miqin Zhang, and Mary L. Disis

INTRODUCTION

Epitope-based cancer vaccination, comprised of minimal immunogenic portions of a cancer antigen, represents an immunotherapy that combines target specificity with long-lasting immunity. Advances in epitope identification and immunogenicity assays, as well as peptide formulation and delivery methods, have bolstered interest in this approach. Increased understanding of the mechanisms of T cell-induced activation and immune tolerance has influenced the design of T cell-epitope vaccines. This chapter discusses the use of T cell-epitope vaccines for cancer.

RATIONALE FOR EPITOPE VACCINES

Among the various vaccine approaches for cancer, including cell-based vaccines (derived from tumor or dendritic cells), and recombinant viral or bacterial vectors, peptide vaccines confer distinct advantages. Peptides can be designed to contain epitopes that induce T helper (Th) or cytotoxic T-lymphocyte (CTL) responses, while avoiding those that induce regulatory T (T_{REG}) responses. Peptides can be administered singly or with immune adjuvants, offering an ideal broad-based approach to prevent or treat cancer. Most importantly, the use of epitopes can override immune tolerance, allowing the induction of T- or B-cell responses against tumor-associated antigens that are also 'self' antigens (1,2).

Epitope-Specific Immune Suppression

Central and peripheral tolerance, while important for preventing autoimmunity, impedes successful cancer immunotherapy (3). In central tolerance, self-antigen expression in the thymus results in clonal deletion or negative selection of developing T cells that are capable of recognizing self antigens with high avidity (4). However, it has been demonstrated that 25–40% of potentially autoreactive T cells with low to intermediate avidity can escape clonal deletion and are released into the periphery (5). There are several peripheral regulatory mechanisms that can control these autoreactive T cells (5). Self antigens encountered in the periphery may be deleted by an antigen-induced apoptosis or induction of a state of anergy of the T cell by incomplete co-stimulation from receptors such as B7, CD80/CD86, and CTLA-4 or by chronic stimulation with tolerogenic immature dendritic cells (DCs). Additionally, a state of ignorance can be induced where naive T cells are limited to where they traffic or when T cells have been activated in the absence of an inflammatory signal. Furthermore, an avidity model of peripheral tolerance has been demonstrated where CD8+ T cells can downregulate self-reactive T cells with intermediate avidity by recognizing the major histocompatibility complex (MHC) class I b (MHCIb) molecule preferentially expressed by T cells with intermediate, but not high, avidity (6,7).

Peripheral tolerance can also be maintained by the activity of T regulatory cells (T_{REGS}), which are present in increased numbers in advanced-stage cancers. CD4+CD25+highFOXP3+ T_{REGS} can be positively selected in the thymus in a regulated equilibrium with self-reactive T cells (8). These naturally occurring T_{REGS} can suppress the immune response in a cell contact–dependent mechanism by mediating the function of CD39, CD73, and LAG-3, or direct killing of antigen-presenting cells (APCs) or activated T cells with granzyme and/or perforin. Adaptively induced T_{REG} cells (Tr1 and Th3 subsets) arise in the periphery and modulate immune responses via secretion of immunosuppressive cytokines interleukin-10 (IL-10) and transforming growth factor-beta (TGF-β) (9–12). IL-10 and TGF-b have been shown to further enhance T_{REG} function by inducing tolerogenic DCs that are able to induce differentiation of antigen-specific CD4$^+$ T cells into immunosuppressive regulatory cells (12). Notably, the removal of T_{REGS} by various mechanisms has led to the generation of antitumor immunity (13).

Despite these numerous regulatory mechanisms, low-avidity self-reactive T cells are allowed to persist and it has been demonstrated that these low-avidity T cells can be potentially activated by high concentrations of self antigen and are involved in anti-tumor and autoimmune responses (14,15). Subdominant epitopes from several tumor antigens have been found to elicit high-avidity T cell responses across multiple MHC class II (MHCII) alleles (16–18).

CTL VACCINES

CTL vaccines have been widely studied, given the importance of CTLs in tumor lysis and eradication. CTLs recognize 8–11 amino acid (aa) peptides of an antigen bound within the MHCI molecule. The binding groove of the MHCI molecule contains deep pockets for binding anchor residues of the cognate peptide (19). The N and C terminus of each peptide are connected to the conserved amino acids of the receptor which confines peptide length (20). Anchor residues typically reside at positions 2 and 3, and the C terminus (21). These characteristics create a receptor with exact specifications for the peptides it binds, but also restricts which epitopes can be identified via the sequence motifs.

Epitope Prediction

Two methods are typically used to identify immunogenic peptides for MHCI peptides: the creation of overlapping peptides for individual testing and the use of predictive modeling to narrow down the putative peptide list to more manageable numbers. Prior to the understanding of the binding characteristics of MHCI molecules, entire sets of overlapping peptides for an antigen were created and tested individually for T-cell reactivity or MHCI tetramer binding. These methods are labor intensive and costly and, in the case of T-cell activation assays, require a great number of lymphocytes, a precious commodity in human studies. These methods, however, help in the identification of all immunogenic and/or MHCI-binding peptides of a protein.

Several methods have been employed to rapidly refine the search for immunogenic peptides. One of these involves combining the groups of peptides into large pools for testing which allows the rejection of large numbers of peptides from a single pool if no activity is observed. Peptide pools that stimulate T cells are then dissected to identify the peptides responsible for the reactivity. This method is advantageous for proteins with few immunogenic epitopes but difficult for those with multiple reactive epitopes since many pools may demonstrate reactivity. Peptide matrices also represent an improvement on the peptide pool methodology where each individual peptide is entered into a grid and pools are created by combining the peptides of each column or row in a manner where each peptide appears in two pools (22).

In addition to overlapping peptide pools, epitope prediction algorithms are widely used to predict immunogenic peptides. These programs aid in the analysis of protein sequences and create putative lists of binding peptides for MHC haplotypes, vastly reducing the number of peptides to be tested. Additionally, these algorithms quickly reveal the peptide candidates, have been widely validated, and reduce utilization of lymphocytes (by decreasing the number of potential epitopes) (23). A major disadvantage of this methodology is that the putative list still requires confirmation by in vitro testing and there exists the possibility of missing immunogenic epitopes not described by these known prediction algorithms.

These algorithms can be divided into three basic classifications depending on the mechanism used to make the predictions: Binding Pattern Recognition, Quantitative Binding Affinity, and Modeling (24). Binding Pattern Recognition methods are qualitative strategies that evaluate the protein sequence for amino acid patterns similar to known binding peptides and predict the probability of whether the putative peptide will bind a particular MHC molecule. Quantitative Binding Affinity algorithms use regression models of the binding affinities of known good binding peptides to the MHC haplotype to predict the probability whether each hypothetical peptide of a protein will bind. Modeling methods use the three-dimensional structure of known haplotypes to evaluate the potential that the amino acid sequence of the peptide will interact with the binding groove to make predictions of its probability to bind the same receptor. Although the first two systems outperform the modeling algorithms, due to intrinsic variability in the data used for any of the methods, one system has yet to demonstrate a uniform superiority over other algorithms.

Confirmation of a peptide as a natural ligand for the MHCI is critical and can involve testing the peptide-binding affinity of MHCI, its ability to stimulate CTLs, and a proof that it is endogenously presented by ensuring that peptide-specific T cells recognize targets pulsed with the entire protein. To measure CTL reactivity multiple methods are used; however, enzyme-linked immunosorbent spot and target cell lysis assays are most frequently used.

Epitope Modification

Based on the fact the anchor residues of CTL peptides are buried deep within the MHC groove and do not interact with the T cell receptor, alteration of the anchor residues of weak-binding peptides to amino acids, a characteristic of the haplotype-binding groove, can increase the affinity and decrease the dissociation rate of the peptide (25,26). These altered peptide ligands (APLs) have been shown to have improved immunogenicity and increase the magnitude of the induced immune response and may be more capable of overcoming tolerance to self peptides (25–27). Early studies included APLs for gp100, while recent studies have revealed "superagonist" APLs capable of activating CTL clones against an epitope of melanoma MART-1 (28,29). Furthermore, APLs have been used in phase I clinical trials of non-small-cell lung cancer (NSCLC) using both the altered peptide of human telomerase reverse transcriptase and the native peptide (30).

Clinical Trials

Various cancer vaccine trials have been conducted [for review, see Ref. (31)]. Among the largest trials for CTL epitope vaccines were the two clinical trials (I-01 and I-02) led by the U.S. Military Cancer Institute Clinical Trials Group, using an 8-mer HER2/neu peptide (p369–377) administered i.d. with granulocyte macrophage colony-stimulating factor (GM-CSF). Enrolling 186 patients, including node-positive and node-negative patients, the study found the vaccine to be safe with minimal toxicities (32). Dose-dependent HER2/neu immunity was observed in both node-negative and node-positive patients. Based on the data, there is interest to evaluate whether the vaccine (E75) can prevent tumor recurrence in disease-free, high-risk breast cancer patients. Most of the other recent and large multisite trials using CTL epitope-based vaccination have been in melanoma. These studies have included the evaluation of gp100 alone or with IL-2, gp100 alone or with ipilimumab (which blocks CTLA-4), and gp96 peptide complexed to tumor-derived heat shock protein (vitespen) with or without adjuvants; clinical results from these studies are mixed as to whether addition of adjuvants to epitope vaccines augments efficacy (33–35).

TH VACCINES

Th1 cells are central to the development of immune responses for protection against malignancy by priming CD8+ T cells and recruiting CD8+ T cells, macrophages, eosinophils, and mast cells to the tumor (36–42). Adoptive transfer of Th cells into tumor-bearing animals has been shown to activate a CTL-mediated anti-tumor response through direct interaction with co-stimulatory molecules present on the surface of the CTL (e.g. CD27, CD134, and MHC). Additionally, activated Th1 cells can secrete inflammatory cytokines such as IL-2, IFNγ, and TNF-α. Recent evidence has demonstrated that multifunctional Th1 cells that simultaneously secrete all three cytokines produce significantly more IFNγ than Th1 cells that produce one or two cytokines, and were more effective at protecting against infection (43). These multifunctional

Th1 cells can modulate the growth and expansion of effector T cells as well as promote the activation and maintenance of memory T cells (42,44,45). As a direct result of activating APCs, antigen-specific Th1 cells have been implicated as the initiators of epitope spreading, a broadening of the immune response to many potential antigens in the tumor. Epitope spreading has been linked with a survival benefit as a result of immunotherapy in patients with melanoma and breast cancer (2,46).

Epitope Prediction

Th epitopes (typically 12 aa or longer) are presented by MHCII proteins on professional APCs (DCs, macrophages, and B cells) and activate Th cells. MHCII proteins consist of three types (human leukocyte antigen-DR [HLA-DR], HLA-DP, and HLA-DQ) with multiple polymorphic alleles for each type in the human population. Since the goal in vaccine development is to generate immunity in a high percent of the treated population, the strategy for Th vaccines involves identifying Th epitopes that are promiscuous binders of multiple MHCII alleles. Due to the expense, limited availability of patient PBMC samples for research, and the workload involved, the identification of Th epitopes experimentally with sets of overlapping peptides is often unrealistic. Instead, the use of in silico tools is favored by many laboratories to screen potential epitopes and narrow down the number peptides to test in vitro. There are several publicly available algorithms for predicting MHCII epitopes that have recently been tested for accuracy in identifying known MHCII-binding peptides (47,48). While no individual algorithm stood out as the most reliable epitope predictor for all MHCII alleles, and all were less accurate than MHCI prediction algorithms, it was demonstrated that the use of consensus results from more than one algorithm improved the accuracy of Th epitope prediction (47).

In our laboratory we have been using a consensus approach with three different algorithms to identify epitopes for HLA-DR alleles to aid in vaccine development (17). Each algorithm identifies and assigns scores for predicted binding peptides within the input protein sequence of a tumor antigen. After normalizing the scores for each algorithm dataset, we calculate the "sum score" at each amino acid position, which is the product of peptide scores from several different HLA-DR alleles, and then multiply that score by the number of HLA-DR alleles predicted to bind peptides at each position, resulting in the "multiple score", which represents the binding strength and promiscuity of the predicted epitopes (17). Figure 10.1 illustrates the identification of five 9–21 aa peptides for HER2/neu (indicated by boxes), based on their "multiple score". Following in silico epitope prediction, synthetic peptides can be assayed in vitro to quantify their ability to induce $CD4^+$ T cell cytokine responses. Sensitivity of detecting responses to tumor antigen epitopes may be improved by manipulations to reduce inhibition by regulatory T cells present in antigen-educated PBMC samples (49,50). By comparing the cytokine profiles elicited by multiple PBMC samples, peptides can be further characterized by their propensity to stimulate Th1 (IFNγ) or Th2 (IL-10) responses within the patient population. Choosing epitopes that preferentially initiate Th1 immunity is desired for cancer vaccine formulations.

Epitope Modification

In practice, it is rare to find highly promiscuous Th epitopes of self antigens that activate $CD4^+$ T cells in a majority of the population. To increase the frequency of immune response within a patient population, several tumor antigen epitopes are often combined in polyepitope peptide or DNA vaccines (51–53). Apart from the rapid advances in adjuvants to promote robust immune responses, a trend toward designing polyepitope cancer vaccines that induce both Th and CTL responses is evident.

Clinical Trials

Many Th peptide vaccine trials, including ours, have focused on eliciting immunity against self antigens, which are often overexpressed or mutated in cancers. Our laboratory has

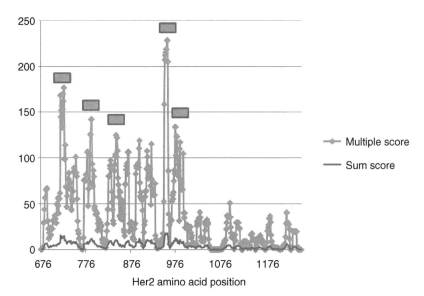

Figure 10.1   HER2/neu C-terminus heatmap for promiscuous T-helper epitopes. Using three different MHC II epitope prediction algorithms, peptides within the HER2 protein are scored for affinity to HLA-DR alleles. Normalized scores from each algorithm are added together at each amino acid position (Sum score, red), and multiplied by the number of HLA-DR allotypes predicted to bind at each position (Multiple score, blue). Boxes indicate 9–21 amino acid regions with the highest multiple scores, representing peptides that are most likely to be promiscuous MHC II epitopes. *Abbreviations*: HLA, human leukocyte antigen; MHC, major histocompatibility complex.

demonstrated that long-lived T cell immunity can be elicited in breast cancer patients against HER2/neu, a self protein, using HER2/neu-derived MHCII Th peptides encompassing HLA-A2-binding motifs (1,16). Vaccines have also targeted epitopes of mutated cancer antigens. Results from a recent phase II, multi-center trial indicated that a vaccine comprised of a 13 aa Th epitope spanning the EGFRvIII mutation increased the overall survival of newly diagnosed glioblastoma patients, compared with the matched control group (54). Recent studies evaluating extended epitopes of HPV-16 oncogenes demonstrated that therapeutic vaccination in patients with high-grade vulvar intraepithelial neoplasia (caused by HPV-16) led to complete responses in nearly 50% of patients (9 of 19) and furthermore, all patients demonstrated vaccine-induced immune responses (55). A shift in the frequency of circulating CD4$^+$ T cells can occur after vaccination, resulting in an increased percentage of FOXP3-negative, Th1-like cells with robust antigen-specific reactivity to cognate peptide, as observed in melanoma patients immunized with a HLA-DQ6-restricted Melan-A peptide (56). Therefore, vaccines can modulate endogenous T$_{REGS}$.

Moreover, induction of a broadened immune response (epitope spreading) is ideal to override mechanisms of epitope-specific immune suppression, mediated by T$_{REGS}$ (discussed in the section "Epitope-Specific Immune Suppression"). Our group recently demonstrated, in a trial of concurrent trastuzumab with Th epitope vaccination, that vaccination promoted the spread of epitopes and that TGF-β, a T$_{REG}$-associated cytokine, decreased in those patients with the greatest magnitude of T cell response (2).

DELIVERY SYSTEMS FOR EPITOPE VACCINATION
Circumventing the Instability of Synthetic Peptides
Peptides have been synthesized with defined chemical modifications that not only serve to mimic natural epitopes but also introduce protease-resistant peptide bonds to protect them

from tissue-specific proteolysis in vivo (57). Other strategies to ensure greater stability include the incorporation of epitopes into DNA-based vectors.

DNA-Based Systems

DNA-based vaccines contain the genetic sequence of the immunizing antigen under the control of a constitutively active promoter, usually in a plasmid or viral vector. Variations employ linear DNA species designed to resist nucleases through phosphorothioate backbones or terminal hairpin loops (58,59). Vaccines have been engineered to encode protein antigens as the entire gene, full-length genes modified to remove oncogenic signaling sites, specific immunogenic regions of the protein, or minimal epitopes (60–64). The MHCI presentation pathway requires proteins to enter the degradation pathway, be processed by the proteasome and bind the MHCI molecules prior to surface presentation. To enhance the processing and presentation of MHCI peptides, strategies that target the encoded protein to degradation pathways have improved to induce immunity. Expressing recombinant antigens containing ubiquitin peptides or endoplasmic reticulum targeting sequence, and adjusting the Kozak sequence to produce a destabilizing arginine amino acid at the start instead of the canonical methionine, have all been shown to increase CD8$^+$ T cell–specific immune responses (65–69). Interestingly, the addition of an ubiquitin molecule to the vaccine can abolish the induction of humoral responses (70). For vaccines composed of tandem minimal epitopes, the addition of three amino acid spacer sequences between epitopes enhanced the generation of reactive CD8$^+$ T cells and efficacy of the induced immunity (65,71,72).

For an MHCII-restricted peptide presentation, antigen is degraded in endolysosomal compartments to peptides and subsequently bound to MHCII molecules. Use of proteins that localize within endolysosomes including LAMP-1, or the cytoplasmic tails of the CD1b molecule has improved the vaccine potency in cancer and infectious disease applications, though this enhancement of immune response has not been seen universally (66,73–75). Insertion of MHCII-restricted peptides with broad haplotype binding specificities has increased the resultant immunity to MHCII restricted epitopes in several models of DNA-based vaccines (69,76,77). Moreover, inclusion of canonical, immunostimulatory CpG sequences in the vaccinating plasmid should theoretically augment induced immune responses; however, the literature contains mixed reports on this subject with some studies showing a benefit and others showing no difference (78,79).

Small vectors (nanoparticles) are also an effective vehicle for epitope vaccination. These nanoparticles must meet several key parameters: (*i*) have a particle size of 20–100 nm diameter, (*ii*) have a highly repetitive and ordered structure, (*iii*) have the ability to display epitopes for activation of innate immunity, and (*iv*) localize in specific areas of the body for efficient immune response (80–82). This has led to the development of virus-like particles (VLPs), which can be engineered from plasmids encoding viral structure proteins. VLPs have been used in vaccination against hepatitis B and human papillomavirus, and currently being explored for vaccination against other diseases, such as arthritis, Alzheimer's, and cancer (83). However, the outcome of VLPs as epitope delivery vehicles remains unpredictable due to undesirable structural perturbations caused by the viral coat protein or epitope, leading to diminished function (84,85). Alternatively, the rapidly advancing field of nanotechnology provides an opportunity to develop safer, more effective, and readily modifiable epitope delivery vehicles for cancer vaccination.

SUMMARY AND FUTURE DIRECTIONS

Pre-clinical and clinical trials using epitope-based cancer vaccines have demonstrated low toxicity and proved that tolerance to self antigens can be broken. Given the plethora of tumor antigens from which multiple epitope-based vaccines can be generated to treat various cancers, the rapid advancement in epitope identification and immune monitoring, and the potential to induce long-term T cell immunity, we predict that the field of epitope-based vaccination will continue to garner interest in years to come. Future efforts to overcome HLA restriction and render epitope-directed vaccines more applicable across wider patient populations will rely on defining appropriate HLA promiscuous epitopes as well as creating multi-component vaccines covering a broad array of appropriate target antigens. The clinical translation of epitope vaccination will remain important for cancer prevention and therapy.

ACKNOWLEDGMENTS

Supporting research grants include NIH Training Grant T32 CA138312 and DOD Breast Cancer Research Program Multidisciplinary Postdoctoral Award W81XWH-06-1-0724 (to VPL), and R01 CA136632, U01 CA141539 and P50 CA083636 (to MLD). We thank Ms. Molly Boettcher for her expert clerical assistance.

REFERENCES

1. Disis ML, Gooley TA, Rinn K, et al. Generation of T-cell immunity to the HER-2/neu protein after active immunization with HER-2/neu peptide-based vaccines. J Clin Oncol 2002; 20: 2624–32.
2. Disis ML, Wallace DR, Gooley TA, et al. Concurrent trastuzumab and HER2/neu-specific vaccination in patients with metastatic breast cancer. J Clin Oncol 2009; 27: 4685–92.
3. Rosenberg SA. Progress in human tumour immunology and immunotherapy. Nature 2001; 411: 380–4.
4. Hogquist KA, Baldwin TA, Jameson SC. Central tolerance: learning self-control in the thymus. Nat Rev Immunol 2005; 5: 772–82.
5. Mueller DL. Mechanisms maintaining peripheral tolerance. Nat Immunol 2010; 11: 21–7.
6. Wu Y, Zheng Z, Jiang Y, et al. The specificity of T cell regulation that enables self-nonself discrimination in the periphery. Proc Natl Acad Sci USA 2009; 106: 534–9.
7. Jiang H, Wu Y, Liang B, et al. An affinity/avidity model of peripheral T cell regulation. J Clin Invest 2005; 115: 302–12.
8. Wing K, Sakaguchi S. Regulatory T cells exert checks and balances on self tolerance and autoimmunity. Nat Immunol 2010; 11: 7–13.
9. Shevach EM. Mechanisms of foxp3+ T regulatory cell-mediated suppression. Immunity 2009; 30: 636–45.
10. Vignali DA, Collison LW, Workman CJ. How regulatory T cells work. Nat Rev Immunol 2008; 8: 523–32.
11. Tang Q, Bluestone JA. The Foxp3+ regulatory T cell: a jack of all trades, master of regulation. Nat Immunol 2008; 9: 239–44.
12. Torres-Aguilar H, Sanchez-Torres C, Jara LJ, et al. IL-10/TGF-beta-treated dendritic cells, pulsed with insulin, specifically reduce the response to insulin of CD4+ effector/memory T cells from type 1 diabetic individuals. J Clin Immunol 2010; 30: 659–68.
13. Zou W. Regulatory T cells, tumour immunity and immunotherapy. Nat Rev Immunol 2006; 6: 295–307.
14. Lustgarten J, Dominguez AL, Cuadros C. The CD8+ T cell repertoire against Her-2/neu antigens in neu transgenic mice is of low avidity with antitumor activity. Eur J Immunol 2004; 34: 752–61.
15. Zehn D, Bevan MJ. T cells with low avidity for a tissue-restricted antigen routinely evade central and peripheral tolerance and cause autoimmunity. Immunity 2006; 25: 261–70.
16. Salazar LG, Fikes J, Southwood S, et al. Immunization of cancer patients with HER-2/neu-derived peptides demonstrating high-affinity binding to multiple class II alleles. Clin Cancer Res 2003; 9: 5559–65.
17. Park KH, Gad E, Goodell V, et al. Insulin-like growth factor-binding protein-2 is a target for the immunomodulation of breast cancer. Cancer Res 2008; 68: 8400–9.
18. Depontieu FR, Qian J, Zarling AL, et al. Identification of tumor-associated, MHC class II-restricted phosphopeptides as targets for immunotherapy. Proc Natl Acad Sci USA 2009; 106: 12073–8.
19. Reche PA, Reinherz EL. Sequence variability analysis of human class I and class II MHC molecules: functional and structural correlates of amino acid polymorphisms. J Mol Biol 2003; 331: 623–41.
20. Matsumura M, Fremont DH, Peterson PA, et al. Emerging principles for the recognition of peptide antigens by MHC class I molecules. Science 1992; 257: 927–34.
21. Zhang C, Anderson A, DeLisi C. Structural principles that govern the peptide-binding motifs of class I MHC molecules. J Mol Biol 1998; 281: 929–47.
22. Precopio ML, Butterfield TR, Casazza JP, et al. Optimizing peptide matrices for identifying T-cell antigens. Cytometry A 2008; 73: 1071–8.

23. Larsen MV, Lundegaard C, Lamberth K, et al. Large-scale validation of methods for cytotoxic T-lymphocyte epitope prediction. BMC Bioinformatics 2007; 8: 424.

24. Lafuente EM, Reche PA. Prediction of MHC-peptide binding: a systematic and comprehensive overview. Curr Pharm Des 2009; 15: 3209–20.

25. Tang Y, Lin Z, Ni B, et al. An altered peptide ligand for naive cytotoxic T lymphocyte epitope of TRP-2(180-188) enhanced immunogenicity. Cancer Immunol Immunother 2007; 56: 319–29.

26. Dionne SO, Myers CE, Smith MH, et al. Her-2/ neu altered peptide ligand-induced CTL responses: implications for peptides with increased HLA affinity and T-cell-receptor interaction. Cancer Immunol Immunother 2004; 53: 307–14.

27. Menez-Jamet J, Kosmatopoulos K. Development of optimized cryptic peptides for immunotherapy. IDrugs 2009; 12: 98–102.

28. Parkhurst MR, Riley JP, Robbins PF, et al. Induction of CD4+ Th1 lymphocytes that recognize known and novel class II MHC restricted epitopes from the melanoma antigen gp100 by stimulation with recombinant protein. J Immunother 2004; 27: 79–91.

29. Abdul-Alim CS, Li Y, Yee C. Conditional superagonist CTL ligands for the promotion of tumor-specific CTL responses. J Immunol 2010; 184: 6514–21.

30. Bolonaki I, Kotsakis A, Papadimitraki E, et al. Vaccination of patients with advanced non-small-cell lung cancer with an optimized cryptic human telomerase reverse transcriptase peptide. J Clin Oncol 2007; 25: 2727–34.

31. Cecco S, Muraro E, Giacomin E, et al. Cancer vaccines in phase II/III clinical trials: state of the art and future perspectives. Curr Cancer Drug Targets 2010; 31: 85–102.

32. Peoples GE, Holmes JP, Hueman MT, et al. Combined clinical trial results of a HER2/neu (E75) vaccine for the prevention of recurrence in high-risk breast cancer patients: U.S. Military Cancer Institute Clinical Trials Group Study I-01 and I-02. Clin Cancer Res 2008; 14: 797–803.

33. Sosman JA, Carrillo C, Urba WJ, et al. Three phase II cytokine working group trials of gp100 (210M) peptide plus high-dose interleukin-2 in patients with HLA-A2-positive advanced melanoma. J Clin Oncol 2008; 26: 2292–8.

34. Hodi FS, O'Day SJ, McDermott DF, et al. Improved survival with ipilimumab in patients with metastatic melanoma. N Engl J Med 2010; 363: 711–23.

35. Testori A, Richards J, Whitman E, et al. Phase III comparison of vitespen, an autologous tumor-derived heat shock protein gp96 peptide complex vaccine, with physician's choice of treatment for stage IV melanoma: the C-100-21 Study Group. J Clin Oncol 2008; 26: 955–62.

36. Baxevanis CN, Voutsas IF, Tsitsilonis OE, et al. Tumor-specific CD4+ T lymphocytes from cancer patients are required for optimal induction of cytotoxic T cells against the autologous tumor. J Immunol 2000; 164: 3902–12.

37. Gao FG, Khammanivong V, Liu WJ, et al. Antigen-specific CD4+ T-cell help is required to activate a memory CD8+ T cell to a fully functional tumor killer cell. Cancer Res 2002; 62: 6438–41.

38. Shedlock DJ, Shen H. Requirement for CD4 T cell help in generating functional CD8 T cell memory. Science 2003; 300: 337–9.

39. Wong SB, Bos R, Sherman LA. Tumor-specific CD4+ T cells render the tumor environment permissive for infiltration by low-avidity CD8+ T cells. J Immunol 2008; 180: 3122–31.

40. Fallarino F, Grohmann U, Bianchi R, et al. Th1 and Th2 cell clones to a poorly immunogenic tumor antigen initiate CD8+ T cell-dependent tumor eradication in vivo. J Immunol 2000; 165: 5495–501.

41. Surman DR, Dudley ME, Overwijk WW, et al. Cutting edge: CD4+ T cell control of CD8+ T cell reactivity to a model tumor antigen. J Immunol 2000; 164: 562–5.

42. Liu Z, Noh HS, Chen J, et al. Potent tumor-specific protection ignited by adoptively transferred CD4+ T cells. J Immunol 2008; 181: 4363–70.

43. Darrah PA, Patel DT, De Luca PM, et al. Multifunctional TH1 cells define a correlate of vaccine-mediated protection against Leishmania major. Nat Med 2007; 13: 843–50.

44. Giuntoli RL, 2nd, Lu J, Kobayashi H, et al. Direct costimulation of tumor-reactive CTL by helper T cells potentiate their proliferation, survival, and effector function. Clin Cancer Res 2002; 8: 922–31.

45. Wu CY, Kirman JR, Rotte MJ, et al. Distinct lineages of T(H)1 cells have differential capacities for memory cell generation in vivo. Nat Immunol 2002; 3: 852–8.

46. Butterfield LH, Ribas A, Dissette VB, et al. Determinant spreading associated with clinical response in dendritic cell-based immunotherapy for malignant melanoma. Clin Cancer Res 2003; 9: 998–1008.

47. Wang P, Sidney J, Dow C, et al. A systematic assessment of MHC class II peptide binding predictions and evaluation of a consensus approach. PLoS Comput Biol 2008; 4: e1000048.

48. Gowthaman U, Agrewala JN. In silico tools for predicting peptides binding to HLA-class II molecules: more confusion than conclusion. J Proteome Res 2008; 7: 154–63.

49. Nuber N, Curioni-Fontecedro A, Matter C, et al. Fine analysis of spontaneous MAGE-C1/CT7-specific immunity in melanoma patients. Proc Natl Acad Sci USA 2010; 107: 15187–92.

50. Tsuji T, Altorki NK, Ritter G, et al. Characterization of preexisting MAGE-A3-specific CD4+ T cells in cancer patients and healthy individuals and their activation by protein vaccination. J Immunol 2009; 183: 4800–8.

51. Perez SA, von Hofe E, Kallinteris NL, et al. A new era in anticancer peptide vaccines. Cancer 2010; 116: 2071–80.

52. Fioretti D, Iurescia S, Fazio VM, et al. DNA vaccines: developing new strategies against cancer. J Biomed Biotechnol 2010; 2010: 174378.

53. Melief CJ, van der Burg SH. Immunotherapy of established (pre)malignant disease by synthetic long peptide vaccines. Nat Rev Cancer 2008; 8: 351–60.

54. Sampson JH, Heimberger AB, Archer GE, et al. Immunologic escape after prolonged progression-free survival with epidermal growth factor receptor variant III peptide vaccination in patients with newly diagnosed glioblastoma. J Clin Oncol 2010; 28: 4722–9.

55. Kenter GG, Welters MJ, Valentijn AR, et al. Vaccination against HPV-16 oncoproteins for vulvar intraepithelial neoplasia. N Engl J Med 2009; 361: 1838–47.

56. Jandus C, Bioley G, Dojcinovic D, et al. Tumor antigen-specific FOXP3+ CD4 T cells identified in human metastatic melanoma: peptide vaccination results in selective expansion of Th1-like counterparts. Cancer Res 2009; 69: 8085–93.

57. Rink R, Arkema-Meter A, Baudoin I, et al. To protect peptide pharmaceuticals against peptidases. J Pharmacol Toxicol Methods 2010; 61: 210–18.

58. Johansson P, Lindgren T, Lundstrom M, et al. PCR-generated linear DNA fragments utilized as a hantavirus DNA vaccine. Vaccine 2002; 20: 3379–88.

59. Schakowski F, Gorschluter M, Junghans C, et al. A novel minimal-size vector (MIDGE) improves transgene expression in colon carcinoma cells and avoids transfection of undesired DNA. Mol Ther 2001; 3: 793–800.

60. Becker JT, Olson BM, Johnson LE, et al. DNA vaccine encoding prostatic acid phosphatase (PAP) elicits long-term T-cell responses in patients with recurrent prostate cancer. J Immunother 2010; 33: 639–47.

61. Norell H, Poschke I, Charo J, et al. Vaccination with a plasmid DNA encoding HER-2/neu together with low doses of GM-CSF and IL-2 in patients with metastatic breast carcinoma: a pilot clinical trial. J Transl Med 2010; 8: 53.

62. Salazar LG, Slota M, Wallace D, et al. A phase I study of a DNA plasmid based vaccine encoding the HER2/neu (HER2) intracellular domain (ICD) in subjects with HER2+ breast cancer. J Clin Oncol 2009; 27: 15s:abstract 3054.

63. Lucansky V, Sobotkova E, Tachezy R, et al. DNA vaccination against bcr-abl-positive cells in mice. Int J Oncol 2009; 35: 941–51.

64. Bei R, Scardino A. TAA polyepitope DNA-based vaccines: a potential tool for cancer therapy. J Biomed Biotechnol 2010; 2010: 102758.

65. Velders MP, Weijzen S, Eiben GL, et al. Defined flanking spacers and enhanced proteolysis is essential for eradication of established tumors by an epitope string DNA vaccine. J Immunol 2001; 166: 5366–73.

66. Dobano C, Rogers WO, Gowda K, et al. Targeting antigen to MHC Class I and Class II antigen presentation pathways for malaria DNA vaccines. Immunol Lett. 2007; 111: 92–102.

67. Rodriguez F, An LL, Harkins S, et al. DNA immunization with minigenes: low frequency of memory cytotoxic T lymphocytes and inefficient antiviral protection are rectified by ubiquitination. J Virol 1998; 72: 5174–81.

68. Bazhan SI, Karpenko LI, Ilyicheva TN, et al. Rational design based synthetic polyepitope DNA vaccine for eliciting HIV-specific CD8+ T cell responses. Mol Immunol 2010; 47: 1507–15.

69. Ishioka GY, Fikes J, Hermanson G, et al. Utilization of MHC class I transgenic mice for development of minigene DNA vaccines encoding multiple HLA-restricted CTL epitopes. J Immunol 1999; 162: 3915–25.

70. Rodriguez F, Zhang J, Whitton JL. DNA immunization: ubiquitination of a viral protein enhances cytotoxic T-lymphocyte induction and antiviral protection but abrogates antibody induction. J Virol 1997; 71: 8497–503.

71. Cardinaud S, Bouziat R, Rohrlich PS, et al. Design of a HIV-1-derived HLA-B07.02-restricted polyepitope construct. AIDS 2009; 23: 1945–54.

72. Wang QM, Sun SH, Hu ZL, et al. Epitope DNA vaccines against tuberculosis: spacers and ubiquitin modulates cellular immune responses elicited by epitope DNA vaccine. Scand J Immunol 2004; 60: 219–25.

73. Vidalin O, Tanaka E, Spengler U, et al. Targeting of hepatitis C virus core protein for MHC I or MHC II presentation does not enhance induction of immune responses to DNA vaccination. DNA Cell Biol 1999; 18: 611–21.
74. Wu TC, Guarnieri FG, Staveley-O'Carroll KF, et al. Engineering an intracellular pathway for major histocompatibility complex class II presentation of antigens. Proc Natl Acad Sci USA 1995; 92: 11671–5.
75. Niazi KR, Ochoa MT, Sieling PA, et al. Activation of human CD4+ T cells by targeting MHC class II epitopes to endosomal compartments using human CD1 tail sequences. Immunology 2007; 122: 522–31.
76. Wu A, Zeng Q, Kang TH, et al. Innovative DNA vaccine for human papillomavirus (HPV)-associated head and neck cancer. Gene Ther 2011; 18: 304–12.
77. Teramoto K, Kontani K, Ozaki Y, et al. Deoxyribonucleic acid (DNA) encoding a pan-major histocompatibility complex class II peptide analogue augmented antigen-specific cellular immunity and suppressive effects on tumor growth elicited by DNA vaccine immunotherapy. Cancer Res 2003; 63: 7920–5.
78. Sato Y, Roman M, Tighe H, et al. Immunostimulatory DNA sequences necessary for effective intradermal gene immunization. Science 1996; 273: 352–4.
79. Yu Q, Li J, Zhang X, et al. Induction of immune responses in mice by a DNA vaccine encoding Cryptosporidium parvum Cp12 and Cp21 and its effect against homologous oocyst challenge. Vet Parasitol 2010; 172: 1–7.
80. Chackerian B. Virus-like particles: flexible platforms for vaccine development. Expert Rev Vaccines 2007; 6: 381–90.
81. Jennings GT, Bachmann MF. The coming of age of virus-like particle vaccines. Biol Chem 2008; 389: 521–36.
82. Ludwig C, Wagner R. Virus-like particles-universal molecular toolboxes. Curr Opin Biotechnol 2007; 18: 537–45.
83. Peek LJ, Middaugh CR, Berkland C. Nanotechnology in vaccine delivery. Adv Drug Deliv Rev 2008; 60: 915–28.
84. Kratz PA, Bottcher B, Nassal M. Native display of complete foreign protein domains on the surface of hepatitis B virus capsids. Proc Natl Acad Sci USA 1999; 96: 1915–20.
85. Tissot AC, Renhofa R, Schmitz N, et al. Versatile virus-like particle carrier for epitope based vaccines. PLoS One 2010; 5: e9809.

11 | Emerging clinical trial design concepts for therapeutic cancer vaccines

Cristina Musselli, Leah Isakov, and Kerry Wentworth

INTRODUCTION

Over the past decade a series of phase III clinical trials in cancer vaccinology has come to an end showing a disappointingly high rate of failure. Irrespective of this lack of success, the promise of cancer vaccine therapy has remained strong and has led various stakeholders (academia, industry, regulators, and so on) to closely examine the reasons for past trial failures. In this process it has become evident that a major limitation rested in the status quo rules for planning and evaluating clinical trials, which was mainly based on the development paradigm from cytoreductive chemotherapy.

Recognizing that new "rules of the road" were needed to support successful cancer vaccine development, a productive debate and collaboration has been growing resulting in mounting literature and interest in creating novel strategies that are specific to the development and evaluation of cancer vaccines. A number of associations (Cancer Immunotherapy Consortium-Cancer Research Institute [CIC-CRI], Association for Cancer Immunotherapy [C-IMT] and Biomarker Consortium) have pursued a series of initiatives leading to the creation of key recommendations in the field. Further to this and most importantly, Food and Drug Administration (FDA) recently published two draft guidelines that serve as crucial references for directing future cancer vaccine development: "Guidance for Industry: Clinical Considerations for Therapeutic Cancer Vaccines" (1) and "Guidance for Industry: Co-Development of Two or More Unmarketed Investigational Drugs for Use in Combination" (2).

In summary, the collective recommendations can be subdivided into three major areas:

1. *Surrogate marker of efficacy*: monitoring cellular immune response as a reliable biomarker. This has proved more difficult than initially anticipated due to intricacies of assay methodologies and variability in results. These issues are actively being addressed through the development of harmonization guidelines, which aim to bring consistency in the application and reporting of immune assays that handles the diversity of cancer vaccine constructs and the complexity of the different immune responses elicited.
2. *Clinical/immunological criteria to evaluate efficacy*: Immunotherapy induces a novel pattern of anti-tumor responses that are not adequately captured in traditional RECIST criteria. To this end, immune-related response criteria (3,4) have been proposed.
3. *Clinical trial designs and statistical methods taking into account the mechanism of action of cancer vaccines*: To this end, there is a strong emphasis on the importance of patient selection criteria, selection of primary and secondary efficacy endpoints, and using the statistical methodology that accounts for the unique efficacy pattern of cancer vaccines.

These recommendations are derived from real-life experience and from the post-hoc analysis of a series of different "failed" clinical trials (5). The challenges today remain in the correct implementation of these guidelines and the use of an ethical and medically correct creative strategy which will allow for the approval of a safe, strongly needed therapy of cancer that cancer vaccines can provide.

IMMUNE RESPONSE: A KEY FEATURE IN CLINICAL TRIALS

The ability to establish a reliable correlation between immune response and clinical efficacy (i.e., establishing a validated surrogate biomarker) will undoubtedly represent a major achievement toward optimizing and streamlining the future of cancer vaccine clinical trials. While their remains debate about the ultimate meaning and value of measuring immune response in the peripheral and local compartments, nonetheless, there is increasing emphasis on the need to incorporate immune measurements across cancer vaccine clinical trials. Only through a continued application of immunoassays will the field ever achieve the ultimate goal of elevating immune response to the level of a validated surrogate biomarker.

Before the above can become a reality, it is first necessary to develop valid assay methodologies to measure immune response. In a series of initiatives led by the Cancer Immunotherapy Consortium, the harmonization of the enzyme-linked immunosorbent spot (ELISPOT) assay (6,7), Tetramer assay, Intracellular Cytokine Staining is on its way. For all assays it would be desirable to define *a priori* the limit of detection, range of positivity, and meaning of response in order to define a true responder to a given vaccine therapy. This is often difficult to implement when the vaccine components cannot be well characterized, such as in the case of autologous vaccines. Hence, the only way to define a range within which an immune response is significant is to obtain samples from vaccinated subjects.

Such a challenge is currently being addressed in a phase 2 trial of tumor-derived HSPPC-96, specifically designed to evaluate immune response over multiple time points in the adjuvant renal cell carcinoma (RCC) setting (NCT 01147536). This trial incorporates a two-part design whereby the first part designates a cohort of 10 patients whose leukapheresis/PBMC samples will be used to establish the immunoassay conditions (the enzyme-linked immunosorbent spot) as well as establish the criteria for defining a "positive immune responder." It is these criteria that will be applied in a prospective manner for determining an immune responder in the second part of the trial. Specifically, the second part of the trial aims to enroll 40 patients who will serve as the main cohort for demonstrating immune response. This patient group will be treated with vaccine for three months at which point the group will then be randomized into two arms: one arm will receive two additional vaccine doses at months 6 and 12 while the other arm will receive placebo injections at months 6 and 12. This mid-study randomized design feature allows for assessing the durability and potential boosting effect of subsequent vaccinations.

This provides an example of, in essence, a two-stage trial design that uses one patient cohort to generate the set of criteria and a second cohort upon which to validate those criteria. This type of trial design could also be useful in investigating the dose and schedule as well as in providing a sense of the time needed to illicit a robust immune response, which could be later contemplated into statistical modeling accounting for delay in treatment effect. At the minimum, a careful study of immune response to a given vaccine should be undertaken (8).

Positive immune response results based on appropriate, qualified assay methodology provides evidence of biological activity and should represent an important evidence-based data point for making a go no-go decision toward embarking into late-phase clinical trials. Further, well-defined immune response criteria established in earlier trials can be carried forward into later phase trials where a correlation with tumor response and clinical response can be definitively tested.

CLINICAL TRIAL DESIGN, SELECTION OF THE RIGHT POPULATION AND EFFICACY ENDPOINTS

Clinical trial design is the basis for the success of the designated treatment. In a scenario of endless resources, one would design multiple early phase studies in parallel in order to answer as many questions as possible before entering the late-phase development. Unfortunately, clinical trials are expensive and often resources face the end quickly, especially in the case of innovative technologies and small biotechnology companies.

In order for cancer vaccines to successfully become available, some key criteria for improving clinical trial outcomes have been identified.

- *Patient selection criteria*. It is generally well accepted that cancer vaccines have the greatest promise as single agents in adjuvant and/or minimal residual disease settings. However, given that trials in adjuvant/minimal residual disease situation can be large, long, and expensive, there remain strong forces that push cancer vaccines to late-stage tumor settings. Thankfully, emerging science in tumor immunology coupled with advancements in the development of targeted antibodies, such as anti-CTLA-4ab, is providing a promising future for successful application of cancer vaccines in combination therapy regimens used in late-stage disease. Therefore, it is vital that any clinical trial design with a cancer vaccine be given a critical thought to the disease setting and decide whether a single agent or a combination strategy is the best. This topic is given further attention in the subsequent text.

- *Choice of control*: Most of the current oncology-based clinical trials employ an active control in their design. In situations where superiority design of single-agent cancer vaccine therapy against an active control is being contemplated, it is important to consider whether time to initiation of treatment could differ between the two arms. For example, in the case of autologous vaccines there is generally a time lag associated with initiating treatment due to manufacturing requirements, which will not likely be the case in the active control arm. This could result in the time taken from randomization to treatment initiation to differ significantly between the two arms. This is further compounded by the fact that once a cancer vaccine is administered it will take time to work. Once again, given the nature of the cancer vaccine and its expected biological activity, it is important to consider in the case of a controlled study design whether a single-agent strategy or a combination strategy is the best. In addition, in order not to bias one of the study arms, careful consideration needs to be given to any time to event calculation to assess whether this should be from randomization, or from surgery (if applicable), or after a period of time sufficient to produce a robust immune response.

- *Choice of efficacy endpoints*: Overall survival is considered the "gold standard" endpoint for oncology trials and is generally the endpoint of choice for assessing the efficacy of cancer vaccines. To this end, use of a dichotomous outcome for proportion of patients surviving at a particular clinically relevant point of time can be a good option; however, for long trials with a lot of censoring, results can be misleading. Recurrence-free survival and time to disease progression are also often used as primary efficacy endpoints, but again have proved to be less successful than overall survival. Widely used in solid tumors, RECIST criteria turn out to be problematic in assessing responses to a cancer vaccine therapy as they do not account for the novel pattern of anti-tumor responses. Instead, immune-related response criteria (3,4,9) have been proposed although not yet widely accepted. In addition, any employment of tumor response criteria is futile in the adjuvant setting as there is generally no measurable disease at the time of initiating vaccine treatment. Until there is a greater acceptance of the proposed irR criteria for assessing tumor responses, the overall survival will likely remain the endpoint of choice.

- *Statistical design*: The time needed to elicit a clinically effective anti-tumor response can lead to a specific violation of proportionality assumption for survival analysis that can occur when the treatment under investigation demonstrates a delayed effect. Standard and widely used statistical survival analysis methods applied without taking delayed treatment effect into account have low power and may underestimate the overall treatment effect. An increase of sample size may help to overcome the issue, but it requires a longer enrollment period and means an additional burden to the sponsor of such a trial. Where it is expected that the treatment under investigation will demonstrate a delayed effect such as in cancer vaccines, during the design of such a trial, considerable care must be taken with the planned statistical analysis as it may involve a much longer follow-up time. Among many proposed models that will apply to trials like these, one could be Cox proportional model with treatment effects modeled as time-dependent covariates. This method demonstrates good operation characteristics. The biggest limitation of this method is that it requires knowledge of time to delayed effect. A nonparametric model that doesn't have this limitation, albeit it has others, is the weighted log rank test which could apply to this clinical design.

Additionally, the current knowledge base around targeted therapies has shed light and imposed a shift in the way the efficacy of treatment is analyzed. This experience has revealed that patients with certain gene profiles may differ in how they respond to treatment. However, it is generally unknown what these profiles will be until the trial is under way. This has made the use of prospective subset analyses more widely accepted, if not imperative, focusing on the qualitative interaction that occurs between a positive drug effect for a subset and a zero drug effect for the complementary set of patients (10,11). Therefore, it is critical to prospectively describe and provide supporting rationale for any envisioned subset analyses.

CONSIDERATIONS FOR COMBINATION VERSUS SINGLE-AGENT CLINICAL TRIAL DESIGNS

As described above, proper patient selection in a cancer vaccine clinical trial is paramount towards its success. No longer is the "all comers" approach viable. Based on where in the continuum of disease one decides to study their cancer vaccine candidate, a determination of whether to study the investigational agent as a monotherapy or in combination needs to be carefully assessed.

A look at the current landscape of cancer vaccine clinical trials reveals that academia and industry have taken heed of past failures and become much smarter about truly optimizing trials for success. To this end two clear pathways have emerged:

1. Single-agent cancer vaccine development strategies have largely shifted away from metastatic disease to the adjuvant/low tumor burden settings. Illustrative of this are the three major randomized phase III trials currently underway: EMD Serono's Stimuvax® in stage III NSCLC (NCT00409188), GSK's vaccine candidate GSK1572932A in adjuvant NSCLC (NCT00480025), and GSK2132231A in patients with melanoma who are rendered disease free subsequent to surgery (NCT00796445). The GSK vaccine candidate is also referred to as the MAGE-A3 vaccine. In addition to optimizing the population through a selection of patient groups with no to low tumor burden, GSK is further narrowing the population to only those who show expression of the MAGE-A3 gene. This strategy of selecting patients on the basis of a potential predictive classifier provides another level of "super-targeting" the population and should only stand to enhance the chances of a successful outcome. The Stivumax® trial selects patients not on the basis of a biological classifier; instead, to enhance the chances of vaccine efficacy through first treating patients with a single infusion of cyclophosphamide.

    While these trial examples adopt many of the lessons learned from the past and represent patient groups where treatment benefit could translate into cures, these do not currently represent viable development strategies for most endeavoring in this field. The statistics are staggering: patient sample sizes range from 1300 to 2300 and trial length spans over 6–10 years. Therefore, it is fair to conclude that the right tools to make this task feasible from a financial and practical point of view still need to be developed. However, much will stand to be learned from the outcomes of these important trials.

2. New combination cancer vaccine development strategies have emerged to encourage trials in late-stage disease. As previously mentioned, emerging science in tumor immunology coupled with advancements in the development of novel targeted antibodies, such as anti-CTLA-4ab, is providing a promising future for successful application of cancer vaccines in combination therapy regimens in late-stage disease. In addition, research on the immune effects of well-established commercially available products, such as cyclophosphamide, temozolomide, and sunitinib, have also helped to advance trials in late-stage settings or in highly aggressive tumor types such as glioma.

    Given that the scientific basis for chemo and targeted agent combinations with cancer vaccines is still in an adolescent phase, there are examples of later-phase trials that are already taking this innovative strategy forward: Immatics is in phase III trials with IMA901 (plus GM-CSF) in combination with sunitinib in metastatic RCC (NCT01265901). The primary endpoint for this trial is overall survival; however, they have clearly described a secondary endpoint to be analyzed based on a subgroup of patients who have a prospectively defined primary bio-marker signature, believed to be predictive of improved clinical outcome with IMA901 (not described). In contrast to the trial size and time demands of an adjuvant trial, the Immatics study describes a sample size of 330 patients with a trial length of four years. In another trial, Argos is following a similar combination strategy with sunitinib with their vaccine candidate AGS-003, but in newly diagnosed metastatic RCC (NCT00678119).

The real explosion in innovative combination clinical trial design and execution is expected when broad commercial access to anti-CTLA-4ab is available. This will provide an exciting "model system" for using cancer vaccines that work through activating T-cells with an agent that directly blocks a key signal, which prevents that activation. Key considerations around trial designs with anti-CTLA-4ab and any other agents will be related to dose and schedule of each agent combined in order to optimize the effect on the immune system.

Anti-CTLA-4ab represents just one of multiple agents that target regulatory T-cell path-ways and potentially offer synergy with cancer vaccines. With the advent of FDA's recently published guidance for industry on the co-development of two or more unmarketed investiga-tional drugs for use in combination (2), there is now a clearer regulatory path to designing trials and setting out the development expectations of combining two investigational agents. Unfor-tunately, a major impediment toward executing combination clinical trials remains on the busi-ness side and will require companies to break out of traditional business development models for the betterment of cancer treatment.

As we look further down the telescope towards the next generation of clinical trial designs, the cancer vaccine field should keep watch on the two initiatives undertaken by the Government/Academia and by the Biomarker Consortium.

In the first case the Department of Defense funded the so called BATTLE – Biomarkers-Integrated Approaches of Targeted Therapy for Lung Cancer Elimination – a series of phase II trials run at MDACC. All the study subjects had metastatic NSCLC refractory to chemother-apy. This initiative uses an adaptive design called "umbrella protocol," which required each patient to undergo biopsy at enrollment and tumor samples to be checked for 11 biomarkers. In all, 255 patients were enrolled and equally random assigned in a first group of 97 subjects and the remaining 158 adaptively randomized to receive one of four treatments for NSCLC (erlotinib, sorafenib, vandetanib, and erlotinib with bexarotene). At the 8 weeks endpoint, patients were assessed for disease control, and statistical analysis was used to determine which biomarkers were associated with benefit. At this stage the adaptive phase was initiated where treatments were based on biomarker testing – that is, patients received a second biopsy and depending on their profile were assigned to drugs that had proven effective in the first phase—patients with similar tumor biomarkers. At the end of 8 weeks, 46% of the patients in the trial experienced disease control versus the historical 30%. This is believed to be the first clinical trial in NSCLC aimed at developing a panel of biomarkers in a real-time fashion, and the inves-tigators at MDACC are planning BATTLE 2 and BATTLE 3 follow-up trials to confirm the encouraging results (12).

The Biomarker Consortium (composed by drug developers as in pharmaceutical and bio-technology companies, NIH, FDA, and patients groups) designed the so called I-SPY trials (13). This initiative is using a highly adaptive clinical design as a way to test in parallel several dif-ferent drugs in women with locally advanced breast cancer in the neoadjuvant setting. To this end, a regimen that shows a high Bayesian predictive probability of being more effective than standard therapy will graduate from the trial with their corresponding biomarker signature. At the same time, regimens that fail will be dropped. In both cases a drug that exits the study will be substituted with a new drug, which depends solely on the patient accrual rate. Drugs that graduate along with their biomarker signature will proceed to be tested in smaller phase III trials and their predictive probability will be provided to the company for all signatures tested.

The overall design will feature two arms of standard neoadjuvant chemotherapy regimen +/– Herceptin depending on HER2 positivity. In the other arms, five new drugs, each being added to the standard therapy, will be tested in parallel. On the basis of statistical modeling, a minimum of 20 patients to a maximum of 120 patients will be tested for each drug. The primary endpoint will be pathologic complete response at surgery, and patients will be also followed for disease-free and overall survival for up to 10 years. The biomarkers used for the purpose, include the standard biomarkers (FDA approved), as well as the qualifying (not yet approved by FDA) and exploratory biomarkers.

A major endeavor taken by this effort relies on the complexity of the adaptive design statistical plan that allows for the selection of an active regimen quickly and to learn over time which profiles predict response to each drug, and the introduction of a sophisticated informatics portal developed for I-SPY 1. This portal is a model of multidisciplinary collaboration that will categorize, integrate, and interpret a massive amount of information (genomics, proteomics, pathology, and imaging) under the auspices of the Center for Biomedical Informatics and Information Technology.

In summary, the aim of the study is to predict drug responsiveness based on the presence or absence of genetic and biological markers in nearly real time; it is also evaluating tumor response to multiple investigational drugs, albeit not in combination but used in series. The success of this project is based upon the commitment by all stakeholders to share the information and openly collaborate in testing different therapies.

This is an example of how a targeted therapy can develop in a more expedite manner. This is also an example of how such a capillary experiment can only be performed in collaboration with several parties and when governmental entities are involved in the coordination and funding of the initiative. A hypothetical initiative that could mirror the I-SPY 2 effort would be in the application of vaccines on top of a series of combination agents that span from chemotherapeutic to other biologics.

We all agree that the ultimate goal is to treat cancer patients safely and possibly find a cure expeditiously. We can only take the I-SPY 2 example as a model for future similar activities involving cancer vaccines.

REFERENCES

1. U.S. Food and Drug Administration. Draft Guidance for Industry: Clinical Considerations for Therapeutic Cancer Vaccines Sept. 2009.
2. U.S. Food and Drug Administration. Guidance for industry - codevelopment of two or more unmarketed investigational drugs for use in combination. Dec. 2010.
3. Wolchok JD, Hoos A, O'Day S, et al. Guidelines for the evaluation of immune therapy activity in solid tumors: immune-related response criteria. Clin Cancer Res 2009; 15: 7412–20.
4. Hoos A, Eggermont AM, Janetzki S, et al. Improved endpoints for cancer immunotherapy trials. J Natl Cancer Inst 2010; 102: 1388–97.
5. Finke LH, Wentworth K, Blumenstein B, et al. Lessons from randomized phase III studies with active cancer immunotherapies--outcomes from the 2006 meeting of the Cancer Vaccine Consortium (CVC). Vaccine 2007; 25(Suppl 2): B97–109.
6. Janetzki S, Panageas KS, Ben-Porat L, et al. Results and harmonization guidelines from two large-scale international Elispot proficiency panels conducted by the Cancer Vaccine Consortium (CVC/SVI). Cancer Immunol Immunother 2008; 57: 303–15.
7. Britten CM, Janetzki S, Ben-Porat L, et al. Harmonization guidelines for HLA-peptide multimer assays derived from results of a large scale international proficiency panel of the Cancer Vaccine Consortium. Cancer Immunol Immunother 2009; 58: 1701–13.
8. Hoos A, Parmiani G, Hege K, et al. A clinical development paradigm for cancer vaccines and related biologics. J Immunother 2007; 30: 1–15.
9. Berry DA. The hazards of endpoints. J Natl Cancer Inst 2010; 102: 1376–7.
10. Schellens JH, Beijnen JH. Novel clinical trial designs for innovative therapies. Clin Pharmacol Ther 2009; 85: 212–16.
11. Simon R. New challenges for 21st century clinical trials. Clin Trials 2007; 4: 167–9; discussion 173–167.
12. Kim ES, et al. The BATTLE trial: personalizing therapy for lung cancer. Cancer Discovery 2011; 1: 1.
13. Barker AD, Sigman CC, Kelloff GJ, et al. I-SPY 2: an adaptive breast cancer trial design in the setting of neoadjuvant chemotherapy. Clin Pharmacol Ther 2009; 86: 97–100.

12 | T-cell immune monitoring assays to guide the development of new cancer vaccines

Cedrik M. Britten, Sylvia Janetzki, Cécile Gouttefangeas, Marij J. P. Welters, Michael Kalos, Christian Ottensmeier, Axel Hoos, and Sjoerd H. van der Burg

INTRODUCTION

The conceptual basis for therapeutic cancer vaccines was first established in studies that dealt with immunogenic tumor cell lines in mice, more than 25 years ago (1). Since then, a large body of data generated from mechanistic studies in animal models has confirmed that both vaccine-induced tumor-specific CD4+ T-helper (Th) type 1 and cytotoxic CD8+ T cells (CTL)—as well as B cells—play a major role in controlling tumor growth. Recent results obtained in patients have confirmed the conclusions from the animal models for the critical role of the immune system's response against tumors (2–4). Further evidence is provided by (*i*) long-term follow-up studies showing an increased incidence of cancer in immune-suppressed patients (5,6), (*ii*) clinical studies that provide evidence of clinical benefit of donor lymphocyte infusions after stem-cell transplantation and adoptive transfer of antigen-specific T cells (7,8), and (*iii*) studies on large numbers of patients with different tumor types showing that the presence of memory CD4+ Th1 and CTL in tumors is predictive of a beneficial clinical outcome (9,10).

The mechanistic data obtained in animal models and cancer patients support two major statements. First, in contrast to cytotoxic reagents, therapeutic cancer vaccines do not affect the tumor directly, but elicit their effect indirectly through the immune system, by immune activation and the resulting anti-tumor activity. Second, vaccine-induced T-cell responses play an important role in controlling tumor growth in vivo. Therefore, the development of novel cancer immunotherapy agents should be accompanied by the rational use of robust immune monitoring assays to evaluate the magnitude, breadth, and quality of vaccine-induced T-cell responses. If performed adequately, immunological monitoring will enable more effective clinical development of immunotherapeutic agents, lead to the identification of biomarkers that serve several clinical purposes, and also potentially allow identification of surrogate endpoints for clinical efficacy.

A SHORT INTRODUCTION TO THE MOST COMMONLY USED T-CELL IMMUNE MONITORING ASSAYS: THE TRIUMVIRATE

A plethora of in vitro assays are available for measuring the frequency and function of antigen-specific T cells. There is currently no gold standard assay for monitoring antigen-specific immune responses, but three assays are widely used: the enzyme linked immunospot (ELISPOT) assay, human leukocyte antigen (HLA) peptide multimer (MULTIMER) staining, and intracellular cytokine staining (ICS) by flow cytometry.

The ELISPOT assay was developed 25 years ago to quantify antigen-specific T cells (11). In most cases, interferon-gamma (IFNγ) secretion is the parameter assessed, although many other cytokines can be evaluated (12,13). The ELISPOT assay is mainly used as a monoparametric screening assay with its main advantages being robustness and sensitivity. Detection of antigen-specific T cells at frequencies of approximately 1 in 15,000–40,000 peripheral blood mononuclear cells (PBMCs) is possible (14–16). The ELISPOT assay and the analysis of raw data can be validated making it a prototype assay for compliance with good laboratory practice (17,18).

MULTIMER staining and ICS are flow cytometric methods used for monitoring vaccine-induced T cells. Both assays can usually detect approximately 1 specific cell in 2000–5000 T cells, with a technical limit of approximately 1 in 10,000 T cells (15,19–21). Test performance depends on various factors such as the quality of the cells, the number of events analyzed, the

Table 12.1 Major Characteristics of the Three Common T-Cell Monitoring Assays

Assay	Detection Range	Advantages	Limitations
IFNγ ELISPOT	0.005–0.002% of PBMC	• Functional assay • High throughput • Cost effective • Objective analysis criteria	• Mono-(Oligo)-parametric • No info on T-cell subset • No single-cell analysis
HLA-peptide MULTIMER	0.01–0.04% of CD8$^+$	• Independent of functional properties • Single-cell analysis • Multi-parametric • Accurate cell sorting	• No functional info • HLA restriction has to be known • Cost intensive • No objective analysis criteria
ICS	0.1–0.04% of CD8$^+$ or CD4$^+$	• Functional assay • Single-cell analysis • Multi-parametric	• Dependent on stimulation conditions • Cytokine production • No objective analysis criteria

Abbreviations: ELISPOT, the enzyme linked immunospot; HLA, human leukocyte antigen; ICS, intracellular cytokine staining; IFNγ, interferon-gamma; PBMC, peripheral blood mononuclear cells.

avidity of the relevant T-cell receptors, and the conditions of cell staining and stimulation (for ICS).

The MULTIMER (tetramer, pentamer, and dextramer) technology has constituted a breakthrough in the T-cell research field (22) and allows the reliable detection of antigen-specific T cells independent of functional attributes independent of prior ex vivo antigen-specific activation. MULTIMERS can be combined with various antibodies for phenotyping T-cell subsets. The technique has an intrinsic limitation that only responses to defined HLA-restricted epitopes can be evaluated. Moreover, HLA-class II MULTIMERS for characterizing CD4$^+$ cells are still rarely used. MULTIMERS are costly reagents and for this reason, they are preferentially used for monitoring small-scale trials that involve few patients and antigens.

ICS is a functional assay, through which the production of specific cytokines by T cells is evaluated following in vitro stimulation (23). In contrast to the MULTIMER staining platform, the antigenic specificities to be assessed are not limited by available detection reagents. As with ELISPOT, IFNγ is the preferred cytokine of measurement (24,25). A recent finding that the production of several cytokines by effector cells is associated with the fact that protective anti-pathogen T-cell immunity is moving the field toward multi-cytokine measurements (26).

In contrast to ELISPOT, an essential hurdle for establishing quality standards for flow cytometry is the subjectivity of the analysis, which until now remains largely dependent on the operator as highlighted by the results of recent proficiency panels (27,28). Initial guidelines have been proposed and an automated analysis of flow data is an active field of research (29,30).

The major advantages and limitations of ELISPOT, MULTIMER staining, and ICS are summarized in Table 12.1.

NEW TECHNOLOGIES AND TRENDS: "GETTING MAXIMUM INFORMATION FROM A SAMPLE"

One current trend in the field of immunological monitoring is to measure T-cell reactivity more comprehensively. Importantly, in most of the published reports, the detection of vaccine-induced T cells could not be directly associated with tumor response, as tested with any of the three basic assays (ELISPOT, MULTIMER, and ICS) alone. For this reason, the parallel use of two or more complementary assays, which aim at detecting different mechanistic aspects of the same biology, should be encouraged (31). A second trend is that scientists seek to obtain as much information per assay as possible. This holds true for all popular T-cell assays including multi-color ELISPOT (32,33) and multi-parametric flow cytometry (34–36). Due to recent technical advances in flow cytometry, which includes new hardware, software as well as innovative fluorochromes, comprehensive phenotyping (cell type and activation status) as well as functional assessment of T cells (cytokines and phosphorylation state of proteins involved in signal transduction) can now be assessed by using up to 18 colors in parallel. A single sample can now be analyzed with a combinatorial approach using 15–24 labeled MULTIMERS simultaneously. Multiplexing of MULTIMERS is reached by coupling each individual MULTIMER at to two positions with different fluorochromes, giving a set of unique dual-color codes. The total number of unique dual-color codes depends on the number of different fluorescent labels used. A set of combinatorial MULTIMERS labeled with four different colors at the first position and six different colors at the second position will allow for 24 unique combinations (4 × 6) using only 10 (4 + 6) different colors (37,38). A multiparametric flow cytometry in combination with a time-of-flight mass spectrometry (also called "single-cell mass cytometry") is being developed as a future assay to analyze a large number of markers (up to 75) in patient samples (39,40). The novelty of this assay is that fluorochromes are replaced by specially designed multi-atom elemental tags which can be detected with high resolution due to their differential chemical nature and avoid spillover and compensation problems inherent to fluorochromes. T-cell monitoring should be extended to the measurement of T-cell types that could interfere with therapy efficacy. One T-cell type that has been associated with vaccine failure is the population of regulatory CD4$^+$ T cells (CD4$^+$ T$_{REGS}$), which can be induced or boosted upon vaccination when these T cells recognize the antigen injected (41–43). Another population consists of antigen-specific CD8$^+$ T$_{REGS}$, which have a high capacity to inhibit the proliferation and function of cytotoxic effector T cells (44).

Finally, the measurement of T-cell reactivity in the circulation may not reflect the local response at the site of injection or inside the tumor; hence a better insight into the local biological events is needed. The use of fine needle aspirations and gene arrays or focused quantitative PCR arrays to assess the local in situ situation will form logical additions to current monitoring strategies. In breast cancer, colorectal cancer, and melanoma certain immunological gene expression signatures found in the tumors were reported to correlate with the clinical efficacy of immunotherapy (45–47).

IMMUNOGUIDING "A CONCEPT TO FACILITATE THE DEVELOPMENT OF IMMUNE THERAPY"

The concept of immunoguiding fosters the systematic use of comprehensive monitoring studies of immunological events in patients to understand the strengths, weaknesses, and efficacy of a new drug entity, and to use these results to steer decisions with respect to developmental aspects of the vaccine (43).

The constant interactions between the immune system and the tumor tissue that occur in any tumor patient shapes and/or edits an individual pre-existing immune state which is different to what can be presumed from animal tumor models. Such "edited" immunity could reflect tumor-specific CD4$^+$ Th1 and CD8$^+$ CTL responses, which are believed to be the most effective anti-tumor responses (47,48), but may also comprise functionally impaired or incorrectly polarized T cells, and even tumor-specific T$_{REGS}$.

Notably, the immunological monitoring should assess the presence, magnitude, and function of all (wanted or unwanted) subsets of T cells expected to respond to a treatment. This array of information, gathered by complementary assays, may explain the reasons for therapy being a success or failure and, consequently, point to weaknesses in the vaccine strategy. A clear example of this comes from a recent trial in which therapeutic vaccination resulted in the complete regression of premalignant high grade lesions of the vulva in about half of the treated patients (49). The combined results of at least four different immune assays show a clear-cut association between clinical success and the kinetics of the wanted immune response. In addition, the presence of vaccine-boosted T$_{REGS}$ could explain why the treatment failed in the other half of the patients (50). Notably, the logistical problems associated with obtaining the necessary materials—especially from target tissues—for such an in-depth immunological monitoring are numerous. Therefore, clinicians and vaccine developers are encouraged to implement the concept of immunoguiding at an early stage of protocol design. Clearly, a set of immune assays may allow the generation of hypotheses explaining why a clinical endpoint was (not) reached. However, immunological monitoring as a whole still lacks predictive power and it can be questioned whether such a point will ever be reached due to the complexity of tumor biology and (genetic) heterogeneity of individual patients. Still, good reasons to embrace the concept of immunoguiding prevail. A proficient understanding of the effects of a vaccine on the patient's immune system may encourage investigators to move forward into bigger randomized trials or to go one step back to optimize the vaccine or strategy used (43). In one example, the observation of immunogenic competition between two co-injected antigens was the rationale to call for a separation of these antigens in a subsequent trial (51). Similarly, the association between vaccine failure, large lesions, and T_{REGS} with each other (49,50) may prompt patient selection or alteration of the treatment strategy. Finally, researchers responsible for immunological monitoring of trials should actively pursue the validation of the most decision-impact assays in later stages of clinical development.

ASSAY HARMONIZATION "ENHANCING THE COMPARABILITY AND REPRODUCIBILITY OF ASSAYS"

The concept of assay harmonization includes the participation of individual laboratories in a consortium-based iterative testing process designed to identify variables which are critical for assay performance. As described earlier, a number of well-established assays are employed in the immune monitoring arena among which are the ELISPOT, MULTIMER staining, and ICS. While the core steps of these assays are being preserved and globally followed, an inevitable divergence in standard operating procedures (SOPs), reagents, and materials has occurred across the field, reflecting necessary adaptation to experimental requirements, local preferences, and availability of reagents, as well as the experience of scientists performing the assay. Not surprisingly, such protocol divergence has led to a high degree of variability in performance across experiments within and between institutions, as demonstrated in recent large proficiency panels conducted by the Cancer Immunotherapy Consortium, a program of the Cancer Research Institute (CIC/CRI) and the Immunoguiding Program of the Association for Cancer Immunotherapy (CIP/CIMT) as well as by others (19,52–55). Data obtained in these panels have pointed to a limited number of specific assay variables that could account for most of the variability observed, providing the opportunity for feasible corrective measures via assay harmonization. Assay parameters such as cell quantity, cell quality, culture media, and background cytokine production have been identified as sources of variation (19,56,57). Further, the introduction of reagents that simplify the assay and thus decrease possible variability including automation steps has been proposed for ICS (58). Central laboratories could also play an effective role in harmonizing T-cell measurements in clinical trials (59). With all these developments, three additional factors influencing the comparability of reported data have to be kept in mind.

1. One complicating factor is the lack of true gold reference standards for T-cell assays. While the use of T-cell clones or lines and PBMC reference samples can aid in precise measurements, they are less standardized than reference samples for assays which utilize solutions with pre-established cytokine concentrations (e.g., ELISA).
2. Data reports from immune monitoring studies can only be as good as the transparency of the report about how the data were obtained. Therefore, a project called, Minimal Information about T Cell Assays (MIATA) has been initiated (60,61), the aim of which is to provide guidelines for the publication of results from T-cell assays and adequate annotations for T-cell data sets for a public database, as envisioned in the Human Immunity Project (62).

3. Finally, the comparison of data from different institutions is also influenced by the criteria used to define T-cell responses. Different statistical and empirical tests are being used by centers for the definition of a positive immune response as measured by a given assay at a given time point. This topic has recently been discussed for ELISPOT and recommendations including an available web tool were given (14).

The variability in the way of reporting immune response measurements contributes to the difficulty in establishing immune response parameters as reliable biomarkers in human trials. The field is currently responding with harmonization strategies which allow laboratories to continue using their specialized assay protocols for T-cell assessment but provide general harmonization guidelines as part of a laboratory SOP to minimize variability (19,27,52,53). In summary, assay harmonization can support assay development and optimization, increase the quality and robustness of immune assays, enable benchmarking of assays and laboratories on a regular basis to ensure test performance within defined margins, and facilitate the comparability of results generated across institutions without mandating the use of a specific test procedure.

ASSAY STANDARDIZATION

Despite its advantages, harmonization efforts are not suited to replace the need for standardizing the assay procedure within each laboratory prior to its use on clinical sample specimens. Assay standardization is the process of developing and agreeing upon a technical standard for a given assay to make sure that a test is performed, interpreted, and documented in a consistent (or "standard") manner. Various publications in peer-reviewed journals and guidelines addressing the topic of standardization of single-cell immune assays give guidance on critical assay components and performance characteristics (25,63–65). The implementation of SOP comprising the standards for (*i*) cell sampling, (*ii*) assay procedure, (*iii*) data acquisition, (*iv*) interpretation of raw data, and (*v*) implementation of quality-supporting laboratory infrastructure should be the initial step to ensure that data derived from assays are meaningful and reliable. Evidence for reproducible test performance following standardization should be provided by data generated on representative sample specimens. Depending on the stage of clinical testing and the context in which data from T-cell assays are being used, a formal assay validation might be premature and even counterproductive (*e.g., in early clinical development, for research use only or when a hypothesis generation is the primary aim*) or a mandatory requirement (*e.g., in advanced clinical testing, to test hypothesis, to support drug licensure, co-marketing of biomarker assay, and drug product*). The context-specific value of full assay validation is a principle reason because of which a general recommendation cannot be made for formal validation.

TECHNICAL VALIDATION OF T-CELL ASSAYS

Assay validation is the formal process by which the specifications are initially defined and subsequently confirmed to ensure that an assay is performing appropriately every time it is utilized. The concept of assay validation has been principally employed in bioanalytical assays to evaluate well-characterized and defined analytes and a guidance document for the validation of bioanalytical assays is available on the United States Food and Drug Administration (U.S. FDA) website www.fda.gov/cder/guidance/index.htm. As described in this document and further expanded on in a recent review (66), validation plans need to first define and subsequently evaluate with statistical significance a list of parameters, summarized in Table 12.2, that commonly define the performance characteristics of an assay.

The assay validation process involves a series of linked but discrete steps. The first step in the process is to define what the assay is intended to measure, how it will be measured, and how each of the validation parameters will be addressed and evaluated. The second step is referred to as the assay qualification or pre-validation stage. During the assay qualification stage, the performance characteristics of each of the validation parameters for the assay are

Table 12.2   Parameters to Be Evaluated During the Assay Validation Process

Parameter	Output
Specificity	The ability to differentiate and quantify the test article in the context of the bioassay components
Accuracy	The closeness of the test results to the true value
Precision (intra-assay)	The closeness of values upon replicate measurement within the same assay
Precision (inter-assay)	The closeness of values upon replicate measurement across independent assays
Upper limit of quantification	The upper range of the standard curve that can be used to quantify test values
Lower limit of quantification	The lower range of the standard curve that can be used to quantify test values
Lower limit of detection	The lowest value that can be reliably detected above the established negative or background value
Robustness	How well the assay transfers to another operator/instrument/laboratory

Table 12.3   Different Stages of the Assay Development Process and Their Primary Objectives

Stage	Primary Objective	Output
Exploratory	Define and explore assay performance characteristics	• Compile a draft standard operating procedure (SOP) • Assemble standards and reference materials • Assemble the Qualification Plan
Pre-validation	Define statistical ranges for assay performance	• Assemble qualification report • Define statistically supported assay performance ranges • Finalize the SOP • Assemble draft assay worksheets • Compile the Validation Plan
Validation	Confirm statistical ranges for assay performance	• Complete the Validation Report • Determine the pass/fail parameters for assay • Compile finalized assay worksheets

evaluated in a rigorous and statistically supported manner. The next step of the process is the assay validation. The primary objective of this stage is to confirm that the statistically determined performance characteristics defined during the qualification stage are appropriate. The final step in the process is to finalize the assay-specific worksheets that are linked to the SOP used during the assay validation process and release them for use (Table 12.3).

In the context of validation of biomarker assays for cancer vaccines, assay validation is constrained by the inherent complexity and variability of both the source and composition of the sample. In addition, the ability to determine assay accuracy in biological assays is often compromised since the "true value" for what is being measured is not known or it changes during the course of treatment. Thus, depending on the biological assay, it may not be possible to validate one or more of the above described validation parameters. There is currently no tailored process for immunological biomarker validation and qualification; however, the core principles for biomarker development, as defined by the U.S. FDA in several guidance documents, can provide general directions for immunological biomarkers and contribute to our current understanding of this evolving process (67,68). For assay method validation, a "fit-for-purpose" approach (69) was recently introduced. Several validation steps were defined: exploratory method validation, pre-study and in-study validation as well as advanced method validation, which include assay robustness, cross-validation, and documentation control. Each subsequent step increases in rigor and provides adaptation of the assay requirements to the advancing clinical purpose (69). The "fit-for-purpose" approach allows sufficient flexibility to accommodate a wide spectrum of biomarker assays and can be synchronized with the clinical qualification part of biomarker development.

CLINICAL VALIDATION/QUALIFICATION OF IMMUNE MONITORING ASSAYS

A biomarker is a biological characteristic that can be objectively measured and evaluated as an indicator of normal or abnormal biologic processes or pharmacologic responses to a therapeutic intervention. Immunological biomarkers as measured through immune monitoring assays can fulfill multiple applications: (*i*) determine whether an immune intervention hits its biological target, (*ii*) define dose and schedule for the intervention, (*iii*) measure synergistic effects for therapeutic combinations, (*iv*) define study populations, (*v*) measure therapeutic effects as biological activity, and (*vi*) predict clinical outcomes as surrogates for clinical benefit (31,70). The utility of a biomarker, in clinical trials and practice, depends on the ability of the marker to meet its intended purpose as well as the underlying assay to provide reproducible measurements in the clinical setting. This is accomplished through the validation process, which integrates biomarker and associated assay discovery, assay method validation, clinical qualification, and the regulatory pathway for drug development. Ideally, both assay method validation (see the previous section) and the clinical qualification run in parallel, are iterative in nature, and the degree of validity is increasing with every iterative step.

Clinical qualification steps can be oriented on FDA guidance on pharmacogenomic data submissions (67), which categorizes exploratory and valid biomarkers. Exploratory biomarkers form a foundation for biomarker development and create a body of evidence that can vouch for validity. In turn, a valid biomarker is measured in an analytical test system with well-established performance characteristics and has an established scientific framework or a body of evidence that elucidates the significance of the test results. Further, valid biomarkers may be "known valid" when they have been accepted in the broad scientific community and "probable valid" when they appear to have predictive value for clinical outcomes, but may not yet be widely accepted or independently verified by other investigators or institutions. Valid biomarkers may be appropriate for regulatory decision making (67). Clinical qualification progresses biomarkers from an exploratory to a valid status. Clinical qualification may be based on a process map, whose steps determine the usefulness of the biomarker in meeting its purpose (e.g., predicting clinical benefits) (71).

At the current stage of immune monitoring assay use, immunological biomarkers resulting from clinical trials must be seen as exploratory. Several steps toward a structured use of immune monitoring assays in clinical trials, which may contribute to their validation, were proposed by the Cancer Vaccine Clinical Trial Working Group, a joint initiative of the CIC and the international Society for Biological Therapy of cancer (31). Biomarker development for clinical use is complex and requires a collaborative effort across the community of stakeholders which is involved in the respective specialty as is amply illustrated throughout this chapter. To improve the cancer biomarker development process, the American Association for Cancer Research, the National Cancer Institute, and FDA have formed the Cancer Biomarkers Collaborative (72). A more specialized approach is taken by the collaborative efforts of the CIC and CIP to address immune monitoring-related biomarker issues for cancer immunotherapy development (19,27,52,53,60,61).

So far no clinically qualified or validated immunological biomarker could be established. This may be in part due to data variability of immunological assays in the exploratory stage of biomarker development. Assay harmonization as discussed above may help overcome this limitation. Given the complex nature of cancer and immunotherapy approaches it is likely that correlative immunological signatures will consist of either a combination of several complementary mono- or oligo-parametric assays or one multi-parametric more complex assay. It is also possible that immunological signatures that correlate with clinical events in one tumor entity, disease stage, or innovative therapy might not apply in other settings. As immune surrogates may be highly context specific and as the field is still searching for clinically validated immune correlates, investigation of the antitumor T-cell response should capture as many immune- and tumor parameters as possible during exploratory development (aim: hypothesis generation). In our view this should at least include a set of complementary assays which allows the measurement of the breadth, magnitude, and quality of vaccine-specific CD4$^+$ and CD8$^+$ T cells, as well as assess the presence and function of potentially inhibitory cells (e.g., T$_{REGS}$, MSDCs, monocytes or neutrophils) and parameters of normal immune function in order to stand a chance to discover potential immune parameters correlated with success or failure of therapy. The most promising assays established in early clinical development should be technically harmonized, validated, and applied in later stage clinical studies (aim: clinical validation).

CONCLUSION

We conclude with the following:

- Rational drug development needs to understand the mechanistic underpinnings of the treatment and link them to clinical outcomes.
- Clinical development of therapeutic vaccines should be accompanied by T-cell immune monitoring assays.
- Monitoring of vaccine-induced immune responses will probably be the key to understand the mode of action of therapeutic vaccines.
- Many scientifically established T-cell assays are available and innovative assays are constantly added to the arsenal of available tools.
- So far no accepted gold-standards for immune assays use exist despite the protocols for any given assay being heterogeneous.
- Performance characteristics for the three most commonly used assays are described in detail and allow a selection of the most appropriate assay.
- The concept of immunoguiding includes the use of a set of complementary assays, screening for wanted and unwanted T-cell immunity and focusing on more than just the peripheral blood compartment in order to mechanistically understand the immune response induced by an immunotherapeutic intervention.
- Harmonization guidelines can support assay development and optimization and can increase comparability of results across experiments within and between institutions.
- Assay harmonization cannot replace the need to standardize assays in phase III trials.
- Effective measures to support assay quality and documented evidence of assay reproducibility should always be in place.
- In contrast, no general recommendation can be given to fully validate immunological assays, as it depends on the stage of clinical development and the context of its use.
- Although the process for validation of analytical assays is clearly defined by existing guidelines it can still be cumbersome for the more complex cellular assay.
- Clinical utility of immune monitoring assays depends on their methodological validation and clinical qualification, which should be integrated parts of the overall clinical immunotherapy development process.

Following the given recommendations and applying the described strategies from early on in the process will enhance the development of new therapeutic cancer vaccines and close the gap in immunotherapy drug development, which results from treating the immune system but measuring clinical outcomes.

REFERENCES

1. Boon T. Antigenic tumor cell variants obtained with mutagens. Adv Cancer Res 1983; 39: 121–51.
2. Cavallo F, Offringa R, van der Burg SH, et al. Vaccination for treatment and prevention of cancer in animal models. Adv Immunol 2006; 90: 175–213.
3. Ostrand-Rosenberg S. CD4+ T lymphocytes: a critical component of antitumor immunity. Cancer Invest 2005; 23: 413–9.
4. Nelson BH. CD20+ B cells: the other tumor-infiltrating lymphocytes. J Immunol 2010; 185: 4977–82.

5. Gutierrez-Dalmau A, Campistol JM. Immunosuppressive therapy and malignancy in organ transplant recipients: a systematic review. Drugs 2007; 67: 1167–98.

6. Bonnet F, Chene G. Evolving epidemiology of malignancies in HIV. Curr Opin Oncol 2008; 20: 534–40.

7. Kolb HJ, Holler E. Adoptive immunotherapy with donor lymphocyte transfusions. Curr Opin Oncol 1997; 9: 139–45.

8. Hunder NN, Wallen H, Cao J, et al. Treatment of metastatic melanoma with autologous CD4+ T cells against NY-ESO-1. N Engl J Med 2008; 358: 2698–703.

9. Pages F, Berger A, Camus M, et al. Effector memory T cells, early metastasis, and survival in colorectal cancer. N Engl J Med 2005; 353: 2654–66.

10. Galon J, Costes A, Sanchez-Cabo F, et al. Type, density, and location of immune cells within human colorectal tumors predict clinical outcome. Science 2006; 313: 1960–4.

11. Czerkinsky C, Andersson G, Ekre HP, et al. Reverse ELISPOT assay for clonal analysis of cytokine production. I. Enumeration of gamma-interferon-secreting cells. J Immunol Methods 1988; 110: 29–36.

12. Bennouna J, Hildesheim A, Chikamatsu K, et al. Application of IL-5 ELISPOT assays to quantification of antigen-specific T helper responses. J Immunol Methods 2002; 261: 145–56.

13. Nowacki TM, Kuerten S, Zhang W, et al. Granzyme B production distinguishes recently activated CD8(+) memory cells from resting memory cells. Cell Immunol 2007; 247: 36–48.

14. Moodie Z, Price L, Gouttefangeas C, et al. Response definition criteria for ELISPOT assays revisited. Cancer Immunol Immunother 2010; 59: 1489–501.

15. Comin-Anduix B, Gualberto A, Glaspy JA, et al. Definition of an immunologic response using the major histocompatibility complex tetramer and enzyme-linked immunospot assays. Clin Cancer Res 2006; 12: 107–16.

16. Samri A, Durier C, Urrutia A, et al. Evaluation of the interlaboratory concordance in quantification of human immunodeficiency virus-specific T cells with a gamma interferon enzyme-linked immunospot assay. Clin Vaccine Immunol 2006; 13: 684–97.

17. Mander A, Chowdhury F, Low L, et al. Fit for purpose? A case study: validation of immunological endpoint assays for the detection of cellular and humoral responses to anti-tumour DNA fusion vaccines. Cancer Immunol Immunother 2009; 58: 789–800.

18. Smith JG, Liu X, Kaufhold RM, et al. Development and validation of a gamma interferon ELISPOT assay for quantitation of cellular immune responses to varicella-zoster virus. Clin Diagn Lab Immunol 2001; 8: 871–9.

19. Britten CM, Gouttefangeas C, Welters MJ, et al. The CIMT-monitoring panel: a two-step approach to harmonize the enumeration of antigen-specific CD8+ T lymphocytes by structural and functional assays. Cancer Immunol Immunother 2008; 57: 289–302.

20. Speiser DE, Pittet MJ, Guillaume P, et al. Ex vivo analysis of human antigen-specific CD8+ T-cell responses: quality assessment of fluorescent HLA-A2 multimer and interferon-gamma ELISPOT assays for patient immune monitoring. J Immunother 2004; 27: 298–308.

21. Horton H, Thomas EP, Stucky JA, et al. Optimization and validation of an 8-color intracellular cytokine staining (ICS) assay to quantify antigen-specific T cells induced by vaccination. J Immunol Methods 2007; 323: 39–54.

22. Altman JD, Moss PA, Goulder PJ, et al. Phenotypic analysis of antigen-specific T lymphocytes. Science 1996; 274: 94–6.

23. Jung T, Schauer U, Heusser C, et al. Detection of intracellular cytokines by flow cytometry. J Immunol Methods 1993; 159: 197–207.

24. Van Tendeloo VF, Van de Velde A, Van Driessche A, et al. Induction of complete and molecular remissions in acute myeloid leukemia by Wilms' tumor 1 antigen-targeted dendritic cell vaccination. Proc Natl Acad Sci USA 2010; 107: 13824–9.

25. Maecker HT, Rinfret A, D'Souza P, et al. Standardization of cytokine flow cytometry assays. BMC Immunol 2005; 6: 1–18.

26. Seder RA, Darrah PA, Roederer M. T-cell quality in memory and protection: implications for vaccine design. Nat Rev Immunol 2008; 8: 247–58.

27. Britten CM, Janetzki S, van der Burg SH, et al. Toward the harmonization of immune monitoring in clinical trials: Quo vadis? Cancer Immunol Immunother 2007; 57: 285–8.

28. Jaimes MC, Maecker HT, Yan M, et al. Quality assurance of intracellular cytokine staining assays: Analysis of multiple rounds of proficiency testing. J Immunol Methods 2010; 363: 143–57.

29. Chattopadhyay PK, Hogerkorp CM, Roederer M. A chromatic explosion: the development and future of multiparameter flow cytometry. Immunology 2008; 125: 441–9.

30. Frelinger J, Ottinger J, Gouttefangeas C, et al. Modeling flow cytometry data for cancer vaccine immune monitoring. Cancer Immunol Immunother 2010; 59: 1435–41.
31. Hoos A, Parmiani G, Hege K, et al. A clinical development paradigm for cancer vaccines and related biologics. J Immunother 2007; 30: 1–15.
32. Gazagne A, Claret E, Wijdenes J, et al. A Fluorospot assay to detect single T lymphocytes simultaneously producing multiple cytokines. J Immunol Methods 2003; 283: 91–8.
33. Boulet S, Ndongala ML, Peretz Y, et al. A dual color ELISPOT method for the simultaneous detection of IL-2 and IFN-gamma HIV-specific immune responses. J Immunol Methods 2003; 320: 18–29.
34. Lovelace P, Maecker HT. Multiparameter intracellular cytokine staining. Methods Mol Biol 2011; 699: 165–78.
35. Lugli E, Roederer M, Cossarizza A. Data analysis in flow cytometry: the future just started. Cytometry A 2010; 77: 705–13.
36. Tesfa L, Volk HD, Kern F. A protocol for combining proliferation, tetramer staining and intracellular cytokine detection for the flow-cytometric analysis of antigen specific T-cells. J Biol Regul Homeost Agents 2003; 17: 366–70.
37. Hadrup SR, Bakker AH, Shu CJ, et al. Parallel detection of antigen-specific T-cell responses by multi-dimensional encoding of MHC multimers. Nat Methods 2009; 6: 520–6.
38. Newell EW, Klein LO, Yu W, et al. Simultaneous detection of many T-cell specificities using combinatorial tetramer staining. Nat Methods 2009; 6: 497–9.
39. Ornatsky O, Bandura D, Baranov V, et al. Highly multiparametric analysis by mass cytometry. J Immunol Methods 2010; 361: 1–20.
40. Maecker HT, Nolan GP, Fathman CG. New technologies for autoimmune disease monitoring. Curr Opin Endocrinol Diabetes Obes 2010; 17: 322–8.
41. Welters MJ, Piersma SJ, van der Burg SH. T-regulatory cells in tumour-specific vaccination strategies. Expert Opin Biol Ther 2008; 8: 1365–79.
42. van der Burg SH, Piersma SJ, de Jong A, et al. Association of cervical cancer with the presence of CD4+ regulatory T cells specific for human papillomavirus antigens. Proc Natl Acad Sci USA 2007; 104: 12087–92.
43. van der Burg SH. Therapeutic vaccines in cancer: moving from immunomonitoring to immunoguiding. Expert Rev Vaccines 2008; 7: 1–5.
44. Andersen MH, Sorensen RB, Brimnes MK, et al. Identification of heme oxygenase-1-specific regulatory CD8+ T cells in cancer patients. J Clin Invest 2009; 119: 2245–56.
45. Gajewski TF, Louahed J, Brichard VG. Gene signature in melanoma associated with clinical activity: a potential clue to unlock cancer immunotherapy. Cancer J 2010; 16: 399–403.
46. Reyal F, van Vliet MH, Armstrong NJ, et al. A comprehensive analysis of prognostic signatures reveals the high predictive capacity of the proliferation, immune response and RNA splicing modules in breast cancer. Breast Cancer Res 2008; 10: R93.
47. Pages F, Kirilovsky A, Mlecnik B, et al. In situ cytotoxic and memory T cells predict outcome in patients with early-stage colorectal cancer. J Clin Oncol 2009; 27: 5944–51.
48. Martorelli D, Muraro E, Merlo A, et al. Role of CD4+ cytotoxic T lymphocytes in the control of viral diseases and cancer. Int Rev Immunol 2010; 29: 371–402.
49. Kenter GG, Welters MJ, Valentijn AR, et al. Vaccination against HPV-16 oncoproteins for vulvar intraepithelial neoplasia. N Engl J Med 2009; 361: 1838–47.
50. Welters MJ, Kenter GG, de Vos van Steenwijk PJ, et al. Success or failure of vaccination for HPV16-positive vulvar lesions correlates with kinetics and phenotype of induced T-cell responses. Proc Natl Acad Sci USA 2010; 107: 11895–9.
51. Kenter GG, Welters MJ, Valentijn AR, et al. Phase I immunotherapeutic trial with long peptides spanning the E6 and E7 sequences of high-risk human papillomavirus 16 in end-stage cervical cancer patients shows low toxicity and robust immunogenicity. Clin Cancer Res 2008; 14: 169–77.
52. Janetzki S, Panageas KS, Ben-Porat L, et al. Results and harmonization guidelines from two large-scale international Elispot proficiency panels conducted by the Cancer Vaccine Consortium (CVC/SVI). Cancer Immunol Immunother 2008; 57: 303–15.
53. Britten CM, Janetzki S, Ben Porat L, et al. Harmonization guidelines for HLA-peptide multimer assays derived from results of a large scale international proficiency panel of the Cancer Vaccine Consortium. Cancer Immunol Immunother 2009; 58: 1701–13
54. Scheibenbogen C, Romero P, Rivoltini L, et al. Quantitation of antigen-reactive T cells in peripheral blood by IFNgamma-ELISPOT assay and chromium-release assay: a four-centre comparative trial. J Immunol Methods 2000; 244: 81–9.

55. Cox JH, Ferrari G, Kalams SA, et al. Results of an ELISPOT proficiency panel conducted in 11 laboratories participating in international human immunodeficiency virus type 1 vaccine trials. AIDS Res Hum Retroviruses 2005; 21: 68–81.

56. Mander A, Gouttefangeas C, Ottensmeier C, et al. Serum is not required for ex vivo IFN-gamma ELISPOT: a collaborative study of different protocols from the European CIMT Immunoguiding Program. Cancer Immunol Immunother 2010; 59: 619–27.

57. Janetzki S, Price L, Britten CM, et al. Performance of serum-supplemented and serum-free media in IFN-gamma Elispot Assays for human T cells. Cancer Immunol Immunother 2009; 59: 609–18.

58. Suni MA, Dunn HS, Orr PL, et al. Performance of plate-based cytokine flow cytometry with automated data analysis. BMC Immunol 2003; 4: 9.

59. Maecker HT, McCoy JP Jr, Amos M, et al. A model for harmonizing flow cytometry in clinical trials. Nat Immunol 2010; 11: 975–8.

60. Janetzki S, Britten CM, Kalos M, et al. "MIATA"-minimal information about T cell assays. Immunity 2009; 31: 527–8.

61. Britten CM, Janetzki S, van der Burg SH, et al. Minimal information about T cell assays: the process of reaching the community of T cell immunologists in cancer and beyond. Cancer Immunol Immunother 2010. [Epub ahead of print].

62. Davis MM. A prescription for human immunology. Immunity 2008; 29: 835–8.

63. Lamoreaux L, Roederer M, Koup R. Intracellular cytokine optimization and standard operating procedure. Nat Protoc 2006; 1: 1507–16.

64. Landay AL, Fleisher TA, Kuus-Reicher K, et al. Performance of Single cell Immune response assays; Approved Guideline. NCCLS Guidelines 2004; 24: 1–84.

65. Janetzki S, Cox JH, Oden N, et al. Standardization and validation issues of the ELISPOT assay. Methods Mol Biol 2005; 302: 51–86.

66. Kalos M. An integrative paradigm to impart quality to correlative science. J Transl Med 2010; 8: 26.

67. US Food and Drug Administration. Pharmacogenomic data submissions. Guidance for industry, 2005.

68. US Food and Drug Administration. Bioanalytical method validation. Guidance for industry, 2001.

69. Lee JW, Devanarayan V, Barrett YC, et al. Fit-for-purpose method development and validation for successful biomarker measurement. Pharm Res 2006; 23: 312–28.

70. Biomarkers Definitions Working Group. Biomarkers and surrogate endpoints: preferred definitions and conceptual framework. Clin Pharmacol Ther 2001; 69: 89–95.

71. Goodsaid F, Frueh F. Biomarker qualification pilot process at the US Food and Drug Administration. AAPS J 2007; 9: E105–8.

72. Khleif SN, Doroshow JH, Hait WN. AACR-FDA-NCI Cancer Biomarkers Collaborative consensus report: advancing the use of biomarkers in cancer drug development. Clin Cancer Res 2010; 16: 3299–318.

13 | A biomarker-based, systems biology approach guiding the development of active immunotherapies and immune monitoring

Glenda Canderan, Peter Wilkinson, John Schatzle, Mark Cameron, and Rafick-Pierre Sekaly

INTRODUCTION

The original concept of immunosurveillance as proposed by Burnet and Thomas (1) has proved to be a key factor in controlling the development of tumors and is now an attractive target as another tool in our arsenal in the battle against cancer. Mounting evidence supports the idea of a spontaneous immune response to tumors that has the potential for exploitation by active immunotherapy (2–5). However, cancer immunotherapies have only had marginal clinical success, probably as a consequence of an incomplete understanding of tumor immunology and a lack of adequate investigation tools.

Indeed, while immune modulation (often in the form of vaccination) has been successful in controlling several infectious pathogens, it has not proved as effective in the eradication of established chronic diseases, such as HIV infection and cancer (6). Since the effectiveness of a vaccine is directly linked to the type and the quality of immune responses it elicits, the identification of correlates of immune protection, which could guide the designing of vaccine, is of primary importance. The recent emergence of genome-wide immune monitoring coupled with a systems biology approach has allowed investigators to better identify and define these correlates of protection. This is a shift from the previous approach to vaccine designing that was largely empirical in nature.

Therefore, any approaches to incorporate what we have learnt from the fields of vaccine study and design into the use of immunotherapy as a cancer treatment regimen must take into account the unique requirements of an effective anti-tumor response by the immune system. Cytolytic T lymphocyte (CTL) cells are thought to be an important part of the immune response against cancer as often tumor-associated antigens (TAAs) are intracellular and not targets for antibodies. Indeed tumor-specific CD8 T-cell responses have been correlated with clinical outcomes (7,8). However, many other players are involved in the generation of a strong immune response to tumors, including CD4 helper T and B cells in the adaptive response and dendritic cells (DCs) and natural killer (NK) cells of the innate response. It is clear that as in the generation of an effective vaccine response, an effective anti-tumor response will likely require the orchestrated integration of these various components. In particular, CD4 T cells seem to have a crucial role for priming long-lived CD8 T-cell memory (9) and they are likely key players in the generation of anti-tumor cytolytic T lymphocyte responses. DCs have been a prime target for immunotherapy and vaccine approaches given their key role in priming CD8 T and CD4 T helper (Th1) cells but also due to their ability to interact with B cells, NK, and NK T cells (10).

Since the immune system is comprised of such a complex network of cells and as each particular disease generates an integrated response, only a global approach, monitoring simultaneously all the components of the immune system, could give a complete understanding of the immune response to cancer. Moreover, as predicted by the cancer immunoediting hypothesis (2), the tumor and the immune system dynamically interact with the immune system, shaping the tumor and its inherent properties and antigenicity, and with the tumor affecting the immune response in an attempt to suppress its functions. This relationship is extremely complex involving multiple interacting cell types in a temporal relationship and can only be completely understood through a study approach based on high-throughput monitoring technologies. Finally, when evaluating therapeutic responses, overall survival and relapse-free time are the obvious and more desired endpoints; however, defined immunological responses are often used as surrogates. These responses are identified through the use of techniques such as the enzyme-linked immunosorbent spot (ELISPOT) assay, cytotoxicity assays, flow cytometry [intracellular cytokine staining (ICS), carboxyfluorescein succinimidyl ester (CFSE) staining for proliferation, and antigen-specific cell enumeration]. Although these all capture individual features of immunity, they fail to provide a complex, integrated picture of a true immune response which has been proved to be vital in predicting the success of immune interventions such as vaccines. The immune responses to tumors will likely be as complicated and comprehensive in nature (if not more so) and therefore will require a similar approach. Moreover, since in vitro assays and animal models are often inadequate in predicting what will happen in vivo, a direct and comprehensive analysis of *ex-vivo* samples should be pursued (11).

In this chapter we discuss systems biology, a relatively new approach to biological research, as a tool for obtaining a comprehensive picture of vaccine-induced responses and for uncovering new biomarkers.

DEFINITION OF SYSTEM BIOLOGY

The concept of systems biology stands in contrast to the classical and dominating reductionist approach to biological research. In the reductionist approach, biological entities such as cells, tissues, and diseases are investigated by the study of their single components. Quite often, this is taken to even the most extreme approach of studying singular molecular components in a biological process in isolation. On the other hand, the systems biology approach aims for a holistic, multi-level analysis of the investigated system. Indeed, a system is not merely the sum of its components and therefore, the isolation and study of its singular components is often not sufficient to predict the behavior of a biological system. In any given system the so-called "emergent properties" arise from the interaction between the various principal components. The reductionist approach of dismantling each entity into single building blocks certainly simplifies the study of a system but at the same time incurs the risk of oversimplification by ignoring the complex interplay of seemingly unconnected components that often contribute to the whole of a biological process. Consequently, the quantitative and qualitative analysis of the system in its entireness becomes necessary to fully understand its biology. For this purpose, a change of perspective is needed. The usual hypothesis-driven approach to research is substituted by a hypothesis-generating approach thanks to our recent ability to rapidly acquire, integrate, and analyze large data sets. Several high-throughput techniques have been introduced in biological research allowing researchers to obtain large amounts of information regarding biological processes. This has greatly enhanced our ability to now focus on a specific biological question, make global observations regarding the biological components involved in a particular process, and integrate these large data sets so as to facilitate the development of new hypotheses and predictions in hopes of answering the original biological question.

All principal components of a biological process including specific cell types, their gene expression profiles, their protein content, and their metabolic profiles can be obtained through these high throughput assays. The so-called "omics" represent those scientific disciplines analyzing the interactions of biological information derived by the various "omes" (genome, transcriptome, proteome, metabolome).

Transcriptomics have focused on investigating the expression profile of a given population of cells or tissues by the use of microarray technology and next-generation sequencing, allowing the analysis of both coding (mRNA) and non-coding (microRNA) RNAs (12,13). Proteomics, on the other hand, portray changes in protein levels and post-translational modifications (such as phosphorylation, acetylation, addition of carbohydrates, and disulfide bond formation) on a large scale, thanks to techniques such as mass spectrometry (14,15), 2D electrophoresis, and bioinformatics (16) (Fig. 13.1).

Immunology is an excellent example of a systems science since it involves a diverse array of components, regulatory pathways, and networks and is also integrative, reactive, and adaptive. Great progress in immunology was made possible by technological advances in flow cytometry where now up to 18 parameters can be routinely analyzed at one time to define cell subsets and their activation status (17). Furthermore, intracellular staining and phosflow

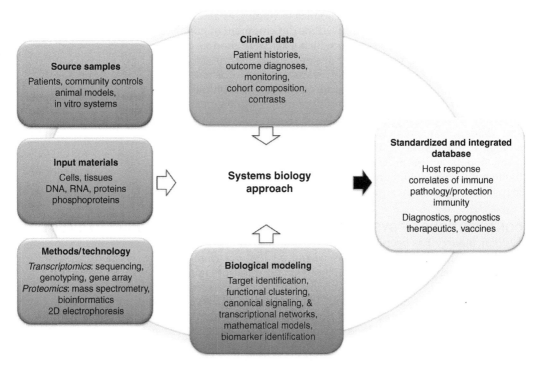

Figure 13.1   Schematic representation of the central nature of a systems biology approach.

protocols (18) help study cell effector functions and intracellular signaling pathways at a cellular level unlike the population based technologies of the past (e.g., Western blot analysis and ELISA); moreover the recent development of multiplex tetramer technology has made the simultaneous detection of several antigen specific T cells easy(19). The combination of these techniques could thus allow an even deeper level of analysis of qualitative and quantitative features of cellular immune responses, as in the case of fluorescence-activated cell sorting (FACS) combined with high-throughput microarray technology, wherein transcription profiles of cell subsets can be analyzed separately. Simultaneous measurement of a wide range of cytokines in a patient's serum or in culture supernatants is possible, thanks to multiplexed cytokine assays, to identify cytokine profiles and monitor clinical responses. Quantitative multiplexed polymerase chain reaction (PCR) analysis enables the simultaneous amplification of many targets of interest in one reaction by using multiple primer sets. Chromatin immunoprecipitation (ChIP)-Chip is a technique that combines chromatin immunoprecipitation with microarray technology while ChIP-Seq combines ChIP with massively parallel DNA sequencing. Both the techniques are powerful methods for the analysis of epigenetic modifications that have also been shown to play a prominent role in the development and function of immune system (20,21).

Furthermore, technological developments pushing the limits of information that we can obtain from smaller and smaller numbers of cells are all allowing the research community access to greater levels of detail about the cellular processes that contribute to biological outcomes.

Another important component of systems biology consists of the computational tools necessary to analyze and integrate the vast amounts of data collected from these high-throughput technologies. The processing of these data requires the combined application of statistics, analysis, database mining, and biological validation to ensure that accurate and relevant biological conclusions are reached. Moreover, since each of these technologies investigates only one layer of a complex network, data need to be integrated into a single model describing the system and predicting its response to perturbation. Systems biology has the capacity to utilize and integrate genomics technologies and generate databases encompassing the whole genome, which has allowed the development of novel transcriptional models. Model building is an iterative process, in which a series of models are constructed and stacked from the simple to the complex using a systems biology approach. A strong collaboration between different areas of expertise (biology, statistics, and informatics) is necessary (Fig. 13.1), along with the integration of good clinical, literature, and online curated database annotation, to bolster researcher-driven model building from simple gene-level correlations, to multi-vector pathways and gene co-expression networks, to biomarker meta-analysis (intra-project scale) and validation of predictive models. The goal of a systems biology analysis is to establish biological models incorporating cross correlations from (*i*) primary data, (*ii*) integration of primary data across multiple experimental modalities, (*iii*) integration of multiple cell and tissue types, and (*iv*) integration and validation against existing biological models to ultimately map the best treatment strategies that will lead to successful patient clinical outcomes.

CONTRIBUTIONS OF SYSTEMS BIOLOGY TO THE FIELD OF IMMUNITY TO INFECTION

Systems biology has been applied successfully to the study of immune response to infections and in turn has revealed some surprising results that change our understanding of what is required to generate a long-lasting protective immunological response. In particular, DNA microarrays have been used to investigate the response to several pathogens. A detailed analysis of the host transcriptional response to smallpox infection was carried out using DNA microarray technology in *Rhesus macaques* (22). Similarly, Djavani et al. recently studied the early transcriptional profile in peripheral blood mononuclear cells (PBMCs) from *macaques* infected with lymphocytic choriomeningitis virus, and their microarray data allowed them to determine gene signatures that can differentiate the response to virulent from avirulent strains of lymphocytic choriomeningitis virus (23). DNA microarrays were used to monitor the RNA levels in PBMC from children with acute measles and convalescent children (24). We and others have used transcriptomics to identify the mechanisms of action of the yellow fever (YF) vaccine (25,26). More recently, signatures of protection for TB disease have been generated and have unraveled the importance of the innate immune response and particularly of neutrophils in protecting from overt disease (27). Over the past few years, our laboratory has developed several applications of transcriptomics to provide a better understanding of the mechanisms of action of vaccines and adjuvants in human subjects and in non-human primate models. Many of the lessons learned from these studies and the implementation of these approaches should be readily applicable to the study of the immune response to cancer. Details regarding the use of systems biology approaches to understanding the immune response to infectious disease or vaccines are described next.

Gene Expression Profiling of Antigen-Specific Responses in Human PBMCs

A major limitation in monitoring vaccine efficacy is the inability of immune monitoring techniques such as ELISPOT or multi-color flow cytometry assays to assess more than a limited number of parameters in the vaccine-specific adaptive response. Gene array analysis of vaccine specific responses, in contrast, has provided a systematic analysis of thousands of parameters simultaneously to characterize antigen-specific responses, and has uncovered many cellular processes as playing a role including metabolic, survival, homing, and effector pathways. Since antigen-specific cells are present at low frequencies, the initial expectation was that in a complex biological sample such as peripheral blood, this would preclude detection of changes in gene expression in population-based studies. However, because of high sensitivity and low dynamic range in the Illumina platform, we could detect gene expression changes in T cells in response to specific antigens, including YF (25) and HIV in vaccines and in natural protection in a mixed population of cells where antigen-specific cells are relatively small in number. As shown in Figure 13.2, an YF17D peptide-specific response could be detected, despite the low frequency of YF17-specific cells, in in-–vitro-stimulated PBMCs. The four peptides used for

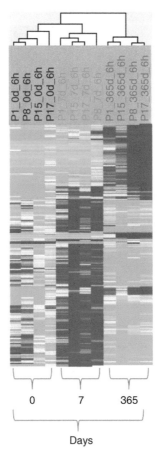

Figure 13.2 Antigen-specific responses can be detected by gene microarray as long as one year post-vaccination. Peripheral blood mononuclear cells from a representative vaccinated volunteer were re-stimulated six hours in vitro with YF17D-derived peptide pools and then processed for microarray analysis. This heat map shows the significant modulation of a distinct panel of genes as a result of vaccination [d7, d365]. Vertical columns represent the four peptide pools used to re-stimulate the cells. Each horizontal row represents a different gene with significant changes: green = downregulation, red = upregulation compared to unstimulated samples.

stimulation induced similar changes in gene expression profiles at day 7 and 365 after vaccination. Most of the genes that were triggered upon vaccination confirmed the commitment of YF17D-stimulated T cells to their differentiation to the Th1/Th2 pathways in terms of effector function. Moreover, these experiments allowed us to capture the memory potential as well as the migration properties of T cells; such features would have never been revealed by conventional assays.

Another example of the usefulness of gene microarray analysis in assessing T-cell response to vaccination is shown in Figure 13.3. The gene transcriptional profiling of HIV-specific responses to a recombinant NYVAC-HIV vaccine shows the upregulation of cytokine, chemokine, and cytokine/chemokine receptor genes including interleukin-15 (IL-15), interferon gamma (IFNγ), CXCL9, CXCL10, and many IFN-induced genes (IFIT3, IFIT2, IFTIM etc.) following vaccination. Thus, instead of measuring a limited number of parameters with conventional immunological analysis techniques such as flow cytometry, a full spectrum of biological responses of peripheral blood cells to vaccination could be assessed and quantified using the gene array analysis.

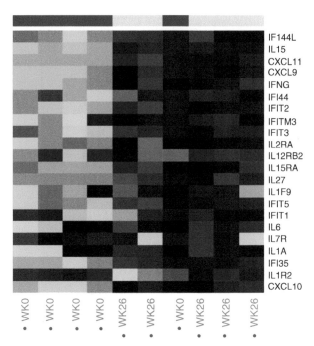

Figure 13.3 Ex vivo stimulation with HIV envelope (env) peptides induces multiple genes in NYVAC-HIV vaccines. Peripheral blood mononuclear cells 0 and 26 weeks after vaccination were incubated with env peptides for six hours and then cells were processed for microarray analysis on the Illumina BeadChip™ platform (Illumina, Inc., San Diego, CA). Using unsupervised clustering, 10 samples were clustered (dendogram not shown). The dark blue rectangle represents week 0 whereas the light blue represents week 26. Red shows the top upregulated genes while green shows downregulated genes. The right axis is a list of genes.

Overall, the transcriptomics of Ag-specific responses demonstrates the ability to measure transcriptional profile changes, across thousands of parameters and biologically important pathways, in vaccine and antigen-specific immune responses of humans. This allows for the identification of novel unsuspected pathways that can predict protective immune responses. Both the sensitivity and the comprehensive nature of the information acquired by using this platform confirm its importance in the monitoring of immune response to chronic viral infections and vaccines.

Use of Transcriptomics to Define Transcriptional Signatures Induced by Adjuvants

Toll-like receptor (TLR) ligands are increasingly tested for their use as vaccine adjuvants in the context of both infectious diseases and cancer. We have used gene array profiling to identify signaling and transcriptional biomarkers and determine the impact of different adjuvants, acting on defined pattern-recognition receptors (PRR). In this work we have been able to observe changes in the gene signatures of cultured blood DCs stimulated by different TLRs (poly-IC [PIC] and Flagellin [Flag] were used as adjuvants). Importantly, we have found that individual TLRs induce unique transcriptional signatures when assessed with the Illumina platform (Fig. 13.4).

Most TLR ligands induce the type-I IFN pathway; however, they differ in their capacity to activate other innate immune response pathways including the inflammasome and the tolerogenic retinaldehyde dehydrogenase pathway (28). With conventional immune monitoring approaches, it would be impossible to reach such data sets and offer a great opportunity for further clinical development of TLR agonists as vaccine adjuvants.

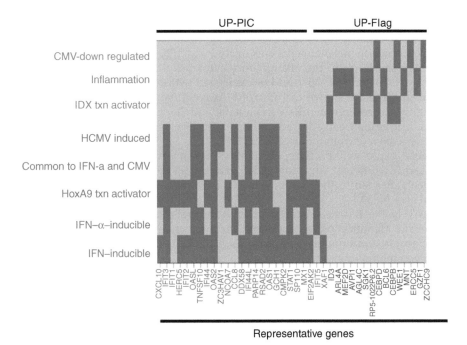

Figure 13.4 A pathway analysis map of some unique pathways in Flag-, and PIC-treated mDCs. On the y-axis are the names of five pathways upregulated by PIC [red] and three upregulated pathways by Flag [blue]. Genes on the x-axis are depicted as top members of each pathway that is upregulated upon TLR ligation. These pathways were identified by Gene Set Enrichment Analysis (GSEA) with p value <0.05. With GSEA, a large number of individual genes are reduced to several defined pathways. *Abbreviations*: Flag, flagellin; PIC, poly-IC; TLR, toll-like receptor.

Overall, transcriptomics has allowed the identification of global transcriptional signatures of innate and antigen-specific adaptive immune responses in both humans and non-human primate models of vaccination and disease. Moreover, systems biology has led to the identification of specific functional biomarker signatures that could guide the development of vaccines and adjuvants.

CONTRIBUTION OF SYSTEMS BIOLOGY TO THE FIELD OF CANCER IMMUNITY

The isolation of effective biomarkers that are capable of guiding cancer therapy is currently a priority. These biomarkers could prove useful for early cancer diagnosis, staging, and progression but also for predicting the outcome of a disease or treatment and for monitoring the effective response to treatment (29). Systems biology has the potential to revolutionize the understanding of cancer and cancer and immune system interactions and could provide the tools for the identification of such biomarkers. The use of quantitative reverse transcription-PCR (QPCR), cytometry and tissue microarrays, for example, led to the identification of a prognostic T-cell signature in colon carcinoma (4). The presence of markers for T-helper 1 (Th1) polarization, cytotoxicity, and memory T cells was strongly correlated with a better prognosis. This signature can be used for the classification of early-stage patients who will benefit from adjuvant therapy to further boost their immune response to the tumor.

While the use of biomarkers for cancer diagnosis and prognosis has been the focus of many research groups recently, few studies have investigated *predictive biomarkers* of the response to immunotherapies of cancer. Sabatino et al. adopted the multiplexed antibody-targeted protein array to study the serum of IL-2-treated metastatic melanoma and renal cancer patients and found that the levels of fibronectin and vascular endothelial growth factor proteins were associated with lack of clinical response and decreased survival (30). Moreover, by a multiplex analysis of serum cytokines in melanoma patients treated with IFN-a2b, Yurkowetsky et al. found that higher pretreatment levels of proinflammatory cytokines (IL-1β, IL-1α, IL-6, and TNF-α) and chemokines (MIP-1α and MIP-1β) could be associated with a longer relapse-free survival (31).

Recent studies have shown that microRNAs could be useful cancer-related biomarkers. In particular, the expression of mIR-26 in patients with hepatocellular carcinoma is associated with survival and response to adjuvant therapy with IFN-α and may be used to select patients who are likely to benefit from the treatment (32).

The gene expression profiling of biopsies taken before treatment with recombinant MAGE-A3 and two different adjuvants (AS15 and AS02B) in unresectable stage III and IV melanoma patients, has led to the identification of a immune-related gene signature associated with clinical benefit (33,34).

Collectively these data suggest that high-throughput technologies should be further exploited for the identification of prognostic and predictive biomarkers in the field of cancer immunotherapy. In addition, these approaches could be used to define in exquisite detail the events involved in immunological responses to cancer.

Systematic Analysis of Tumor Microenvironment and its Impact on the Tumor-Specific Immune Response

Most studies evaluate the impact of vaccination in cancer by examining tumor-specific immune responses in circulating lymphocytes. However, positive immune responses in these peripheral lymphocytes often could not be correlated with tumor regression or better clinical prognosis. Quite likely, the local immune response is very different from what is observed in the periphery. This holds true for responses to infectious diseases, and logic dictates the same would be observed for immune responses to tumors. Therefore, an analysis of the tumor microenvironment and cells resident in that environment could prove useful to providing a more complete picture of the response to vaccination or immunotherapy.

This is supported by studies wherein the group of Marincola used repeated fine needle aspirates combined with gene array analysis to study the response to IL-2 treatment and TAA vaccination in melanoma. They demonstrated that melanoma metastases undergoing regression after peptide vaccination and IL-2 treatment had a different transcription profile than those not responding, with responding lesions showing over-expression of many immune related genes (T1A-1, IL-10, and IRF-1) (35). Moreover, the analysis of melanoma metastases in patients undergoing systemic IL-2 administration demonstrated how treatment had only minimal effects on the migration, activation, and proliferation of T cells. The immediate effect of IL-2 administration was instead the transcriptional activation of genes associated with monocyte function. In particular, the study showed the activation of antigen-presenting monocytes, the production of chemoattractants (as MIG and PARC), and the activation of cytolytic mechanisms in monocytes (calgranulin and grancalcin) and NK cells (NKG5, NK4), suggesting that IL-2 administration may induce inflammation at the tumor site and promote the migration and activation of T cells in situ (36). The expression profile of basal cell cancer lesions treated with the TLR7 ligand, Imiquimod, which predominantly targets pDCs, induced not only type I IFN-related IFN- stimulated genes but also other genes involved in the activation of cellular innate and adaptive immune-effector mechanisms (i.e., IFNγ, granzyme, perforin, granulysin, NK-4, C1QA, and STAT1) (37,38). Gajewski et al. analyzed fresh tumor biopsies obtained before tumor antigen vaccination, and by doing gene expression profiling showed that patients who responded clinically were characterized by having an inflammatory tumor microenvironment precedent to the initiation of vaccination (33,39). Moreover, by the analysis of melanoma metastases they showed that tumors could be segregated according to the presence of T cell–associated transcripts. The presence of lymphocytes correlated with the expression of defined chemokine genes such as CCL2, CCL3, CCL4, CCL5, CXCL9, and CXCL10 (40). A gene expression profile (biomarker signature) that includes T-cell markers and specific chemokines was associated with clinical benefit in a DC-based vaccine trial which included both class I and II HLA-binding peptides (41). Collectively, these data and future studies could shed light on the immunoregulatory environment encountered at the tumor site. This information may be crucial in determining the potential effectiveness of current and future cancer immunotherapies.

Gene Expression Profiles Could Reveal Mechanisms of Tumor Immune Escape

While these studies demonstrate the presence of immune effectors at the tumor site, the analysis of gene array data of melanoma metastasis has also shown the presence of in situ transcripts that encode immune regulatory factors as indoleamine 2,3-diooxygenase, PD-L1, and Fox-P3 and the lack of expression of co-stimulatory ligands as B7-1 and B7-2 (42). Moreover, the expression profile comparison of immune-susceptible cell lines with highly resistant variants could give hints on new mechanism of tumor escape as in the case of the ectopic expression of vascular cell adhesion molecule-1 (VCAM-1) (43). T-cell dysfunction in cancer patients has been extensively demonstrated and represents one of the main reasons for the failure of vaccination strategies. Monsurro et al. showed in a model of tumor antigen immunization, the presence of a quiescent phenotype lacking ex vivo cytotoxic and proliferative potential. The transcription profile comparison of these quiescent cells with that of in vitro sensitized, TAA-specific T cells showed that they were deficient in the expression of genes associated with T-cell activation, proliferation, and effector function possibly explaining the observed lack of correlation between the frequency of vaccine-induced T cells and tumor regression (44). Gene expression profiles could in the future prove useful in determining the immuno-suppressive mechanism present in the tumor microenviroment allowing specific interventions to overcome them.

High-Throughput Technologies Can Also Be Applied to Antigen Discovery

The development of successful immunotherapeutic approaches requires the identification and characterization of tumor antigens that will be recognized by the host immune system. High-throughput technologies have been successfully applied to tumor antigen discovery. Proteomics approaches as serological analysis of recombinant cDNA expression libraries (SEREX), serological proteome analysis (SERPA), and protein microarrays make use of the humoral response to TAAs in cancer patients for the screening of cDNA expression libraries or proteins derived from fresh tumour specimens as a means of identifying novel TAAs (45). Antigens such as NY-ESO-1 (46) and CAGE-1 (47) were identified by SEREX. In particular, protein microarrays could prove useful not only for the detection of new immunotherapy targets but also for the development of diagnostic chips which could allow early cancer detection (48).

Candidate tumor antigens can also be isolated by DNA sequencing and DNA chip–microarray analysis, with an approach called "reverse immunology," as the candidates are identified by comparative expression profiling of tumors and corresponding normal tissue and only in a second step evaluated for their immunogenicity. Potentially this strategy could be used for the design of patient-tailored vaccination (49).

Wide Scale Monitoring of Immune Response to Therapy

Systems biology can also be used for monitoring immunotherapy responses, especially in cases where it is not feasible to monitor antigen-specific responses, as in the case of vaccines made of whole tumor cells [GVAX (50) is one example] where the relevant TAA is not known. A systems biology approach aimed at trying to identify therapies mimicking responses shown to be protective for vaccines or infectious disease models could aid in the design of more specific therapies in the treatment of cancer. In addition, monitoring the full repertoire of B and T cells in physiological, pathological, or therapeutic settings is currently possible thanks to deep sequencing technologies. Boyd et al. (51) showed that parallel DNA sequencing of rearranged immune receptor loci could allow the tracking of the repertoire of B cell lymphocytes, both in physiological and pathological conditions (such as the evaluation of clonal malignancies and of minimal residual disease). This technology could allow a better understanding of repertoire dynamics in response either to disease or specific therapies.

STRATEGY

Systems biology has not only a great potential for the dissection of immune responses to both infectious disease and cancer but it could also prove to be of great value for guiding the development of effective immunotherapies. To better exploit the advantage of using this approach in biological research some basic guidelines should be followed. (*i*) Studies should be designed or analyzed to minimize the variability derived from ethnic affiliation, gender, age, other medical treatments or clinical complications, and disease status. These confounding variables could indeed prevent an effective conclusion from the data; therefore, studied groups should be as homogeneous as possible. (*ii*) When possible, pure populations of cellular subsets should be analyzed. High-throughput analyses of total PBMCs, for example, are of great value, but when possible the separation of the different immune subsets (e.g., T, B, NK, and monocyte subpopulations) should be pursued. Furthermore, with the advances in our understanding of immunology it is increasingly evident that our current definitions of cell subsets can be further divided into smaller subgroups with different functional properties as in the case of T cells which can be separated in different memory, naïve, and effectors subsets and DCs divided into plasmacytoid and myeloid subsets. An example of how a separation of complex cell populations into different immune subsets can reveal otherwise a hidden association is given in Figure 13.5. Using the microarray technology combined with fluorescent activated cell sorting, we could resolve the differential pattern of gene expression confined in CD8 T cells and missed when examining whole blood or PBMC in HIV-1 infected subjects versus their uninfected partner. (*iii*) Studies should contain as many biological replicates as possible. As such, systems biology should aim at collecting more information not only on a single individual but also about more individuals. Larger study populations allow for better statistical power and minimize some of the confounding variables related to specific individuals. Genetic variability could indeed account for differences in disease and treatment response. Moreover, since our immune system is characterized by being able to adapt to the several pathogens an individual could encounter during lifetime, differences originated by a different history of exposure should be taken in consideration as well as different lifestyles and environments. The studies should be designed for being sufficiently large and randomized leading to conclusive information about the effectiveness of a treatment and the isolation of reliable biomarkers. (*iv*) Multiple validation steps should be integrated in the overall strategy to confirm the obtained results using an array of techniques spanning from PCR to proteomics and genome-wide small interfering RNA (siRNA). An important step of systems biology is the validation of the data obtained by high-throughput technologies. While microarrays provide a semi-quantitative estimate of levels of expression, multiplex RNA PCR technologies allow highly quantitative estimates of gene expression. Moreover, the recent development of multiplex single-cell gene expression assays (from Fluidigm) (52) overcomes the heterogeneity that characterizes the immune system as it is now possible to define several single cells in a population. One should not lose the perspective that both population and single-cell analysis provide important information. FACS-based deconvolution strategies are currently available that collect complementary data on the relative contributions of different cell types and/or cell viability and comparing that data to the gene expression profiles derived from the traditional microarray of mixed tissues or cell types. For example, a FACS panel measuring the relative contribution of T cells, B cells, NK cells, monocytes, and DCs in a mixed cell population or tissue can be used to define standardized specific gene expression changes attributed to monocyte, DC, B-cell, and T-cell specific activity in the subjects and deconvolute the dataset using the recently published cell type–specific significance analysis of microarrays (csSAM) algorithm (53). Moreover, protein validation and functional validation using genome-wide siRNA approaches should be an integral component of

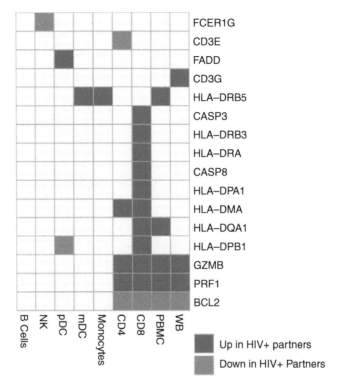

Figure 13.5 Differential gene modulation between whole blood and cell subset populations. This heat map shows the significant modulation of a panel of differentially regulated genes (horizontal row) whose expression is confined to the CD8 compartment and not whole blood (WB) when comparing partners from HIV-discordant couples (Sekaly and Lingappa unpublished data). *Abbreviation*: PBMC, peripheral blood mononuclear cell.

any strategy aimed at defining gene expression signatures that are specific for multiple disease states or different treatment modalities. (*v*) Greater efforts should be put into developing new assays that are multiparametric, high throughput, and highly sensitive and invested in the harmonization of techniques and protocols used. Standardized operating procedure and reagents could indeed help in controlling variations in studies conducted in different laboratories encouraging cross comparison of data and resulting in an acceleration of biomarker identification and cancer immunotherapy development.

CONCLUSIONS

Given the exquisite specificity of the immune system, immunotherapy has the potential of being the most tumour-specific treatment that can be devised to fight cancer. However, this will only be realized when we have a sufficient understanding of the patient and system-level components that contribute to a successful anti-tumor immune response.

This must include information not only about the cells of the immune system as they are the active players in this process but the environment in which they function and the contribution of the tumor itself to the eventual outcome of the therapy. Most of the successful vaccines have indeed been developed empirically (YF being one example) but the recent employment of more sophisticated and high-throughput technologies can provide us with the information we need for a more rational design of vaccines. Not only do we desire a clearer picture of the types of immune responses we need to elicit protection, but we also want to understand how to specifically elicit that response. Systems biology approaches have allowed us to obtain some

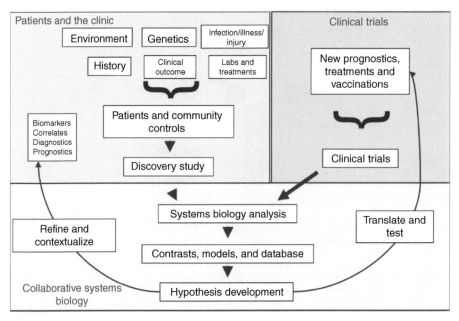

Figure 13.6 Collaborative workflow for a systems biology approach to modeling human illness. This figure demonstrates the potential routes for samples and information in and out of a collaborative systems biology center. (*Top left panel*): Doctors and clinical study coordinators can provide a myriad of necessary information about the ill patient or matched community control, including natural history of the illness or injury, the history of the patient, the clinical lab profiles, treatment regimens, and the course of disease and outcome. Through a discovery immune modeling study, the systems biology center (*bottom panel*) can conduct the analysis based on the compare-and-contrast goals of the study (e.g., patients of different outcomes or relationships with controls), model and database the immune or host responses, and develop preliminary hypotheses. These hypotheses can be refined or contextualized and fed back to the discovery study to develop more detailed biomarker-based goals or eventually translated from the database against other cohorts and tested in clinical trials (*top right panel*) in the form of new prognostics, treatments, or vaccines.

answers regarding what constitute a protective immune response and these approaches are also allowing us the opportunity to test and evaluate novel therapies based on lessons learned. Data and biomarkers obtained by this integrated approach can be used to prioritize research, defining appropriate treatments for specific patient groups, and provide targets for future therapeutics (54). However, we should not forget that not all the vaccines generate the same kind of immune response and their efficacy could be based on different signatures, depending on specific mechanisms that they employ to generate effective immunity. So, a one-size-fits-all approach may not be possible and an iterative process of novel therapeutics and trials followed by intense and comprehensive immune monitoring that is then followed by improved therapeutics and more monitoring may be implemented.

Investigating cancer and its interaction with the immune system involves dealing with the complex nature of this relationship in humans where the heterogeneity of a particular response is due not only to its intrinsic stochastic characteristics but also to genetic polymorphism adding to this relationship another layer of complexity of possible clinical relevance. Immunogenetic profiling could prove useful for better understanding differences in responses to the disease and treatment in patient populations.

Another main challenge derives from the necessity of integrating large amounts of data in a single system capable of portraying the immune status and its response as an integrated whole. To reach this goal, a greater degree of collaboration and integration among various clinical and scientific disciplines is essential (Fig. 13.6). However, a correct balance must be kept among the need of being interdisciplinary and the one of having broad specialist knowledge in the area of interest. Moreover, data integration and collaboration among different laboratories and clinical entities should be pursued, possibly with the creation of common curated databases.

It must be kept in mind that systems biology will not replace the reductionist approach to immunology research but rather it should integrate it into the whole study, as global approaches are often incapable of revealing mechanistic details. A balance between the two different approaches should be kept, with high-throughput technologies generating hypothesis that should be validated and tested by conventional reductionist analysis that should then be placed in the perspective of the whole system.

However, as well described by Benoist elsewhere (55), systems biology should not be focused only in generating hypothesis or answering defined immunological questions which are then validated by conventional approaches, because the intrinsic value of the systems approach resides in the possibility of making global comparisons, to assess similarities and differences of systems in their wholeness. This kind of perspective in data analysis requires a concerted effort as the data sets are complex and the analysis often difficult when comparing data at a higher order. The paradox of this approach is that it often generates more questions than it answers.

Finally, systems biology approaches could prove useful in defining correlates of response to treatment, biomarkers which could help the evaluation of vaccine efficacy, and rapid identification of patients likely to respond to specific treatments as well as those unlikely to respond (who can then be enrolled in treatments more appropriate for their response profile). Systems biology therefore holds the promise of leading to a personalized therapy approach that might just be what is needed in the fight against a disease so personalized as cancer.

REFERENCES

1. Burnet M. Cancer; a biological approach. I. The processes of control. Br Med J 1957; 1: 779–86.
2. Dunn GP, Bruce AT, Ikeda H, et al. Cancer immunoediting: from immunosurveillance to tumor escape. Nat Immunol 2002; 3: 991–8.
3. van der Bruggen P, Traversari C, Chomez P, et al. A gene encoding an antigen recognized by cytolytic T lymphocytes on a human melanoma. Science 1991; 254: 1643–47.
4. Galon J, Costes A, Sanchez-Cabo F, et al. Type, density, and location of immune cells within human colorectal tumors predict clinical outcome. Science 2006; 313: 1960–4.
5. Koebel CM, Vermi W, Swann JB, et al. Adaptive immunity maintains occult cancer in an equilibrium state. Nature 2007; 450: 903–7.
6. Liu MA. Immunologic basis of vaccine vectors. Immunity 2010; 33: 504–15.
7. Lonchay C, van der Bruggen P, Connerotte T, et al. Correlation between tumor regression and T cell responses in melanoma patients vaccinated with a MAGE antigen. Proc Natl Acad Sci USA 2004; 101(Suppl 2): 14631–8.
8. Camus M, Tosolini M, Mlecnik B, et al. Coordination of intratumoral immune reaction and human colorectal cancer recurrence. Cancer Res 2009; 69: 2685–93.
9. Sun JC, Bevan MJ. Defective CD8 T cell memory following acute infection without CD4 T cell help. Science 2003; 300: 339–42.
10. Banchereau J, Palucka AK. Dendritic cells as therapeutic vaccines against cancer. Nat Rev Immunol 2005; 5: 296–306.
11. Khalil IG, Hill C. Systems biology for cancer. Curr Opin Oncol 2005; 17: 44–8.
12. Hoheisel JD. Microarray technology: beyond transcript profiling and genotype analysis. Nat Rev Genet 2006; 7: 200–10.
13. Wang Z, Gerstein M, Snyder M. RNA-Seq: a revolutionary tool for transcriptomics. Nat Rev Genet 2009; 10: 57–63.
14. Choudhary C, Mann M. Decoding signalling networks by mass spectrometry-based proteomics. Nat Rev Mol Cell Biol 2010; 11: 427–39.
15. Schiess R, Mueller LN, Schmidt A, et al. Analysis of cell surface proteome changes via label-free, quantitative mass spectrometry. Mol Cell Proteomics 2009; 8: 624–38.
16. Zhu H, Bilgin M, Snyder M. Proteomics. Annu Rev Biochem 2003; 72: 783–812.

17. Chattopadhyay PK, Hogerkorp CM, Roederer M. A chromatic explosion: the development and future of multiparameter flow cytometry. Immunology 2008; 125: 441–9.
18. Schulz KR, Danna EA, Krutzik PO, Nolan GP. Single-cell phospho-protein analysis by flow cytometry. Curr Protoc Immunol 2007; Chapter 8: Unit 8 17.
19. Hadrup SR, Bakker AH, Shu CJ, et al. Parallel detection of antigen-specific T-cell responses by multidimensional encoding of MHC multimers. Nat Methods 2009; 6: 520–6.
20. Wei G, Wei L, Zhu J, et al. Global mapping of H3K4me3 and H3K27me3 reveals specificity and plasticity in lineage fate determination of differentiating CD4+ T cells. Immunity 2009; 30: 155–67.
21. Reiner SL. Epigenetic control in the immune response. Hum Mol Genet 2005; 14 Spec No 1: R41–6.
22. Rubins KH, Hensley LE, Jahrling PB, et al. The host response to smallpox: analysis of the gene expression program in peripheral blood cells in a nonhuman primate model. Proc Natl Acad Sci USA 2004; 101: 15190–5.
23. Djavani MM, Crasta OR, Zapata JC, et al. Early blood profiles of virus infection in a monkey model for Lassa fever. J Virol 2007; 81: 7960–73.
24. Zilliox MJ, Moss WJ, Griffin DE. Gene expression changes in peripheral blood mononuclear cells during measles virus infection. Clin Vaccine Immunol 2007; 14: 918–23.
25. Gaucher D, Therrien R, Kettaf N, et al. Yellow fever vaccine induces integrated multilineage and polyfunctional immune responses. J Exp Med 2008; 205: 3119–31.
26. Querec TD, Akondy RS, Lee EK, et al. Systems biology approach predicts immunogenicity of the yellow fever vaccine in humans. Nat Immunol 2009; 10: 116–25.
27. Berry MP, Graham CM, McNab FW, et al. An interferon-inducible neutrophil-driven blood transcriptional signature in human tuberculosis. Nature 2010; 466: 973–7.
28. Manicassamy S, Ravindran R, Deng J, et al. Toll-like receptor 2-dependent induction of vitamin A-metabolizing enzymes in dendritic cells promotes T regulatory responses and inhibits autoimmunity. Nat Med 2009; 15: 401–9.
29. Copier J, Whelan M, Dalgleish A. Biomarkers for the development of cancer vaccines: current status. Mol Diagn Ther 2006; 10: 337–43.
30. Sabatino M, Kim-Schulze S, Panelli MC, et al. Serum vascular endothelial growth factor and fibronectin predict clinical response to high-dose interleukin-2 therapy. J Clin Oncol 2009; 27: 2645–52.
31. Yurkovetsky ZR, Kirkwood JM, Edington HD, et al. Multiplex analysis of serum cytokines in melanoma patients treated with interferon-alpha2b. Clin Cancer Res 2007; 13: 2422–8.
32. Ji J, Shi J, Budhu A, et al. MicroRNA expression, survival, and response to interferon in liver cancer. N Engl J Med 2009; 361: 1437–47.
33. Gajewski TF, Louahed J, Brichard VG. Gene signature in melanoma associated with clinical activity: a potential clue to unlock cancer immunotherapy. Cancer J 2010; 16: 399–403.
34. Louahed J, Gruselle O, Gaulis S, et al. Expression of defined genes identified by pre-treatment tumor profiling: association with clinical response to the GSK MAGE-A3 immunotherapeutic in metastatic melanoma patients. J Clin Oncol 2008; 26: Abstract 9045.
35. Wang E, Miller LD, Ohnmacht GA, et al. Prospective molecular profiling of melanoma metastases suggests classifiers of immune responsiveness. Cancer Res 2002; 62: 3581–6.
36. Panelli MC, Wang E, Phan G, et al. Gene-expression profiling of the response of peripheral blood mononuclear cells and melanoma metastases to systemic IL-2 administration. Genome Biol 2002; 3: RESEARCH0035.
37. Bedognetti D, Wang E, Sertoli MR, Marincola FM. Gene-expression profiling in vaccine therapy and immunotherapy for cancer. Expert Rev Vaccines 2010; 9: 555–65.
38. Panelli MC, Stashower ME, Slade HB, et al. Sequential gene profiling of basal cell carcinomas treated with imiquimod in a placebo-controlled study defines the requirements for tissue rejection. Genome Biol 2007; 8: R8.
39. Gajewski TF, Meng Y, Harlin H. Chemokines expressed in melanoma metastases associated with T cell infiltration. J Clin Oncol 2007; 25: Abstract 8501.
40. Harlin H, Meng Y, Peterson AC, et al. Chemokine expression in melanoma metastases associated with CD8+ T-cell recruitment. Cancer Res 2009; 69: 3077–85.
41. Gajewski TF, Zha Y, Thurner B, Schuler G. Association of gene expression profile in metastatic melanoma and survival to a dendritic cell-based vaccine. J Clin Oncol 2009; 27: Abstract 9002.
42. Gajewski TF, Fuertes M, Spaapen R, et al. Molecular profiling to identify relevant immune resistance mechanisms in the tumor microenvironment. Curr Opin Immunol 2011; 23: 286–92.
43. Lin KY, Lu D, Hung CF, et al. Ectopic expression of vascular cell adhesion molecule-1 as a new mechanism for tumor immune evasion. Cancer Res 2007; 67: 1832–41.

44. Monsurro V, Wang E, Yamano Y, et al. Quiescent phenotype of tumor-specific CD8+ T cells following immunization. Blood 2004; 104: 1970–8.
45. Gunawardana CG, Diamandis EP. High throughput proteomic strategies for identifying tumour-associated antigens. Cancer Lett 2007; 249: 110–19.
46. Chen YT, Scanlan MJ, Sahin U, et al. A testicular antigen aberrantly expressed in human cancers detected by autologous antibody screening. Proc Natl Acad Sci USA 1997; 94: 1914–18.
47. Park S, Lim Y, Lee D, et al. Identification and characterization of a novel cancer/testis antigen gene CAGE-1. Biochim Biophys Acta 2003; 1625: 173–82.
48. Casiano CA, Mediavilla-Varela M, Tan EM. Tumor-associated antigen arrays for the serological diagnosis of cancer. Mol Cell Proteomics 2006; 5: 1745–59.
49. Mocellin S, Lise M, Nitti D. Tumor immunology. Adv Exp Med Biol 2007; 593: 147–56.
50. Hege KM, Jooss K, Pardoll D. GM-CSF gene-modifed cancer cell immunotherapies: of mice and men. Int Rev Immunol 2006; 25: 321–52.
51. Boyd SD, Marshall EL, Merker JD, et al. Measurement and clinical monitoring of human lymphocyte clonality by massively parallel VDJ pyrosequencing. Sci Transl Med 2009; 1: 12ra23.
52. Flatz L, Roychoudhuri R, Honda M, et al. Single-cell gene-expression profiling reveals qualitatively distinct CD8 T cells elicited by different gene-based vaccines. Proc Natl Acad Sci USA 2011; 108: 5724–9.
53. Shen-Orr SS, Tibshirani R, Khatri P, et al. Cell type-specific gene expression differences in complex tissues. Nat Methods 2010; 7: 287–9.
54. Bindea G, Mlecnik B, Fridman WH, et al. Natural immunity to cancer in humans. Curr Opin Immunol 2010; 22: 215–22.
55. Benoist C, Germain RN, Mathis D. A plaidoyer for 'systems immunology'. Immunol Rev 2006; 210: 229–34.

14 | Targeting regulatory T cells and other strategies to enable cancer vaccines

Christopher Paustian, Shawn M. Jensen, Sarah Church, Sachin Puri, Chris Twitty, Hong-Ming Hu, Brendan D. Curti, Walter J. Urba, Raj K. Puri, and Bernard A. Fox

INTRODUCTION

Cancer vaccines are designed to initiate an effector response from patient lymphocytes that will both assist in clearing the tumor and retain memory of the disease so that disease recurrence is prevented. However, certain subsets of the very lymphocytes targeted by immunotherapies develop suppressor functions after being subverted by the patient's tumor. These subsets include regulatory CD4 T cells, suppressor CD8 T cells, and regulatory B cells. Many current clinical trials testing cancer vaccines include concomitant treatments designed to delete, inactivate, or convert these suppressor cells so that they no longer prevent the development of a therapeutic immune response. This chapter summarizes suppressor lymphocyte subsets and their functions, the mechanisms by which they regulate immune responses, and promising strategies that might overcome these immunologic barriers.

TYPES OF SUPPRESSOR LYMPHOCYTES

Lymphocytic suppression of cancer vaccines has been attributed to three distinct subpopulations of cells. Regulatory CD4 T (T_{REG}) cells have been extensively studied in recent years and a number of ways to delete or inhibit these cells have been investigated. Suppressor CD8 cells have been characterized and studied in relation to their effects on tumor therapies, though not as extensively as CD4 T_{REG} cells. The newly characterized B_{REG} cells, including interleukin-10 (IL-10) secreting B10 cells, have recently been associated with resistance to autoimmune diseases; however, their role in cancer immunotherapy remains a new field of investigation.

Regulatory leukocytes that limit anti-tumor immunity are not confined to the lymphocyte compartment; myeloid-derived suppressor cells (MDSCs) confound anti-tumor immunity through a variety of means. MDSC precursors leave the bone marrow with the potential to mature into macrophages or dendritic cells (DCs), but instead get caught up in the immunosuppressive environment of the tumor and persist as immature myeloid cells. MDSCs are a heterogeneous group of cells that quiesce anti-tumor immunity primarily through the metabolism of L-arginine, which serves as a substrate for two enzymes: inducible-nitric oxide synthase and arginase 1 (1). In addition to starving T cells for arginine, the enzymatic by-products of arginine have immunosuppressive powers of their own, resulting in anergy, T-cell receptor inactivation, or even the formation of new T_{REG} (2). A number of agents are currently being investigated to target MDSCs in cancer patients, but few have translated out of preclinical models.

One candidate approved for clinical use is sunitinib, a broad-spectrum receptor tyrosine-kinase inhibitor that has experienced relative clinical success (3). Significant reductions in circulating MDSCs have been reported in patients treated with sunitinib therapy (4,5). Importantly, MDSC reduction induced by sunitinib correlated with lower numbers of T_{REGS} in the periphery and increased Th1 responsiveness in some cancer patients (5). However, tumors obtained from sunitinib-treated patients have shown no significant declines in MDSC numbers, an observation attributed to the MDSC-protective effects of granulocyte-macrophage colony-stimulating factor found in sunitinib-resistant tumor cultures (6). Research is underway to develop new therapies directly targeting MDSC generation or mechanisms of suppression that may enhance the effectiveness of immune-based therapies.

CD4 T_{REG} Cells

CD4 T_{REG} is an umbrella term that currently comprises four types of suppressor cells generated under different conditions: (*i*) thymic-derived "natural" T_{REGS} (nT_{REG}) and (*ii*) peripherally induced T_{RE} (iT_{REG}) which include (*iii*) Tr1, and (*iv*) Th3 subsets (7) (Fig. 14.1). Roughly 60–70%

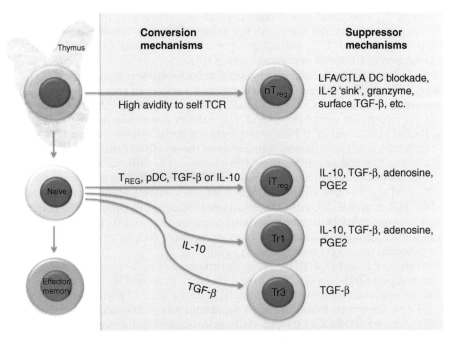

Figure 14.1 CD4$^+$ T regulatory (T$_{REG}$) cell subsets. T$_{REGS}$ can originate from the thymus as T cells with high avidity to self antigens (nT$_{REG}$) or as peripherally induced T$_{REGS}$ that arise from naive precursors (iT$_{REG}$). Two subsets of iT$_{REGS}$ have been identified, Tr1 and Th3. In general, nT$_{REGS}$ mediate tolerance by the contact-dependent mechanisms listed while iT$_{REGS}$ are known for their generation of various immunosuppressive soluble factors. *Abbreviations*: CTLA, cytotoxic T lymphocyte-associated antigen; DC, dendritic cell; IL-10, interleukin-10; LFA, leukocyte function-associated antigen; PGE2, prostaglandin 2; TCR, T-cell receptor; TGF-β, transforming growth factor beta.

of T$_{REGS}$ in mice and humans are nT$_{REG}$ (8) which arise from the thymus as a distinct lineage of CD4$^+$CD25$^+$ T cells with a T-cell receptor (TCR) repertoire characterized by high avidity toward self antigens (9). These cells appear to play an important role in preventing autoimmunity. They are distinguished by high expression of CD25, the alpha chain of the IL-2 receptor, as well as the transcriptional regulator FoxP3 (10). Expression of FoxP3 in these cells is stabilized by demethylation of a CpG-rich non-coding region in the FoxP2 locus and appears to be critical to their function (11).

Naturally occurring T$_{REGS}$ suppress the proliferation of other T cells primarily in a contact-dependent and antigen-specific manner (12). The first mechanism proposed to explain this phenomenon was the most obvious—since T$_{REGS}$ were first defined by high expression of CD25, a part of the IL-2 receptor complex, it was proposed that they acted as a "cytokine sink" absorbing the cytokine necessary for T-cell expansion and function (13). T$_{REGS}$ can also directly eliminate effector cells in a granzyme-dependent manner (14). Several models of autoimmunity have demonstrated that T$_{REG}$ surface expression of transforming growth factor beta (TGF-β) was necessary for the prevention of disease (15,16). A recent study elucidated another important mechanism, the suppression of dendritic cell (DC) function, when co-culturing dye-labeled T$_{REG}$ cells with naïve T cells and DCs (17). In the presence of anti-CD3 they observed T$_{REGS}$ clustering about the DCs, outcompeting the naïve cells in accessing antigen/major histocompatibility complex (MHC). Using lineage specific knockouts (KO) as well as blocking antibodies, they determined that leukocyte function-associated antigen-1 was necessary for T$_{REG}$ aggregation, while cytotoxic T lymphocyte-associated antigen 4 (CTLA-4) was responsible for downregulating the expression of co-stimulatory molecules CD80/86 on DCs. Taken together, they proposed a core mechanism of T_{REG}-mediated cell contact-dependent suppression in which antigen-activated T_{REG} cells act in two distinct steps: (*i*) the initial leukocyte function-associated antigen-1–dependent adherence of T_{REGS} on antigen-presenting DCs and (*ii*) the CTLA-4-dependent downmodulation of CD80/86 expressed on DCs (17).

iT$_{REGS}$ induced in the periphery arise from naïve precursors activated by TCR stimulation in a tolerogenic cytokine milieu (7). A heterogeneous subset of some in-vivo converted iT$_{REGS}$ expresses similar amounts of CD25 and FoxP3 to nT$_{REGS}$. In the past this has made the differentiation of the two major peripheral blood T_{REG} subsets essentially impossible in most mouse models. Recent identification of Helios as a transcriptional marker of thymic lineage in FoxP3 positive cells may ease the differentiation between these cells in future studies (8), although its intracellular location makes purification of live human cells difficult. Regardless, the induction of T_{REGS} from naïve T cells results in a population of suppressors that work very differently from thymic T_{REGS}. iT$_{REGS}$ mediate suppression in a largely contact-independent manner, secreting factors like TGF-β and IL-10, with the additional influence of prostaglandin E2 (PGE2) and adenosine playing roles in tumor-associated suppression (18,19). Both nT$_{REG}$ and iT$_{REG}$ are known to induce "infectious tolerance", converting naïve cells to induced T_{REGS} which in turn have the potential to convert more naïve T_{REGS} (20).

Activation of human CD4+ T cells in the presence of IL-10 results in anergic T_{REG}, called T regulatory type 1 (Tr1) cells (21,22). These cells go on to secrete IL-10 in an autocrine fashion, which helps to maintain their own anergic state; blocking of IL-10 partially restores proliferation (23,24). Tr1 cells have been found to play a significant role in tolerance to head and neck squamous cell carcinoma (HNSCC) (21), especially in the case of cyclooxygenase-2 (COX-2) positive tumors secreting PGE2, a factor which allows for the expansion of these cells (25,26). Mechanisms of suppression are contact independent and include IL-10, TGF-β, adenosine, and PGE2 (23,24,26). While TGF-β may play a small role in the generation of Tr1 cells, another T helper subtype, Th3 is absolutely dependent on it (27). TGF-β plays a central role in oral tolerance as both the inducer of Th3 and primary mechanism of suppression by these cells. Th3 cells also help in IgA production and have suppressive properties for Th1 and other immune cells (28).

Certainly the question of which regulatory cells protect cancers is of interest to immunotherapists. One study examining the dynamics of both nT$_{REG}$ and iT$_{REG}$ in a murine tumor model found that naïve cells were converted by antigen-presenting cells (APC), under the tumor's influence, into iT$_{REG}$ while nT$_{REG}$ proliferated in response to the tumor vaccine. While kinetics and mode of action differed, both sets of T_{REGS} contributed to inhibition of tumor-specific Th1 responses (29). The emerging knowledge of the different mechanisms of action, tissue infiltration by different T-cell populations and consequent TCR specificities inherent in each T_{REG} subset will allow for a more strategic vaccine design in the future, a concept discussed in the conclusion of this chapter.

CD8 T$_{REG}$ Cells

Infiltration of tumors by CD8 T cells is a well-known favorable prognostic indicator, as they are thought to be key players in anti-tumor responses (30–32). Yet, CD8 cells with suppressive function have also been identified in the tumor or draining lymph nodes of most of the human cancers (33–35). These cells are defined by FoxP3 and CD25 expression as well as the absence of the co-stimulatory molecule CD28 (35,36). Mechanisms of suppression include contact-dependent (35) as well as contact-independent suppression of effector-cell proliferation and function (36). Although CD8 T$_{REG}$ have been generated in vitro by co-culture with immature DC and tolerized endothelial cells (37,38) the exact means by which tumors convert these cells is a subject of ongoing research.

B$_{REG}$ Cells

Regulatory B cells have been shown to inhibit autoimmunity and inflammation through IL-10 production in mice and humans (39,40). This newly characterized B cell subset is most commonly identified by the co-expression of CD1d and CD5, and represents 1–3% of adult mouse spleen B cells. In vitro activation of these cells to produce IL-10 commonly involves lipopolysaccharide (LPS), phorbol 12-myristate 13-acetate plus ionomycin stimulation; however, prolonged LPS or CD40 stimulation will induce additional adult spleen B_{REG} cells to secrete IL-10 (39). This indicates that T-cell help in the form of CD40L stimulation may play a role in effective suppression by B_{REGS}, a finding confirmed in systemic lupus erythematosus patients (40). CD20 is a B-cell marker and the target of the monoclonal antibodies such as rituximab, ibritumomab tiuxetan, and tositumomab. The latter two are often conjugated to radioisotopes while rituximab depletion is mediated by Fc receptor-bearing macrophages (41). All are actively used in the treatment of B-cell lymphomas and leukemias, but their utility in the treatment of other human cancers through B_{REG} modulation has not yet been investigated. CD20 mAbs are able to deplete malignant B cells in mouse models (41), but melanoma-bearing mice treated with rituximab accelerated melanoma growth and impaired T-cell responses of CD4 and CD8 (42).

The first set of studies examining the influence of B_{REG} in the tumor environment was conducted in a B-cell KO model. When two out of three tumors analyzed showed IL-10-producing B cells compromised therapeutic anti-tumor immunity, it was proposed that B-cell depletion could enhance anti-tumor immune responses to certain tumors (43). In contrast, subsequent studies using rituximab have not confirmed this finding (44). Possible explanations might include that CD20 does not delineate the B_{REG} subset with enough specificity or that the cellular and innate immune systems in B cell KO mice compensate for the lack of humoral immunity by enhanced efficacy, or that undifferentiated thymocytes fill the B cell gap and are capable of innate killing much like those found in the thymus of mice with severe combined immunodeficiency diseases (45). An additional cautionary note for researchers seeking to inhibit B_{REG} for non-lymphoid tumors, a recent study found that activated B cells from tumor draining lymph nodes could synergize when adoptively transferred with T cells in a metastatic pulmonary mouse model (46) highlighting their ability to help induce cellular immune responses.

THREE STRATEGIES TO DEAL WITH SUPPRESSOR LYMPHOCYTES

In the normal course of immune activation, regulatory cells balance inflammation precisely in order to allow for pathogen clearance and prevent induction of autoimmunity. The basic principle of cancer vaccines is to "fool" the immune system into recognizing malignant tissue as foreign. However, activating a therapeutic immune response to tissue previously identified as self by tumor-primed regulatory cells presents a sizable hurdle since it amounts to inducing autoimmunity for these cells, the very scenario that regulatory cells have evolved to deliberately prevent. Thus, specific targeting of regulatory cells may be necessary to induce a therapeutic response in most of the cases. The three strategies to do so are to (*i*) eliminate the relevant suppressor population during treatment, (*ii*) inactivate the relevant suppressor population during treatment, (*iii*) or convert the suppressors into effectors. Table 14.1 and Figure 14.2 summarize these strategies.

Subset Deletion Therapies

The most direct route to breaking tumoral tolerance will be to identify specific markers on regulatory cells and delete them with targeted antibodies or toxin-conjugated ligands prior to vaccination. Unfortunately, the most specific marker of regulatory function, FoxP3, is an intracellular transcription factor and thus not accessible to current cellular depletion strategies. Furthermore, FoxP3 is transiently expressed on effector cells in humans, albeit at lower levels than in regulatory cells. While the problem of selectively identifying regulatory cells remains, several interventions in clinical trials have been promising.

Table 14.1 T_{REG} Interventions

Target	Agent	T_{REG} Effect	Refs
CD25	Denileukin diftitox	Antibody-toxin conjugate mediated deletion	(49)
	Daclizumab	Antibody-mediated deletion (ADCC)	(47)
	Ex-vivo depletion		(149)
CD4	Zanolimumab	Antibody mediated deletion (ADCC)	(55)
Chemotherapy	Cyclophosphamide	Crosslinks DNA	(60)
	Paclitaxel	Microtubule stabilization	
	Gemcitabine	Nucleoside analogue	
	Cisplatin	Cross-links DNA	
	Temozolomide	Guanine methylation on DNA	
GITR	TRX518	GITR agonist antibody	NCT01239134
CTLA-4	Ipilimumab	Co-stimulator blockade	(79)
	Tremelimumab	Co-stimulator blockade	NCT00313794
OX40	OX86	OX40 agonist antibody	(150)
TGF-beta	AP12009	Anti-sense oligonucleotide to TGF-β	(100)
	GC1008	Humanized anti-TGF-β	(97)
	LY2157299	Small-molecule serine/threonine TGF-β receptor I kinase inhibitor	
PGE2	Celecoxib	Selective COX-2 inhibitor	(108)
CD39	ARL67156	ATP analog	(121)
A2 receptor	ZM241385	Selective A2a/A2b receptor antagonist	(120)
TLR	Resiquimod	T_{REG} inactivation/conversion	(142)
APC	Activated monocyte?	T_{REG} inactivation/conversion	(131)
IDO	1-methyl-D-tryptophan	Tryptophan analogue blocks enzyme	(147)

Abbreviations: ADCC, antibody-dependent cell-mediated cytotoxicity; APC, antigen-presenting cell; COX-2, cyclooxygenase-2; CTLA, cytotoxic T lymphocyte-associated antigen; IDO, indoleamine 2,3-dioxygenase; GITR, glucocorticoid-induced TNFR-related protein; PGE2 prostaglandin; TGF-β, transforming growth factor beta; TLR, toll-like receptor.

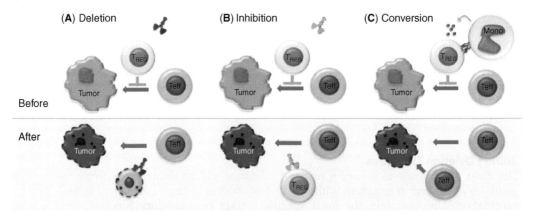

Figure 14.2 Three strategies to enhance vaccines by addressing regulatory cells. Cancers enlist the aid of regulatory cells to escape immune-mediated rejection. In order to enhance vaccine efficiency in therapeutic settings researchers seek ways to either (**A**) kill these immunosuppressive cells, (**B**) render them functionally inactive, or (**C**) convert them to effector cell function that they might assist in priming a cytotoxic T-cell response. *Abbreviations:* Teff, T effector cells; T_{REGS}, T regulatory cells.

CD25

Since CD25 is highly expressed on the surface of regulatory cells, it represents an obvious target for a depletion strategy. However, CD25 is also upregulated on T effector cells during their IL-2-dependent expansion as well as on activated DC. This makes timing a key aspect for targeting CD25.

Daclizumab is a humanized antibody directed against CD25. A phase I study, while using this agent for depleting T_{REG}s prior to a peptide-based breast cancer vaccine, found that Fox P3- positive cells were reduced out to five weeks after treatment (47). Unfortunately, another study using daclizumab found that CD25$^+$ effector cells induced by a peptide-pulsed DC vaccine for metastatic melanoma were deleted as well, and that this impaired vaccine-specific T cells from acquiring effector functions (48). While further studies are needed to confirm these findings, the results indicate that vaccination during depletion by this agent may be ill advised, at least at the dose of 0.5 mg/kg used in that study.

Denileukin diftitox is an engineered protein combining IL-2 and diphtheria toxin, which binds to CD25 on T_{REG} and introduces the diphtheria toxin into the cells, blocking protein production and causing cell death. The adverse events reported in patients who received denileukin diftitox were hypoalbuminemia, fever, chills, acute hypersensitivity reactions, nausea, vomiting, asthenia, and vascular leak syndrome (49). In a phase I study of advanced cancer patients depletion of FoxP3$^+$ T_{REGS} with multiple denileukin diftitox treatments appeared to augment the development of T-cell responses to carcinoembryonic antigen at early time points after administration of a DC vaccine (50); however, patients who did not receive denileukin diftitox exhibited the strongest carcinoembryonic antigen-specific interferon gamma (IFNγ) responses at the completion of the study. Additional trials with this drug are underway and should help determine the utility of this agent in a multiple vaccine setting in which the agent may target both T_{REG} and tumor-specific T cells that are activated by vaccination.

Another strategy involves *ex vivo* depletion during non-myeloablative chemotherapy. In a preclinical model the depletion of CD25$^+$ cells from the lymphocytes that were used to reconstitute lymphopenic tumor-bearing mice recovered the priming of tumor-specific effector T cells and therapeutic efficacy in an adoptive immunotherapy studies. (51). Add-back experiments confirmed the suppressive function of the tumor-induced CD25$^+$ T_{REG} cells. In patients with metastatic melanoma who underwent leukapheresis prior to low-dose chemotherapy followed by reinfusion of the CD25-depleted apheresis product there was a rapid T_{REG} cell repopulation with a high percentage of peripheral CD4$^+$ T cells expressing FoxP3 shortly after cell infusion. Patients in that study received high-dose intravenous IL-2 following infusion of the CD25 depleted cell product, a therapy to which those patients had already proven refractory. Thus the selection criterion may have compromised the results (52). Also, a high-dose IL-2 therapy may not coordinate well with such a strategy since IL-2 plays an important role in the generation and maintenance of T_{REG} cells (53). Another trial attempted to deplete CD25 off a reinfusion product with renal cell carcinoma patients and found that while T_{REG} numbers were down two weeks following treatment, they came back to normal levels by week 4 and grew to twice the proportion of before by week 8 before tapering back down to normal levels (54). No vaccination was given following treatment in that trial, but the investigators considered these results proof of concept. Based on the work of Poehlein and colleagues (51), reconstitution of non-myeloablated patients infused with CD25-depleted peripheral blood mononuclear cells and vaccinated may augment the anti-cancer immune response. A clinical trial of this strategy in metastatic melanoma is currently underway.

CD4

In a recent study on the effect of multiple vaccinations with a granulocyte-macrophage colony-stimulating factor (GM-CSF) secreting melanoma cell line in cyclophosphamide treated mice that were reconstituted with naïve splenocytes it was found that a single vaccination primed tumor-specific T cells with therapeutic efficacy in adoptive immunotherapy experiments, but T cells from mice that had received multiple vaccinations were not therapeutic. Subsequent experiments showed that multiple vaccinations preferentially expanded T_{REG} cells in this model. However, partial depletion of CD4 T cells with anti-CD4 antibody prior to receiving booster vaccines restored the therapeutic efficacy of T cells obtained from multiply vaccinated mice (55).

Several phase I/II trials of zanolimumab, an anti-CD4 depleting antibody currently used to treat T cell lymphomas, found that the drug was well tolerated (56). The adverse events reported most frequently included low-grade infections and eczematous dermatitis (57). Zanolimumab also influences CD4$^+$ T cells by inhibiting TCR signaling in addition to Fc-mediated deletion, which was found to selectively affect CD45RO$^+$ cells more than CD45RA$^+$ cells (58). Since CD4 help is necessary for the development of functional CD8 T-cell memory but dispensable in some scenarios for recall responses (59,60), use of a CD4 depleting antibody may translate well to clinical trials of solid tumor vaccines, as long as it is not used during the initial priming phase. A strategy reducing CD4 T cell numbers, leaving 30–50% of the population intact, may be sufficient to reduce T_{REG} function while providing sufficient help to support memory responses.

Chemotherapy

The mechanism by which chemotherapy kills tumor cells has traditionally been viewed as direct cytotoxicity of aggressively dividing cells, with immunosuppression being an unwanted but unavoidable complication of therapy. Recent studies have shown that the unintended consequence of immunomodulation may in fact be partly responsible for tumor regression. Non-myeloablative chemotherapies have been found to modulate tumor immunogenicity, inducing immunogenic apoptosis as well as activating DCs and inducing a homeostatic proliferative burst of lymphocytes that can "reboot" the exhausted immune system (61). Likewise, some chemotherapy treatments seem to have preferential effects on T_{REG} cells.

Preclinical models indicate that T_{REG}s are more sensitive to low-dose lympho-depleting chemotherapy regimens than T effector cells and thus may be selectively depleted to enhance anti-tumor immunity (62,63). Cisplatin decreased relative T_{REG} numbers in peripheral blood and spleens of tumor-bearing mice, thus help rejecting tumors in a DNA vaccine model (64). Other studies have found that T_{REG} activity is diminished in mice treated with metronomic (i.e., many periodic low-concentration doses of chemotherapy) cyclophosphamide, paclitaxel, or temozolamide (55–67).

In patients with metastatic solid tumors metronomic cyclophosphamide resulted in fewer CD4$^+$ CD25$^+$ FoxP3$^+$ T_{REG} and heightened effector lymphocyte function one month into therapy (68). Following paclitaxel-based chemotherapy, non-small-cell lung carcinoma patients showed a selective decrease in the number and suppressive capacity of T_{REG} without measurably affecting effector T cells (69). Gemcitabine combined with FOLFOX4, prior to GM-CSF and IL-2 significantly reduced the number of T_{REG} in 65% of colorectal cancer patients resulting in a 70% objective response rate (70,71). The old adage "the dose makes the poison" was never truer than in immunomodulatory chemotherapies. A recent study employed a factorial study design to determine the optimum dosing of combined therapy with cyclophosphamide and doxorubicin; the highest dose of doxorubicin tested (35 mg/m^2) enhanced patients' humoral responses to a HER-2 (human epidermal growth factor receptor 2) vaccine while the lowest dose of cyclophosphamide best increased HER-2 antibody responses of the patients. Cyclophosphamide doses more than 200 mg/m^2 abrogated both cellular and humoral responses (72). These findings were observed in the context of a dual chemotherapy regimen; therefore, extrapolating to single-agent treatment studies is tenuous. Since most trials of cyclophosphamide have given doses of 250–300 mg/m^2 to reduce T_{REGS}, further investigation of this phenomena and combined dose-ranging studies with specific immunological monitoring of lymphocyte subtypes is certainly warranted.

Inhibiting the Mechanisms of Suppression

While the plethora of mechanisms by which regulatory T cells mediate suppression give researchers many targets for intervention, it also implies a functional redundancy such that the blockade of any one pathway will not completely compromise immune regulation. Some mechanisms have proven to be particularly important in constraining anti-tumor responses and their blockade has proven to be therapeutic. A combined treatment may be necessary to overcome this mechanistic redundancy and is currently a hot topic when discussing the next generation of clinical trials.

CTLA-4

CTLA-4 is constitutively expressed on T_{REG} cells. It is also expressed by recently activated T cells and is a crucial regulator of the early stages of T-cell expansion by opposing the actions of CD28-mediated co-stimulation. In mice, a KO of CTLA-4 results in a lymphoproliferative disorder characterized by T-cell infiltration of multiple organs and lethality within weeks after birth (73), showing how important CTLA-4 is for lymphocyte regulation.

Tremelimumab and ipilimumab are two human anti-CTLA-4 monoclonal antibodies currently used in advanced clinical trials; ipilimumab is currently under review for Food and Drug Administrationapproval. Their mechanism of action seems to be the inhibition of negative signals leading to enhanced co-stimulation and activation of effector T cells (74,75). Recent work has revealed that ipilimumab blocks both the inhibitory regulation of effector T cell expansion as well as the contact-dependent suppression of T_{REG}, leading to a synergistic effect in tumor rejection (76). Clinical trials with ipilimumab have shown promising results in the treatment of late-stage metastatic melanoma (77–80) and renal cancer (81). The most frequently observed side effects are skin rash, diarrhea often with autoimmune colitis as well as occasional reports of hypophysitis, hepatitis, iridocyclitis, or lupus nephritis (82).

GITR

Glucocorticoid-induced TNFR-related protein (GITR) is expressed at low levels on resting responder T lymphocytes and is upregulated after activation, though it is more highly expressed on T_{REG} cells. GITR signaling abrogates the suppressive activity of T_{REG} cells and co-stimulates responder T cells, making GITR an attractive target for immunotherapy (83). Additionally, GITR is expressed on CD8 T_{REGS} isolated from healthy donors and is upregulated in vitro in response to IL-2 and IL-10 (84).

A monoclonal anti-GITR antibody, DTA-1, has been found to assist in tumor rejection by suppressing T_{REG} function through agonist activity in preclinical experiments (85,86). It was also proposed to have depleting function since DTA-1 is IgG2b, an isotype shared by a large panel of in vivo depleting mAbs (87). Later experiments found that T_{REG} cells isolated from DTA-1-treated mice were as suppressive as those from untreated mice in vitro, indicating that in vivo GITR ligation does not disable T_{REG} cells. Furthermore, DTA-1 treatment of Foxp3-GFP knock-in mice resulted in a reduction of circulating T_{REGS}, implying that DTA-1 is a depleting monoclonal antibody (88). In contrast, a later study using the same FoxP3-GFP mouse model has concluded that GITR ligation leads to a loss of FoxP3 expression by T_{REGS} that results in a loss of suppressive capacity (89). While confusion surrounding the mechanism in these pre-clinical models still exists, all agree on efficacy; as it has led to the development of TRX518, a humanized Fc-disabled (non-depleting) anti-human GITR monoclonal antibody is currently being evaluated for safety in phase I trials.

OX40

OX40 (CD134) is a T-cell co-stimulatory molecule that belongs to the TNF/TNFR superfamily. It is induced for two to eight days after T-cell activation and is highly expressed on T_{REGS} (90). Activated T effector cells that express OX40 and CD40 stimulate CD40 ligand–positive DC, which in turn induces the OX40 ligand (OX40L) expression on DC. The resultant OX40-OX40L signaling acts as a positive feedback loop that induces cytokine secretion and co-stimulatory molecule expression from DC while reinforcing survival, proliferation, and resistance to infectious tolerance for the effector T cell (91–94). OX40 signaling on T_{REG} can abrogate their ability to suppress T effector–cell proliferation, IFNγ production, and T effector cell–mediated allograft rejection (93). However, this effect on T_{REGS} is actually quite complex. If OX40 agonist antibody is given to healthy naive mice it will drive T_{REG} expansion (95). Minimal levels of the cytokines IFNγ or IL-4, which skew T cells to helper phenotypes, are needed to ensure T_{REG} do not proliferate to OX40 stimulation, indicating OX40 serves very different purposes during steady state and inflammation. Timing plays a key role as well since an OX40 antibody given during antigen priming in an EAE model results in an inhibition of disease while treatment at disease onset worsens symptoms (95). This highlights the general principle that tinkering with co-stimulatory molecules requires impeccable timing to achieve the desired results. OX40 signaling has also been reported to be instrumental in the homeostatic proliferation of T_{REG} cells following transfer into lymphopenic mice (92).

Preclinical mouse models are able to reject tumors of varying immunogenicity following administration of OX40 agonists (96). OX40 agonists can synergize with cyclophosphamide treatment resulting in anti-tumor immunity causing regression of established, poorly immunogenic B16 melanoma tumors. This effect is coincident with a reduction of tumor-infiltrating T_{REG} and T_{REG} cell-specific apoptosis (97). Importantly, in a factorial experiment design with tumor-bearing Rag1KO mice reconstituted with (*i*) T_{REG} cells and (*ii*) effector T cells from (*a*) OX40 KO or (*b*) WT mice both T_{REG} and effector T cells require OX40 stimulation for the tumor to be rejected (90). Such promising preclinical results have spurred a phase I clinical trial of agonist mouse anti-human OX40 monoclonal antibody 9B12, with work underway to develop a humanized antibody to facilitate multiple treatments.

TGF-β

TGF-β is a pleiotropic cytokine involved in apoptosis, homeostasis, angiogenesis, and wound healing (98). In addition to these necessary functions, TGF-β plays an important role in the generation, maintenance, and suppressive function of T_{REGS} (99). The roles of TGF-β and T_{REGS} in cancer are illustrated in a preclinical model where tumor-sensitized T_{REGS} from tumor-bearing mice block the generation of tumor-specific T cells in reconstituted lymphopenic mice. However, if tumor-sensitized T_{REGS} are transferred from tumor-bearing mice insensitive to TGF-β due to the expression of the dominant-negative TGF-βRII in T cells, the reconstituted lymphopenic mice then mount an effective anti-tumor response (100). Thus TGF-β blockade may improve the generation of therapeutic immune responses in patients with cancer by limiting the generation of new tumor-sensitized T_{REGS}.

Three TGF-β inhibition strategies are currently in use in early phase clinical trials. An anti-sense oligonucleotide to TGF-β, AP12009, is being employed in clinical trials for advanced-stage glioblastoma multiforme and anaplastic astrocytoma; preliminary results indicate increased survival with lower toxicity than standard chemotherapy (temozolomide or procarbazine/lomustine/vincristine) (101). The anti-TGF monoclonal antibody, GC1008, and a small-molecule serine/threonine TGF-β receptor I kinase inhibitor, LY2157299, are both currently used in phase I trials (98).

PGE2

COX-2 is a key enzyme in converting arachidonic acid into the immunosuppressive molecule PGE2. Selective COX-2 inhibitors inhibit inflammation and pain. Selectivity for COX-2 reduces the risk of peptic ulcers, and is the main advantage of celecoxib, rofecoxib, and other members of this class. However, COX-2 selectivity seems to induce other adverse effects, highlighted by the withdrawl of rofecoxib from the market in 2004, due to an increased risk of myocardial infarction and stroke (102).

Tumor-derived COX-2/PGE2 can induce FoxP3 expression of CD4$^+$ CD25- T cells and increase T$_{REG}$ suppresive activity (18). Furthermore, these induced T$_{REG}$ cells can in turn promote 'infectious tolerance' via their own PGE2 production (26). Treatment of naive mice with a COX-2 inhibitor skews splenocytes toward a type 1 cytokine response, inducing IFNγ, IL-12, and IP-10 which when combined with vaccination enhanced the rejection of tumors upon challenge (103).

Though not intended as T$_{REG}$ inhibition strategies, several large-scale clinical trials examined whether rofecoxib could reduce cancer incidence, with conflicting results. In a placebo-controlled randomized trial enrolling 2587 subjects with a recent history of colorectal adenomas, a precursor to colorectal cancer, rofecoxib significantly reduced the incidence of subsequent adenomas, but at the expense of serious toxicity (104). Another placebo-controlled randomized trial involving 2327 stage II and III colorectal cancer patients found rofecoxib did not improve overall survival or protect from recurrence (105).

A more well-tolerated COX-2 inhibitor, celecoxib, has shown an ability to synergize with immunotherapies in several mouse models (106–108), making it a promising candidate to accompany cancer vaccines. One caveat being that celecoxib has been shown to mediate anti-tumor effects in vitro in a COX-2-independent manner (109), complicating interpretations of regulatory cell effects in models and patients. However, if model systems are to be believed, use of this drug may really be a win-win-win situation; killing tumors directly, relaxing T$_{REG}$ inhibition of anti-tumor immunity, and reducing pain as well.

Adenosine

Adenosine, a product of ATP's enzymatic degradation by sequential activation of CD39 and CD73 on T$_{REG}$ cells, has been shown to suppress T cell–mediated inflammation (110). CD39 hydrolyzes ATP into AMP while CD73 creates adenosine from AMP; adenosine can inhibit T-cell proliferation (111,112), synthesis of IL-2, IFNγ and TNF-α (113–115), as well as perforin and Fas ligand expression (111,116). These potentially immunosuppressive effects are mediated primarily by the A2a and A3 adenosine receptors that are highly expressed on human T lymphocytes (117–119). While both A2a and A3 adenosine receptors appear to inhibit T cell–mediated immunity, they each control different aspects of T-cell biology. A2a impairs IL-2 responsiveness and effector molecule expression (112,116), while A3 interrupts TCR-mediated proliferation (111) and adhesion of activated cells to tumor cells (120).

The frequency of CD39-positive T$_{REG}$ cells and associated adenosine-mediated suppression are significantly increased in HNSCC patients (121). T$_{REGS}$ from the patients could hydrolyze ATP at higher rates than T$_{REG}$ from normal controls. The increased frequency and enzymatic activity of CD4$^+$CD39$^+$ cells correlated with the increased suppression of effector T cells, which was partly inhibited by ARL67156, a structural analogue of ATP and a CD39 inhibitor. Likewise, ARL67156 recovered T cell IL-17 production suppressed by ovarian cancer–associated T$_{REG}$ cells (122), hinting at novel therapeutic applications for CD39 antagonists. Blocking the adenosine-mediated suppression with the CD39 inhibitor ARL67156 appeared to be equally as effective as using the selective A2a/A2b receptor antagonist ZM241385 in HNSCC patient material (121). Current research is being conducted regarding the use of these pharmacological agents to modulate adenosine-mediated suppression by directly inhibiting the adenosine receptors or antagonizing CD39.

Lymphocyte Plasticity

The old dogma of lymphoid commitment toward terminally differentiated Th1/Th2 cells has been challenged by the recently described FoxP3$^+$ T$_{REG}$ and RORγt$^+$ Th17 subsets. Human T$_{REGS}$ cultured in IL-2 and IL-15 can be converted to Th17 cells by adding IL-1β, IL-23, and IL-21 in vitro. This change in phenotype and functional capacity is mirrored by the loss of FoxP3 expression and gain of RORγt, the key regulator of Th17-associated genes (123). Furthermore, some Th17 cells can be converted to a dual Th1/Th17 phenotype after exposure to IL-12 (124).

Whether human T_{REG} cells can be induced to differentiate and pass through the Th17 state ultimately to take on a Th1 effector function remains to be seen, but recent mouse models suggest that that might be possible.

Using mice expressing a Foxp3-GFP fusion reporter in a vaccine model depending on CD4 cells that help for cross-presentation to naïve CD8 T cells, researchers found that many T_{REG} cells had acquired the ability to produce IL-2, TNF-α, and IL-17 (125). While the Foxp3-GFP fusion reporter knockin allowed these cells to be tracked up to four days post vaccination, intracellular staining of FoxP3 using flow cytometry was lost in direct proportion to the concentration of CpG (a Toll-like receptor [TLR] agonist simulating double-stranded pathogenic DNA) an adjuvant in the vaccine. Further investigation found that IL-6-dependent upregulation of CD40L on the converted T_{REG} was necessary for cross-priming of cytotoxic T cells and ultimately clearance of tumor burden.

While the extent of T_{REG} plasticity that occurs in vivo remains controversial (126,127) many studies are finding IL-6 is a key player in mouse studies of this phenomenon. Murine Th17 cells develop in response to IL-6 and TGF-β while human Th17 cells originate in response to IL-1β and IL-23 (128). This discrepancy is important to keep in mind for translational research, since IL-6 has been shown to mediate T_{REG}-to-Th17 plasticity in mice but not in humans. While demethylation of the upstream region of FoxP3 is associated with T_{REG} function (11), remethylation of that same region in response to IL-6 was found to accompany a loss of FoxP3 expression in former murine T_{REG} cells (129). Furthermore, a knock-in model designed to overexpress IL-6 in vivo found Helios⁻ but not Helios⁺ T_{REG} generation was impaired (130) confirming the hints from an earlier paper that these Helios⁻iT_{REG} were far more plastic than their nT_{REG} counterparts (8). Taken together these data illustrate a phenomenon where iT_{REG} in the periphery might regulate immune responses to self, food or, particularly, commensal antigens while retaining the ability to revert to a more inflammatory phenotype should commensals become pathogens. This plasticity has the potential to be employed as a tool for immunotherapy.

APC-Induced T_{REG} Conversion

Although conversion of T_{REG} to a more inflammatory subtype may be accomplished in the absence of APCs through the addition of a large array of cytokines (123,131), most studies of T_{REG} plasticity have found that conversion can be achieved relatively simply with stimulated APCs. While DCs have been in clinical trials for years, their limited therapeutic benefit in most trials has lowered expectations in the field. These recent studies of T_{REG} plasticity now call into question the basic precepts of what constitutes an effective APC vaccine.

While DCs differentiated in GM-CSF and IL-4 (GM4 DC) have been the APCs of choice in the vast majority of clinical trials, these are not the cells reported in the literature to convert T_{REGS} into effectors. One in vitro study found TCR stimulation in the presence of LPS-activated monocytes and IL-2 induced the conversion of human T_{REG} into Th17 cells while GM4 DC activated with LPS did not (132). Another group used allogeneic monocytes combined with anti-CD3, anti-CD28, low- dose IL-2, and human serum to convert T_{REGS} into Th17 cells (133). Since IL-23 played a role in the conversion process in these studies and others (123,131,134) and it has been shown that the presence of IL-4 in human monocyte culture can have suppressive effects on IL-23 production (135), perhaps future DC vaccines should focus initially on the generation of IL-23-secreting APC as illustrated in Figure 14.3. DC engineered to produce IL-23 can induce a potent anti-tumor immune response after intra-tumor implantation in mice (136). It remains to be seen whether TLR-activated monocytes will be efficient in converting tumor-induced T_{REG} into effector T cells in humans.

TLR Agonists

Another attractive intervention is the use of TLR agonists as vaccine adjuvants. TLR agonists initiate a cytokine cascade from APC that can abolish the suppressive function of CD25 CD4 T_{REG} (137). Although commonly thought of as APC sensory molecules, TLR2, TLR4,

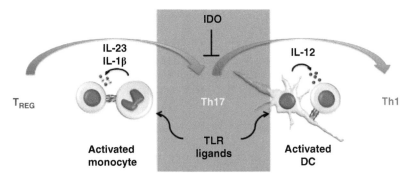

Figure 14.3 APC-mediated conversion of human T_{REG}. While evidence mounts that T_{REG} can be converted to anti-tumor effector cells in mice, proof of concept in humans is lacking. Yet, in vitro studies indicate that properly activated monocytes can turn FoxP3⁺ T_{REGS} into Th17 cells. Th17 cells in turn have been shown to exhibit Th1 function when influenced by IL-12. Thus, the possibility exists that human tumor-infiltrating T_{REGS} might be converted to effector function. *Abbreviations*: APC, antigen-presenting cells; DC, dendritic cell; IDO, indoleamine 2,3-dioxygenase; IL-10, interleukin-10; Th, T helper; TLR, toll-like receptor; T_{REG}, T regulatory cell.

TLR5, TLR7, and TLR8 are all expressed on human T_{REG} cells and, depending on the TLR ligand used, their direct ligation can either enhance or attenuate the suppressive action of these cells (138).

While in vitro TLR4 and TLR5 activation of purified human T_{REG} increased FoxP3 expression and suppressive capacity compared with unstimulated T_{REG} (139,140), TLR2 activation of human T_{REG} resulted in functional inactivation in the presence of concurrent TCR and IL-2 stimulation (141). One study found that squamous cell carcinomas treated with imiquimod, a topical TLR7 agonist, had T-cell infiltrates with less FoxP3, CD39, CD73, IL-10, and TGF-β and a reduced suppressive activity (142). TLR8 stimulation of purified human CD4 T_{REG} inhibits their suppressive function and an adoptive transfer of TLR8 agonist-stimulated T_{REG} cells into tumor-bearing mice enhances anti-tumor immunity (143), implying that direct conversion to an inflammatory Th1 or Th17 phenotype may be possible by T_{REG} TLR ligation. TLR8 agonists are also capable of inhibiting CD8 T_{REG}-mediated suppression of naïve CD4 proliferation in a co-culture assay devoid of APCs; however, the effects of TLR agonists on responder cells was not isolated in that experiment (35). Additional off-target effects of TLR8 agonists include their ability to synergize with other TLR agonists in maturing DCs enhancing Th1-type responses (144,145). Resiquimod gel is a TLR8 activator that is currently being investigated as a topical adjuvant in six different NIH-funded clinical trials.

IDO

The immunoregulatory enzyme indoleamine 2,3-dioxygenase (IDO) is an inducible enzyme that catalyzes tryptophan. The depletion of tryptophan and accumulation of its resultant toxic catabolites in the tumor microenvironment inactivate effector T cells and render DCs immunosuppressive. IDO helps maintain a suppressive phenotype for T_{REGS} within tumor draining lymph nodes (146) and can convert purified human CD4+ CD25- T cells into suppressive CD4+ CD25+ cells (147). Human plasmacytoid DCs (pDC) express high levels of IDO and triggering TLR 9 with CpG activating human pDCs to increase the expression of IDO resulting in T_{REG} induction (148).

One inhibitor of IDO, 1-methyl-D-tryptophan (1MT), is currently used in phase I clinical trials as adjuvant therapy of solid tumors; other higher-avidity inhibitors are also in development. Blocking IDO activity in vitro with 1MT abrogates human pDC-dependent T_{REG}

generation and suppressor cell function (148). In a mouse model of metastatic melanoma IDO inhibition by 1MT has induced conversion of T_{REG}s to a Th17 phenotype (146). In a later report with the same model system 1MT when used alone limited the tumor growth more than when 1MT was with concurrent T_{REG}-specific depletion, attesting to the potential power of converted T_{REG} to activate an anti-tumor response (125). If the same activity seen in preclinical models is found in clinical trials, the excitement surrounding this therapy will definitely be justified.

CONCLUSIONS

Clinical investigators seeking to enhance the efficacy of cancer vaccines and immunotherapy are currently faced with a variety of alternatives to target T_{REGS}. The most obvious question that will come to mind is which one is the best? The answer may not be as simple as the question presumes. Optimal therapeutic efficacy in tumor immunology may depend on pairing the right vaccine with an appropriate T_{REG} depletion strategy. While more work needs to be done to define those regulatory subsets which are more closely associated with different cancers, current knowledge may allow for educated guesses in combining therapies. For example, vaccines that focus on normal self antigens that will be encountered in the thymus must overcome a strong component of contact-dependent antigen-specific nT_{REG} suppression. Thus, ipilimumab may coordinate well in such a scenario by blocking the CTLA-4-dependent suppression of antigen-specific DCs (17). Likewise, vaccines against altered or oncofetal tumor antigens will not be expected to be inhibited by an antigen-specific nT_{REG} response for initial priming, but instead have to overcome the effect of iT_{REG} cells and the soluble factors they secrete. Inhibiting TGF-β in such a scenario may result in an augmented priming response. Of course, tumors will express all types of antigens and are infiltrated with both natural and induced T_{REGS} that cooperate in their suppressive functions (29). However, focusing on deterring antigen-specific suppression to a mono-antigen vaccine may prove crucial for priming a therapeutic response in some strategies.

The better question might be, "What intervention works best with which cancers?" Different cancers may necessitate different regulatory interventions irrespective of the vaccine used. For example FoxP3+CD8 cells were reported to be potent suppressors infiltrating prostate cancers (35). While mechanisms of suppression were both contact dependent and independent, they relied neither on CTLA-4 for the former nor on TGF-β and/or IL-10 for the latter. Though confirming reports will make decision making more certain, the available evidence suggests that a locally delivered TLR8 agonist (35) or anti-GITR therapy (84) will merit testing. Percentages of circulating T_{REGS} in patients vary widely and may be a prognostic indicator of how amenable a patient might be to these therapies. Likewise, variations in the phase of immunoediting, equilibrium, or escape (149) or whether metastases have arisen from or invaded mucosal epithelia may impact T_{REG}-targeting strategies in ways researchers have yet to decipher. It is possible that some therapeutic responses will not be seen until individualized T_{REG} targeting strategies are the norm.

Finally, combining different therapies to target T_{REGS} may be necessary for some highly tolerogenic diseases, but this adds another layer of complexity. One must ask which of these therapies will be complementary and which won't be? Will dual depletion strategies complement one another or will they prove redundant and serve only to increase the cost associated with an already expensive disease? Might opposing strategies be paired in a clinically useful sense? It seems like a depletion strategy paired with a conversion strategy would be a poor choice, but if they were timed so that conversion accompanied the priming vaccination while boosts were preceded by a depletion strategy, then vaccine enhancement might be achieved. Never before have cancer immunotherapists possessed such a plethora of means for the purpose of cancer cures. The next big step may not be a new therapy, but rather figuring out how to best coordinate the ones we have now at hand.

ACKNOWLEDGMENTS

This work was supported by CA080964 (BAF), CA119123 (BAF), CA123864 (WJU), CA141278 (H-MH), CA109563 (BDC), the Chiles Foundation, Robert W. Franz, the Prostate Cancer Foundation, the Kuni Foundation, the Providence Medical Foundation, and the Murdock Trust. We regret the point that we could not cite many investigators' significant research due to space limitations.

REFERENCES

1. Bronte V, Zanovello P. Regulation of immune responses by L-arginine metabolism. Nat Rev Immunol 2005; 5: 641–54.
2. Youn JI, Gabrilovich DI. The biology of myeloid-derived suppressor cells: the blessing and the curse of morphological and functional heterogeneity. Eur J Immunol 2010; 40: 2969–75.
3. Motzer RJ, Rini BI, Bukowski RM, et al. Sunitinib in patients with metastatic renal cell carcinoma. JAMA 2006; 295: 2516–24.
4. van Cruijsen H, van der Veldt AA, Vroling L, et al. Sunitinib-induced myeloid lineage redistribution in renal cell cancer patients: CD1c+ dendritic cell frequency predicts progression-free survival. Clin Cancer Res 2008; 14: 5884–92.
5. Ko JS, Zea AH, Rini BI, et al. Sunitinib mediates reversal of myeloid-derived suppressor cell accumulation in renal cell carcinoma patients. Clin Cancer Res 2009; 15: 2148–57.
6. Ko JS, Rayman P, Ireland J, et al. Direct and differential suppression of myeloid-derived suppressor cell subsets by sunitinib is compartmentally constrained. Cancer Res 2010; 70: 3526–36.
7. Curotto de Lafaille MA, Lafaille JJ. Natural and adaptive foxp3+ regulatory T cells: more of the same or a division of labor? Immunity 2009; 30: 626–35.
8. Thornton AM, Korty PE, Tran DQ, et al. Expression of Helios, an Ikaros transcription factor family member, differentiates thymic-derived from peripherally induced Foxp3+ T regulatory cells. J Immunol 2010; 184: 3433–41.
9. Hsieh CS, Liang Y, Tyznik AJ, et al. Recognition of the peripheral self by naturally arising CD25+ CD4+ T cell receptors. Immunity 2004; 21: 267–77.
10. Hori S, Nomura T, Sakaguchi S. Control of regulatory T cell development by the transcription factor Foxp3. Science 2003; 299: 1057–61.
11. Baron U, Floess S, Wieczorek G, et al. DNA demethylation in the human FOXP3 locus discriminates regulatory T cells from activated FOXP3(+) conventional T cells. Eur J Immunol 2007; 37: 2378–89.
12. Sakaguchi S, Wing K, Onishi Y, Prieto-Martin P, Yamaguchi T. Regulatory T cells: how do they suppress immune responses? Int Immunol 2009; 21: 1105–11.
13. Gershon RK, Cohen P, Hencin R, Liebhaber SA. Suppressor T cells. J Immunol 1972; 108: 586–90.
14. Gondek DC, Lu LF, Quezada SA, Sakaguchi S, Noelle RJ. Cutting edge: contact-mediated suppression by CD4+CD25+ regulatory cells involves a granzyme B-dependent, perforin-independent mechanism. J Immunol 2005; 174: 1783–6.
15. Nakamura K, Kitani A, Strober W. Cell contact-dependent immunosuppression by CD4(+)CD25(+) regulatory T cells is mediated by cell surface-bound transforming growth factor beta. J Exp Med 2001; 194: 629–44.
16. Shevach EM, Tran DQ, Davidson TS, Andersson J. The critical contribution of TGF-beta to the induction of Foxp3 expression and regulatory T cell function. Eur J Immunol 2008; 38: 915–17.
17. Onishi Y, Fehervari Z, Yamaguchi T, Sakaguchi S. Foxp3+ natural regulatory T cells preferentially form aggregates on dendritic cells in vitro and actively inhibit their maturation. Proc Natl Acad Sci USA 2008; 105: 10113–18.
18. Sharma S, Yang SC, Zhu L, et al. Tumor cyclooxygenase-2/prostaglandin E2-dependent promotion of FOXP3 expression and CD4+ CD25+ T regulatory cell activities in lung cancer. Cancer Res 2005; 65: 5211–20.
19. Deaglio S, Dwyer KM, Gao W, et al. Adenosine generation catalyzed by CD39 and CD73 expressed on regulatory T cells mediates immune suppression. J Exp Med 2007; 204: 1257–65.
20. Cobbold SP, Castejon R, Adams E, et al. Induction of foxP3+ regulatory T cells in the periphery of T cell receptor transgenic mice tolerized to transplants. J Immunol 2004; 172: 6003–10.
21. Bergmann C, Strauss L, Zeidler R, Lang S, Whiteside TL. Expansion and characteristics of human T regulatory type 1 cells in co-cultures simulating tumor microenvironment. Cancer Immunol Immunother 2007; 56: 1429–42.

22. Groux H, Bigler M, de Vries JE, Roncarolo MG. Interleukin-10 induces a long-term antigen-specific anergic state in human CD4+ T cells. J Exp Med 1996; 184: 19–29.
23. Bacchetta R, Bigler M, Touraine JL, et al. High levels of interleukin 10 production in vivo are associated with tolerance in SCID patients transplanted with HLA mismatched hematopoietic stem cells. J Exp Med 1994; 179: 493–502.
24. Groux H, O'Garra A, Bigler M, et al. A CD4+ T-cell subset inhibits antigen-specific T-cell responses and prevents colitis. Nature 1997; 389: 737–42.
25. Bergmann C, Strauss L, Zeidler R, Lang S, Whiteside TL. Expansion of human T regulatory type 1 cells in the microenvironment of cyclooxygenase 2 overexpressing head and neck squamous cell carcinoma. Cancer Res 2007; 67: 8865–73.
26. Mandapathil M, Szczepanski MJ, Szajnik M, et al. Adenosine and prostaglandin E2 cooperate in the suppression of immune responses mediated by adaptive regulatory T cells. J Biol Chem 2010; 285: 27571–80.
27. Faria AM, Weiner HL. Oral tolerance and TGF-beta-producing cells. Inflamm Allergy Drug Targets 2006; 5: 179–90.
28. Weiner HL. Oral tolerance: immune mechanisms and the generation of Th3-type TGF-beta-secreting regulatory cells. Microbes Infect 2001; 3: 947–54.
29. Zhou G, Levitsky HI. Natural regulatory T cells and de novo-induced regulatory T cells contribute independently to tumor-specific tolerance. J Immunol 2007; 178: 2155–62.
30. Naito Y, Saito K, Shiiba K, et al. CD8+ T cells infiltrated within cancer cell nests as a prognostic factor in human colorectal cancer. Cancer Res 1998; 58: 3491–4.
31. Schumacher K, Haensch W, Roefzaad C, Schlag PM. Prognostic significance of activated CD8(+) T cell infiltrations within esophageal carcinomas. Cancer Res 2001; 61: 3932–6.
32. Mlecnik B, Tosolini M, Kirilovsky A, et al. Histopathologic-based prognostic factors of colorectal cancers are associated with the state of the local immune reaction. J Clin Oncol 2011; 29: 610–18.
33. Filaci G, Fenoglio D, Fravega M, et al. CD8+ CD28- T regulatory lymphocytes inhibiting T cell proliferative and cytotoxic functions infiltrate human cancers. J Immunol 2007; 179: 4323–34.
34. Wei S, Kryczek I, Zou L, et al. Plasmacytoid dendritic cells induce CD8+ regulatory T cells in human ovarian carcinoma. Cancer Res 2005; 65: 5020–6.
35. Kiniwa Y, Miyahara Y, Wang HY, et al. CD8+ Foxp3+ regulatory T cells mediate immunosuppression in prostate cancer. Clin Cancer Res 2007; 13: 6947–58.
36. Filaci G, Fravega M, Negrini S, et al. Nonantigen specific CD8+ T suppressor lymphocytes originate from CD8+CD28- T cells and inhibit both T-cell proliferation and CTL function. Hum Immunol 2004; 65: 142–56.
37. Dhodapkar MV, Steinman RM. Antigen-bearing immature dendritic cells induce peptide-specific CD8(+) regulatory T cells in vivo in humans. Blood 2002; 100: 174–7.
38. Manavalan JS, Kim-Schulze S, Scotto L, et al. Alloantigen specific CD8+CD28- FOXP3+ T suppressor cells induce ILT3+ ILT4+ tolerogenic endothelial cells, inhibiting alloreactivity. Int Immunol 2004; 16: 1055–68.
39. Yanaba K, Bouaziz JD, Matsushita T, Tsubata T, Tedder TF. The development and function of regulatory B cells expressing IL-10 (B10 cells) requires antigen receptor diversity and TLR signals. J Immunol 2009; 182: 7459–72.
40. Lemoine S, Morva A, Youinou P, Jamin C. Human T cells induce their own regulation through activation of B cells. J Autoimmun 2011; 36: 228–38.
41. Minard-Colin V, Xiu Y, Poe JC, et al. Lymphoma depletion during CD20 immunotherapy in mice is mediated by macrophage FcgammaRI, FcgammaRIII, and FcgammaRIV. Blood 2008; 112: 1205–13.
42. DiLillo DJ, Matsushita T, Tedder TF. B10 cells and regulatory B cells balance immune responses during inflammation, autoimmunity, and cancer. Ann NY Acad Sci 2010; 1183: 38–57.
43. Inoue S, Leitner WW, Golding B, Scott D. Inhibitory effects of B cells on antitumor immunity. Cancer Res 2006; 66: 7741–7.
44. DiLillo DJ, Yanaba K, Tedder TF. B cells are required for optimal CD4+ and CD8+ T cell tumor immunity: therapeutic B cell depletion enhances B16 melanoma growth in mice. J Immunol 2010; 184: 4006–16.
45. Garni-Wagner BA, Witte PL, Tutt MM, et al. Natural killer cells in the thymus. Studies in mice with severe combined immune deficiency. J Immunol 1990; 144: 796–803.
46. Li Q, Teitz-Tennenbaum S, Donald EJ, Li M, Chang AE. In vivo sensitized and in vitro activated B cells mediate tumor regression in cancer adoptive immunotherapy. J Immunol 2009; 183: 3195–203.

47. Rech AJ, Vonderheide RH. Clinical use of anti-CD25 antibody daclizumab to enhance immune responses to tumor antigen vaccination by targeting regulatory T cells. Ann NY Acad Sci 2009; 1174: 99–106.
48. Jacobs JF, Punt CJ, Lesterhuis WJ, et al. Dendritic cell vaccination in combination with anti-CD25 monoclonal antibody treatment: a phase I/II study in metastatic melanoma patients. Clin Cancer Res 2010; 16: 5067–78.
49. Figgitt DP, Lamb HM, Goa KL. Denileukin diftitox. Am J Clin Dermatol 2000; 1: 67–72; discussion 3.
50. Morse MA, Hobeika AC, Osada T, et al. Depletion of human regulatory T cells specifically enhances antigen-specific immune responses to cancer vaccines. Blood 2008; 112: 610–18.
51. Poehlein CH, Haley DP, Walker EB, Fox BA. Depletion of tumor-induced Treg prior to reconstitution rescues enhanced priming of tumor-specific, therapeutic effector T cells in lymphopenic hosts. Eur J Immunol 2009; 39: 3121–33.
52. Powell DJ, Jr, de Vries CR, Allen T, Ahmadzadeh M, Rosenberg SA. Inability to mediate prolonged reduction of regulatory T Cells after transfer of autologous CD25-depleted PBMC and interleukin-2 after lymphodepleting chemotherapy. J Immunother 2007; 30: 438–47.
53. Malek TR, Bayer AL. Tolerance, not immunity, crucially depends on IL-2. Nat Rev Immunol 2004; 4: 665–74.
54. Thistlethwaite FC, Elkord E, Griffiths RW, et al. Adoptive transfer of T(reg) depleted autologous T cells in advanced renal cell carcinoma. Cancer Immunol Immunother 2008; 57: 623–34.
55. Lacelle MG, Jensen SM, Fox BA. Partial CD4 depletion reduces regulatory T cells induced by multiple vaccinations and restores therapeutic efficacy. Clin Cancer Res 2009; 15: 6881–90.
56. d'Amore F, Radford J, Relander T, et al. Phase II trial of zanolimumab (HuMax-CD4) in relapsed or refractory non-cutaneous peripheral T cell lymphoma. Br J Haematol 2010; 150: 565–73.
57. Kim YH, Duvic M, Obitz E, et al. Clinical efficacy of zanolimumab (HuMax-CD4): two phase 2 studies in refractory cutaneous T-cell lymphoma. Blood 2007; 109: 4655–62.
58. Rider DA, Havenith CE, de Ridder R, et al. A human CD4 monoclonal antibody for the treatment of T-cell lymphoma combines inhibition of T-cell signaling by a dual mechanism with potent Fc-dependent effector activity. Cancer Res 2007; 67: 9945–53.
59. Shedlock DJ, Shen H. Requirement for CD4 T cell help in generating functional CD8 T cell memory. Science 2003; 300: 337–9.
60. Sun JC, Bevan MJ. Defective CD8 T cell memory following acute infection without CD4 T cell help. Science 2003; 300: 339–42.
61. Emens LA. Chemoimmunotherapy. Cancer J 2010; 16: 295–303.
62. Ghiringhelli F, Larmonier N, Schmitt E, et al. CD4+CD25+ regulatory T cells suppress tumor immunity but are sensitive to cyclophosphamide which allows immunotherapy of established tumors to be curative. Eur J Immunol 2004; 34: 336–44.
63. Lutsiak ME, Semnani RT, De Pascalis R, et al. Inhibition of CD4(+)25+ T regulatory cell function implicated in enhanced immune response by low-dose cyclophosphamide. Blood 2005; 105: 2862–8.
64. Tseng CW, Hung CF, Alvarez RD, et al. Pretreatment with cisplatin enhances E7-specific CD8+ T-Cell-mediated antitumor immunity induced by DNA vaccination. Clin Cancer Res 2008; 14: 3185–92.
65. Banissi C, Ghiringhelli F, Chen L, Carpentier AF. Treg depletion with a low-dose metronomic temozolomide regimen in a rat glioma model. Cancer Immunol Immunother 2009; 58: 1627–34.
66. Chen CA, Ho CM, Chang MC, et al. Metronomic chemotherapy enhances antitumor effects of cancer vaccine by depleting regulatory T lymphocytes and inhibiting tumor angiogenesis. Mol Ther 2010; 18: 1233–43.
67. Hermans IF, Chong TW, Palmowski MJ, Harris AL, Cerundolo V. Synergistic effect of metronomic dosing of cyclophosphamide combined with specific antitumor immunotherapy in a murine melanoma model. Cancer Res 2003; 63: 8408–13.
68. Ghiringhelli F, Menard C, Puig PE, et al. Metronomic cyclophosphamide regimen selectively depletes CD4+CD25+ regulatory T cells and restores T and NK effector functions in end stage cancer patients. Cancer Immunol Immunother 2007; 56: 641–8.
69. Zhang L, Dermawan K, Jin M, et al. Differential impairment of regulatory T cells rather than effector T cells by paclitaxel-based chemotherapy. Clin Immunol 2008; 129: 219–29.
70. Correale P, Cusi MG, Tsang KY, et al. Chemo-immunotherapy of metastatic colorectal carcinoma with gemcitabine plus FOLFOX 4 followed by subcutaneous granulocyte macrophage colony-stimulating factor and interleukin-2 induces strong immunologic and antitumor activity in metastatic colon cancer patients. J Clin Oncol 2005; 23: 8950–8.
71. Correale P, Tagliaferri P, Fioravanti A, et al. Immunity feedback and clinical outcome in colon cancer patients undergoing chemoimmunotherapy with gemcitabine + FOLFOX followed by subcutaneous

granulocyte macrophage colony-stimulating factor and aldesleukin (GOLFIG-1 Trial). Clin Cancer Res 2008; 14: 4192–9.

72. Emens LA, Asquith JM, Leatherman JM, et al. Timed sequential treatment with cyclophosphamide, doxorubicin, and an allogeneic granulocyte-macrophage colony-stimulating factor-secreting breast tumor vaccine: a chemotherapy dose-ranging factorial study of safety and immune activation. J Clin Oncol 2009; 27: 5911–18.

73. Waterhouse P, Penninger JM, Timms E, et al. Lymphoproliferative disorders with early lethality in mice deficient in Ctla-4. Science 1995; 270: 985–8.

74. Maker AV, Attia P, Rosenberg SA. Analysis of the cellular mechanism of antitumor responses and autoimmunity in patients treated with CTLA-4 blockade. J Immunol 2005; 175: 7746–54.

75. Kavanagh B, O'Brien S, Lee D, et al. CTLA4 blockade expands FoxP3+ regulatory and activated effector CD4+ T cells in a dose-dependent fashion. Blood 2008; 112: 1175–83.

76. Peggs KS, Quezada SA, Chambers CA, Korman AJ, Allison JP. Blockade of CTLA-4 on both effector and regulatory T cell compartments contributes to the antitumor activity of anti-CTLA-4 antibodies. J Exp Med 2009; 206: 1717–25.

77. Hodi FS, Mihm MC, Soiffer RJ, et al. Biologic activity of cytotoxic T lymphocyte-associated antigen 4 antibody blockade in previously vaccinated metastatic melanoma and ovarian carcinoma patients. Proc Natl Acad Sci USA 2003; 100: 4712–17.

78. Phan GQ, Yang JC, Sherry RM, et al. Cancer regression and autoimmunity induced by cytotoxic T lymphocyte-associated antigen 4 blockade in patients with metastatic melanoma. Proc Natl Acad Sci USA 2003; 100: 8372–7.

79. Ribas A, Camacho LH, Lopez-Berestein G, et al. Antitumor activity in melanoma and anti-self responses in a phase I trial with the anti-cytotoxic T lymphocyte-associated antigen 4 monoclonal antibody CP-675,206. J Clin Oncol 2005; 23: 8968–77.

80. Hodi FS, O'Day SJ, McDermott DF, et al. Improved survival with ipilimumab in patients with metastatic melanoma. N Engl J Med 2010; 363: 711–23.

81. Yang JC, Hughes M, Kammula U, et al. Ipilimumab (anti-CTLA4 antibody) causes regression of metastatic renal cell cancer associated with enteritis and hypophysitis. J Immunother 2007; 30: 825–30.

82. Kaehler KC, Piel S, Livingstone E, et al. Update on immunologic therapy with anti-CTLA-4 antibodies in melanoma: identification of clinical and biological response patterns, immune-related adverse events, and their management. Semin Oncol 2010; 37: 485–98.

83. Nocentini G, Riccardi C. GITR: a modulator of immune response and inflammation. Adv Exp Med Biol 2009; 647: 156–73.

84. Negrini S, Fenoglio D, Balestra P, et al. Endocrine regulation of suppressor lymphocytes: role of the glucocorticoid-induced TNF-like receptor. Ann NY Acad Sci 2006; 1069: 377–85.

85. Fontenot JD, Rasmussen JP, Williams LM, et al. Regulatory T cell lineage specification by the forkhead transcription factor foxp3. Immunity 2005; 22: 329–41.

86. Ko K, Yamazaki S, Nakamura K, et al. Treatment of advanced tumors with agonistic anti-GITR mAb and its effects on tumor-infiltrating Foxp3+CD25+CD4+ regulatory T cells. J Exp Med 2005; 202: 885–91.

87. Shevach EM, Stephens GL. The GITR-GITRL interaction: co-stimulation or contrasuppression of regulatory activity? Nat Rev Immunol 2006; 6: 613–18.

88. Coe D, Begom S, Addey C, et al. Depletion of regulatory T cells by anti-GITR mAb as a novel mechanism for cancer immunotherapy. Cancer Immunol Immunother 2010; 59: 1367–77.

89. Cohen AD, Schaer DA, Liu C, et al. Agonist anti-GITR monoclonal antibody induces melanoma tumor immunity in mice by altering regulatory T cell stability and intra-tumor accumulation. PLoS One 2010; 5: e10436.

90. Piconese S, Valzasina B, Colombo MP. OX40 triggering blocks suppression by regulatory T cells and facilitates tumor rejection. J Exp Med 2008; 205: 825–39.

91. Ohshima Y, Tanaka Y, Tozawa H, et al. Expression and function of OX40 ligand on human dendritic cells. J Immunol 1997; 159: 3838–48.

92. Takeda I, Ine S, Killeen N, et al. Distinct roles for the OX40-OX40 ligand interaction in regulatory and nonregulatory T cells. J Immunol 2004; 172: 3580–9.

93. Vu MD, Xiao X, Gao W, et al. OX40 costimulation turns off Foxp3+ Tregs. Blood 2007; 110: 2501–10.

94. So T, Croft M. Cutting edge: OX40 inhibits TGF-beta- and antigen-driven conversion of naive CD4 T cells into CD25+Foxp3+ T cells. J Immunol 2007; 179: 1427–30.

95. Ruby CE, Yates MA, Hirschhorn-Cymerman D, et al. Cutting Edge: OX40 agonists can drive regulatory T cell expansion if the cytokine milieu is right. J Immunol 2009; 183: 4853–7.

96. Sadun RE, Hsu WE, Zhang N, et al. Fc-mOX40L fusion protein produces complete remission and enhanced survival in 2 murine tumor models. J Immunother 2008; 31: 235–45.

97. Hirschhorn-Cymerman D, Rizzuto GA, Merghoub T, et al. OX40 engagement and chemotherapy combination provides potent antitumor immunity with concomitant regulatory T cell apoptosis. J Exp Med 2009; 206: 1103–16.

98. Korpal M, Kang Y. Targeting the transforming growth factor-beta signalling pathway in metastatic cancer. Eur J Cancer 2010; 46: 1232–40.

99. Bluestone JA, Abbas AK. Natural versus adaptive regulatory T cells. Nat Rev Immunol 2003; 3: 253–7.

100. Petrausch U, Jensen SM, Twitty C, et al. Disruption of TGF-beta signaling prevents the generation of tumor-sensitized regulatory T cells and facilitates therapeutic antitumor immunity. J Immunol 2009; 183: 3682–9.

101. Bogdahn U, Hau P, Stockhammer G, et al. Targeted therapy for high-grade glioma with the TGF-beta2 inhibitor trabedersen: results of a randomized and controlled phase IIb study. Neuro Oncol 2011; 13: 132–42.

102. Martinez-Gonzalez J, Badimon L. Mechanisms underlying the cardiovascular effects of COX-inhibition: benefits and risks. Curr Pharm Des 2007; 13: 2215–27.

103. Sharma S, Zhu L, Yang SC, et al. Cyclooxygenase 2 inhibition promotes IFN-gamma-dependent enhancement of antitumor responses. J Immunol 2005; 175: 813–19.

104. Baron JA, Sandler RS, Bresalier RS, et al. A randomized trial of rofecoxib for the chemoprevention of colorectal adenomas. Gastroenterology 2006; 131: 1674–82.

105. Midgley RS, McConkey CC, Johnstone EC, et al. Phase III randomized trial assessing rofecoxib in the adjuvant setting of colorectal cancer: final results of the VICTOR trial. J Clin Oncol 2010; 28: 4575–80.

106. Dovedi SJ, Kirby JA, Davies BR, Leung H, Kelly JD. Celecoxib has potent antitumour effects as a single agent and in combination with BCG immunotherapy in a model of urothelial cell carcinoma. Eur Urol 2008; 54: 621–30.

107. Basu GD, Tinder TL, Bradley JM, et al. Cyclooxygenase-2 inhibitor enhances the efficacy of a breast cancer vaccine: role of IDO. J Immunol 2006; 177: 2391–402.

108. Mukherjee P, Basu GD, Tinder TL, et al. Progression of pancreatic adenocarcinoma is significantly impeded with a combination of vaccine and COX-2 inhibition. J Immunol 2009; 182: 216–24.

109. Schonthal AH. Direct non-cyclooxygenase-2 targets of celecoxib and their potential relevance for cancer therapy. Br J Cancer 2007; 97: 1465–8.

110. Dwyer KM, Deaglio S, Gao W, et al. CD39 and control of cellular immune responses. Purinergic Signal 2007; 3: 171–80.

111. Hoskin DW, Butler JJ, Drapeau D, Haeryfar SM, Blay J. Adenosine acts through an A3 receptor to prevent the induction of murine anti-CD3-activated killer T cells. Int J Cancer 2002; 99: 386–95.

112. Huang S, Apasov S, Koshiba M, Sitkovsky M. Role of A2a extracellular adenosine receptor-mediated signaling in adenosine-mediated inhibition of T-cell activation and expansion. Blood 1997; 90: 1600–10.

113. Lappas CM, Sullivan GW, Linden J. Adenosine A2A agonists in development for the treatment of inflammation. Expert Opin Investig Drugs 2005; 14: 797–806.

114. Butler JJ, Mader JS, Watson CL, et al. Adenosine inhibits activation-induced T cell expression of CD2 and CD28 co-stimulatory molecules: role of interleukin-2 and cyclic AMP signaling pathways. J Cell Biochem 2003; 89: 975–91.

115. Raskovalova T, Lokshin A, Huang X, et al. Inhibition of cytokine production and cytotoxic activity of human antimelanoma specific CD8+ and CD4+ T lymphocytes by adenosine-protein kinase A type I signaling. Cancer Res 2007; 67: 5949–56.

116. Koshiba M, Kojima H, Huang S, Apasov S, Sitkovsky MV. Memory of extracellular adenosine A2A purinergic receptor-mediated signaling in murine T cells. J Biol Chem 1997; 272: 25881–9.

117. Koshiba M, Rosin DL, Hayashi N, Linden J, Sitkovsky MV. Patterns of A2A extracellular adenosine receptor expression in different functional subsets of human peripheral T cells. Flow cytometry studies with anti-A2A receptor monoclonal antibodies. Mol Pharmacol 1999; 55: 614–24.

118. Mirabet M, Herrera C, Cordero OJ, et al. Expression of A2B adenosine receptors in human lymphocytes: their role in T cell activation. J Cell Sci 1999; 112: 491–502.

119. Gessi S, Varani K, Merighi S, et al. Expression of A3 adenosine receptors in human lymphocytes: up-regulation in T cell activation. Mol Pharmacol 2004; 65: 711–19.

120. MacKenzie WM, Hoskin DW, Blay J. Adenosine inhibits the adhesion of anti-CD3-activated killer lymphocytes to adenocarcinoma cells through an A3 receptor. Cancer Res 1994; 54: 3521–6.

121. Mandapathil M, Szczepanski MJ, Szajnik M, et al. Increased ectonucleotidase expression and activity in regulatory T cells of patients with head and neck cancer. Clin Cancer Res 2009; 15: 6348–57.

122. Kryczek I, Banerjee M, Cheng P, et al. Phenotype, distribution, generation, and functional and clinical relevance of Th17 cells in the human tumor environments. Blood 2009; 114: 1141–9.

123. Koenen HJ, Smeets RL, Vink PM, et al. Human CD25highFoxp3pos regulatory T cells differentiate into IL-17-producing cells. Blood 2008; 112: 2340–52.

124. Annunziato F, Cosmi L, Santarlasci V, et al. Phenotypic and functional features of human Th17 cells. J Exp Med 2007; 204: 1849–61.

125. Sharma MD, Hou DY, Baban B, et al. Reprogrammed foxp3(+) regulatory T cells provide essential help to support cross-presentation and CD8(+) T cell priming in naive mice. Immunity 2010; 33: 942–54.

126. Rubtsov YP, Niec RE, Josefowicz S, et al. Stability of the regulatory T cell lineage in vivo. Science 2010; 329: 1667–71.

127. Zhou X, Bailey-Bucktrout SL, Jeker LT, et al. Instability of the transcription factor Foxp3 leads to the generation of pathogenic memory T cells in vivo. Nat Immunol 2009; 10: 1000–7.

128. Annunziato F, Cosmi L, Liotta F, Maggi E, Romagnani S. Human Th17 cells: are they different from murine Th17 cells? Eur J Immunol 2009; 39: 637–40.

129. Lal G, Zhang N, van der Touw W, et al. Epigenetic regulation of Foxp3 expression in regulatory T cells by DNA methylation. J Immunol 2009; 182: 259–73.

130. Fujimoto M, Nakano M, Terabe F, et al. The influence of excessive IL-6 production in vivo on the development and function of Foxp3+ regulatory T cells. J Immunol 2011; 186: 32–40.

131. Valmori D, Raffin C, Raimbaud I, Ayyoub M. Human RORgammat+ TH17 cells preferentially differentiate from naive FOXP3+Treg in the presence of lineage-specific polarizing factors. Proc Natl Acad Sci USA 2010; 107: 19402–7.

132. Deknuydt F, Bioley G, Valmori D, Ayyoub M. IL-1beta and IL-2 convert human Treg into T(H)17 cells. Clin Immunol 2009; 131: 298–307.

133. Voo KS, Wang YH, Santori FR, et al. Identification of IL-17-producing FOXP3+ regulatory T cells in humans. Proc Natl Acad Sci USA 2009; 106: 4793–8.

134. Osorio F, LeibundGut-Landmann S, Lochner M, et al. DC activated via dectin-1 convert Treg into IL-17 producers. Eur J Immunol 2008; 38: 3274–81.

135. Roses RE, Xu S, Xu M, et al. Differential production of IL-23 and IL-12 by myeloid-derived dendritic cells in response to TLR agonists. J Immunol 2008; 181: 5120–7.

136. Hu J, Yuan X, Belladonna ML, et al. Induction of potent antitumor immunity by intratumoral injection of interleukin 23-transduced dendritic cells. Cancer Res 2006; 66: 8887–96.

137. Pasare C, Medzhitov R. Toll pathway-dependent blockade of CD4+CD25+ T cell-mediated suppression by dendritic cells. Science 2003; 299: 1033–6.

138. Dai J, Liu B, Li Z. Regulatory T cells and Toll-like receptors: what is the missing link? Int Immunopharmacol 2009; 9: 528–33.

139. Milkova L, Voelcker V, Forstreuter I, et al. The NF-kappaB signalling pathway is involved in the LPS/IL-2-induced upregulation of FoxP3 expression in human CD4+CD25high regulatory T cells. Exp Dermatol 2010; 19: 29–37.

140. Crellin NK, Garcia RV, Hadisfar O, et al. Human CD4+ T cells express TLR5 and its ligand flagellin enhances the suppressive capacity and expression of FOXP3 in CD4+CD25+ T regulatory cells. J Immunol 2005; 175: 8051–9.

141. Oberg HH, Ly TT, Ussat S, et al. Differential but direct abolishment of human regulatory T cell suppressive capacity by various TLR2 ligands. J Immunol 2010; 184: 4733–40.

142. Clark RA, Huang SJ, Murphy GF, et al. Human squamous cell carcinomas evade the immune response by down-regulation of vascular E-selectin and recruitment of regulatory T cells. J Exp Med 2008; 205: 2221–34.

143. Peng G, Guo Z, Kiniwa Y, et al. Toll-like receptor 8-mediated reversal of CD4+ regulatory T cell function. Science 2005; 309: 1380–4.

144. Napolitani G, Rinaldi A, Bertoni F, Sallusto F, Lanzavecchia A. Selected Toll-like receptor agonist combinations synergistically trigger a T helper type 1-polarizing program in dendritic cells. Nat Immunol 2005; 6: 769–76.

145. Paustian C, Caspell R, Johnson T, et al. Effect of multiple activation stimuli on the generation of Th1-polarizing dendritic cells. Hum Immunol 2011; 72: 24–31.

146. Sharma MD, Hou DY, Liu Y, et al. Indoleamine 2,3-dioxygenase controls conversion of Foxp3+ Tregs to TH17-like cells in tumor-draining lymph nodes. Blood 2009; 113: 6102–11.

147. Curti A, Pandolfi S, Valzasina B, et al. Modulation of tryptophan catabolism by human leukemic cells results in the conversion of CD25- into CD25+ T regulatory cells. Blood 2007; 109: 2871–7.

148. Chen W, Liang X, Peterson AJ, Munn DH, Blazar BR. The indoleamine 2,3-dioxygenase pathway is essential for human plasmacytoid dendritic cell-induced adaptive T regulatory cell generation. J Immunol 2008; 181: 5396–404.
149. Dunn GP, Old LJ, Schreiber RD. The three Es of cancer immunoediting. Annu Rev Immunol 2004; 22: 329–60.

15 | Molecular targeting of cancer stem cells

Zhenhua Li, Debraj Mukherjee, Jang-Won Lee, and John S. Yu

INTRODUCTION

WHO grade 3 (anaplastic astrocytoma, anaplastic oligodendroglioma, and anaplastic oligoas-trocytoma) and grade 4 gliomas (glioblastoma multiforme and gliosarcoma) are collectively referred to as malignant gliomas. Glioblastoma multiforme (GBM) has an infiltrative tissue pattern in which a complete surgical resection is not possible. Currently, the standard treatment for GBM is surgical resection followed by a combination of radiotherapy and chemotherapy. Varying modes of chemotherapy have been used for decades in neuro-oncology; however, there is an increasing concern about its limited efficacy as well as significant side effects noted in clinical trials. Recently, molecularly targeted therapies for malignant gliomas have been investigated in clinical trials, but to date only bevacizumab (Avastin®, Genentech, South San Francisco, CA) has been approved for clinical use by the Food and Drug Administration (FDA) (1). The median survival of GBM patients is about 15 months despite aggressive conventional therapies (2). According to data from National Cancer Institute, there were approximately 62,930 newly diagnosed cases of brain tumor, with 13,000 deaths, in the year 2010. Among all the newly diagnosed cases, 22,070 cases will be primary malignant brain tumors, representing 1.5% of all primary malignant cancers expected to be diagnosed annually in the United States (www.cancer.gov).

GBM usually recurs within 12 months post resection, with a subsequent poor prognosis. A fundamental challenge presented in glioma patients is the propensity for tumors to invade distant brain tissue. Invasive tumor cells escape surgery, radiation exposure, and chemotherapy. Temozolomide (TMZ), an oral methylator, is currently considered a standard adjuvant therapy because it has proved to be beneficial when used concurrently with radiation therapy (3). Hegi et al. reported that the susceptibility of tumor cells and the therapeutic benefit of TMZ correlated with the epigenetic silencing of the DNA repair enzyme O(6)-methylguanine-DNA-methyltransferase (MGMT) (4); patients with a methylated MGMT promoter exhibited a more favorable therapeutic response when treated with temozolomide and in those lacking the MGMT promoter (5).

No significant increase in survival of patients suffering from this disease has been achieved during the past 30 years. Thus, novel therapeutic strategies to target and kill GBM cells are desperately needed. Recent advances in the understanding of the cellular and molecular mechanisms of cancer initiation and propagation have demonstrated the presence of cancer stem cells (CSCs) in various cancers, including GBM. These advanced have provided valuable insights into the underlying biological features of GBM and into the development of novel targeting strategies to improve the survival profiles of GBM patients.

GLIOMA CANCER STEM CELLS AND RELATED MARKERS

The hypothesis that tumors may develop from a small population of stem-like cells was proposed in the late 19th century (6); however, evidence of presence of this kind of cell was only first demonstrated by Lapidot et al. in 1994 (7). Building upon this initial work, Bonnet et al. further characterized the acute myelogenous leukemia stem cell (LSC), demonstrating that only a small subset of blast cells was able to reconstitute multi-lineage leukemic cell populations when transplanted into immunodeficient mice (8). Following the accumulating evidence that showed LSCs were responsible for the maintenance and transfer of blood cancers, researchers attempted to confirm the existence of an analogous cell type in solid tumors. In 2003, an influential report describing the prospective identification of human breast CSCs changed the landscape of breast cancer research (9). The investigators reported that a small population of $CD44^+/CD24^-/Lin^-$ human breast cancer cells were enriched for tumorigenic potential using human tumor samples (eight pleural effusions and one primary tumor), which were xenografted into the mammary glands of non-obese diabetic/severe combined immunodeficient (NOD/SCID) mice.

These studies provided fundamental evidence for the definition of a "cancer stem cell" as that of a single cell is able to reconstitute heterogeneous cell populations in vivo. Other studies of other hematological malignancies, for example, chronic myeloid leukemia (CML) (10) and acute lymphoblastic leukemia (11), further supported a hierarchical model of tumorigenesis, whereby CSCs had the ability to generate diverse progenies leading to the heterogeneous cell populations characteristic of "liquid" tumors. For brain cancer, several groups isolated glioma cancer stem cells (gCSC) from primary tumors based on the criteria mentioned earlier as well as on the ability to form neurospheres composed of normal neural stem cells (NSCs) (12–15).

Recently, increasing evidence has shown that CSCs share some characteristics with normal NSCs such as (1) the capacity to remain quiescent; (2) generation of an amplification hierarchy; (3) resistance to chemotherapy; and (4) enhanced tumorigenicity in mice models (16–19). gCSCs also exhibit significant differences from normal stem cells in frequency, proliferation, and aberrant expression of differentiation. The potent tumorigenic capacity of CSCs, coupled with radioresistance and chemoresistance, suggests that CSCs contribute to tumor maintenance and recurrence. Hence, targeting CSCs may offer new avenues for therapeutic intervention.

CSCs have been identified in various other malignant primary tumors and cancer cell lines using different cell-surface markers (Table 15.1) (20). Cell surface markers currently used to identify human CSCs in solid tumors include CD44, CD133, epithelial surface antigen (ESA), and CD24. Specifically, the CD44+ phenotype is positively correlated with colon, breast, prostate, and pancreatic cancer initiator cells (21,22). CD133+ cells have been shown to initiate human glioblastoma and colon, prostate, and pancreatic cancers in mice (12,18,21). Pancreatic and breast cancer–initiating cells express ESA+ markers (23). Additionally, CD24 is known to be positively correlated with tumorigenicity in pancreatic cancer (19) but negatively correlated with tumorigenicity in breast cancer (9); however, CD24+ cells are associated with invasive breast cancer (24).

One of the major hurdles in studying brain tumor stem cells is lack of specific cell surface markers that enable reliable purification of brain CSCs. Among gCSCs-associated markers, CD133, nestin, and A2B5 are currently the most accredited markers for the identification of gCSCs. Their use in gCSCs research has been fundamental to reveal the biological properties of gCSCs, such as tumor progression and resistance to ionizing radiation or chemotherapy.

CD133

CD133 (prominin-1) is one of two members of a pentaspan transmembrane glycoprotein family identified in both mice and humans, originally classified as a marker of primitive hematopoietic and neural stem cells.

Human CD133 is a transmembrane glycoprotein of 865 amino acids (aa) with a total molecular weight of 120 kDa (858 aa and 115 kDa in mice). Prominin-1 has a unique structure consisting of an N-terminal extracellular domain, five transmembrane domains with two large extracellular loops, and a 59-aa cytoplasmic domain. Analysis of the prominin-1 aa sequence shows eight potential N-glycosylation sites: five on the first extracellular loop and three on the second. CD133 has been confirmed as a marker of hematopoietic stem cells for human allogeneic transplantation and is regarded as one of the most useful tools for isolating hematopoietic stem cells. The AC133 epitope of prominin-1 can serve as a substitute for CD34 as a marker in hematopoietic stem cell isolation. Transplanted AC133+/CD34− cells develop similar repopulating potentials as CD34+ cells and can differentiate into AC133+/CD34+ cells with hematopoietic and endothelial capacity (25). Following hematopoietic stem cell transplantation, early clinical studies show slightly improved engraftments with AC133+ cells compared to CD34+ cells (26).

Table 15.1 Summary of Identified Cancer Stem Cells from Different Primary Tumors and Tumor Cell Lines (20)

Tumor	Type	Isolation Markers
Acute myeloid leukemia	Primary tumors	CD34$^+$CD38$^-$
Breast	Primary tumors	CD44$^+$CD24$^{-/low}$
Brain	Primary tumors	CD133$^+$
	Cell lines	CD133$^+$/sphere formation
	Cell lines	Side population(SP)
Colon	Primary tumors	CD133$^+$
	Primary tumors	CD133$^+$CD44$^+$
	Cell lines	CD133$^+$
Laryngeal	Cell lines	CD133$^+$
Leukemia	Primary tumors	CD34$^+$CD10$^-$
Liver	Primary tumors/Cell lines	CD90$^+$CD44$^+$
Lung	Primary tumors	ALDH1
	Primary tumors	CD133$^+$
Melanoma	Primary tumors	ABCB5$^+$
	Primary tumors	CD133$^+$ABCG2$^+$
Ovarian	Primary tumors	CD133$^+$
Pancreas	Primary tumors	CD133$^+$
	Cell lines	CD133$^+$
Prostate	Primary tumors	CD133$^+$

In addition, CD133 represents a marker of tumor-initiating cells in a number of human cancers. Results and in vivo proliferation assays and in vivo tumor initiation studies have provided evidence for the existence of CD133$^+$ CSCs in various cancers, including prostate, colon, lung, hepatocellular, laryngeal, ovarian, pancreatic, and breast cancers, as well as in melanoma and osteosarcoma (27). It may be possible to develop future therapies targeting CSCs based on this marker. The development of such therapies will be aided by understanding the molecular mechanisms and signaling pathways that regulate the behavior of CD133$^+$ cells, and also by new data interconnecting the roles of regulation of Wnt, Notch, and bone morphogenetic protein (BMP) signaling pathways in CD133$^+$ CSCs.

The CD133 antigen has been identified as a putative stem cell marker in malignant brain tissues. In gliomas, it is used to enrich a subpopulation of highly tumorigenic cancer cells. The CD133$^+$ cell population in brain tumors has been described to be highly tumorigenic after xeno-transplantation in NOD/SCID (28). It is reported that CD133$^+$ gCSCs are more resistant to multiple chemotherapeutic agents than their CD133$^-$ counterparts (29). CD133$^+$ gCSCs also expressed higher levels of mRNA for the drug transporter gene ABCG2 (BCRP), DNA repair protein, methylguanine DNA methyltransferase (MGMT) mRNA, and several other genes that inhibit apoptosis, including FLIP (FLICE-like inhibitory protein), Bcl-2, Bcl-X, and some IAP (inhibitor of apoptosis proteins) family genes. These cells were significantly more resistant to chemotherapeutic agents when compared with autologous CD133$^-$ cells (30). Under irradiation, the CD133$^+$ gCSCs could preferentially activate the DNA damage checkpoint response, which is dependent on Chk1 and Chk2 checkpoint kinases (31). Currently, CD133 is still highly efficient in the identification and isolation of gCSCs. Moreover, intensive studies are being conducted to determine whether CD133 can be treated as a prognosis factor and whether brain tumors may be cured by eradicating CD133$^+$ gCSCs. The expression of CD133 can be a useful tool for the enrichment of gCSCs. However, the low CD133 expression in some tumors suggests that additional markers need to be explored. Currently, CD133 markers may still be used in combination with other markers or methods to isolate gCSCs.

Nestin

Nestin is an intermediate filament (IF) protein originally described in 1990 as a neuronal stem cell/progenitor cell marker during the development of central nervous system (CNS) (32). Nestin is expressed in dividing cells during the early stages of development in the CNS, peripheral nervous system, and in myogenic and other tissues. It may be involved in the organization of the cytoskeleton, cell signaling, organogenesis, cell metabolism, proliferation, migration and multi-differentiated characteristics of multi-lineage progenitor cells (33). Recent work has shown that nestin is also expressed in follicle stem cells. Their immediate, differentiated progeny, and the hair follicle bulge area, has been noted as an easily accessible source of actively growing pluripotent adult stem cells (34). In neural cytogenesis, nestin is able to identify stem cells, glial-restricted precursors, and oligodendrocyte-type 2 astrocyte (O2A) progenitors (35). Dahlstrand et al. demonstrated that nestin is greatly expressed in highly malignant tumors, such as GBM, when compared to less anaplastic glial tumors (36). This study identified nestin as a potential prognostic marker for glioblastoma. Thus, nestin expression in tumor cells may be related to their dedifferentiated status, enhanced cell motility, invasive potential, and increased malignancy. In addition, the nestin protein expression has also been identified in the cell nucleus of tumor cell lines obtained from GBM patients (37,38).

A2B5

A2B5, a ganglioside cell-surface epitope expressed on neural precursors, has also been suggested as a marker for identifying tumor-initiating cells from human glioblastoma (39). It has been reported that A2B5-defined white matter progenitor cells yield neurospheres, and these spheres generate all major neural phenotypes, as well as glia *in vivo* and *in vitro* (40). Maric et al. utilized the expression of A2B5 and JONES (anti-9-O-acetylated GD3) protein as a positive marker of neuroglial progenitor cells in multiepitope labeling of E13 rat telencephalon to investigate dynamically changing anatomical distributions of neural progenitors at the beginning of neurogenesis (41). Ogden et al. demonstrated that a large percentage of A2B5$^+$ cells were present in tested glioma specimens and identified a subset of glioma cells with tumorigenic properties (39). Recently, Tchoghandjian et al. isolated A2B5$^+$ cells from human GBM and demonstrated that these cells display neurosphere-like, self-renewing, asymmetrical cell division properties and have multipotency capability (42). A2B5$^+$/CD133$^+$ and A2B5$^+$/CD133$^-$ cell fractions displayed a high proliferative potential to generate spheres and produced tumors in nude mice. Additional evidence showed co-expression of CD133 and the interleukin-13 (IL-13) receptor with A2B5 in addition to abnormal DNA content within the A2B5 population of certain tumors.

L1-CAM

L1-cell adhesion molecule (L1-CAM) is a cell adhesion receptor of the immunoglobulin superfamily, known for its roles in regulating neural cell-growth, -survival, and -migration, as well as axonal outgrowth and neurite extension during CNS development (43). Recently, Bao et al. demonstrated that L1-CAM is important for the survival of gCSCs (44). The siRNA targeting of L1CAM expression in vivo suppressed tumor growth and increased the survival of CD133$^+$ glioma cells both in vitro and in vivo. Thus, L1-CAM may represent a cancer stem cell specific therapeutic target for improving the treatment of malignant gliomas and other brain tumors.

SIGNALING PATHWAYS IN GLIOBLASTOMA STEM CELLS

Numerous signaling pathways, such as Notch, Hedgehog, and Wnt connected with the self-renewal of CSCs have been identified. CSCs share these signaling pathways with normal neural stem cells (NSCs). It has been reported that these pathways are involved in the balance between the self-renewal and differentiation of CSCs and NSCs (45). Understanding the genetic basis for cancer development and the molecular pathways that regulate growth, survival, and metastasis of CSCs is an important step in the development of novel targeting therapies for CSCs.

Notch Signaling

Notch signaling has a critical role in regulating cell-to-cell cross talk during embryogenesis, cellular proliferation, differentiation, and apoptosis (46). Notch proteins include the four members (Notch 1–4), which mediate a short-range cellular communication through interaction with ligands. Recently, the role and function of Notch signaling in CSCs was identified in malignant GBM. Fan et al. reported that Notch blockade by gamma-secretase inhibitors (GSIs) reduced neurosphere growth and clonogenicity *in vitro*, whereas expression of an active form of Notch2 increased the tumor growth (47). The expression of putative CSCs markers such as CD133, Nestin, BMI1, and Olig2 decreased following the Notch blockade, which impaired the tumorigenic potential of these cells. These results demonstrate that Notch pathway blockade depletes stem-like cells in GBMs, suggesting that GSIs may be useful as chemotherapeutic reagents to target CSCs in malignant gliomas. Wang et al. reported that Notch signaling has been linked to radioresistance of gCSCs, suggesting that inhibition of Notch signaling may not only disrupt the maintenance of gCSCs but also reduce the radioresistance of gCSCs (48).

Hedgehog Signaling

The Hedgehog pathway, an essential signaling pathway in embryonic development, is critical for maintaining tissue polarity and stem cell populations. The initial link between Hedgehog signaling and human cancers was based on the discovery that mutations of the human *PTCH1* gene were associated with a rare and hereditary form of basal cell cancer (BCC) basal cell nevus syndrome (49,50). Some tumor types, including colon, ovarian, prostate, and pancreatic adenocarcinomas, have been shown to exhibit Hedgehog pathway activation caused by Hedgehog ligand overexpression (51,52). A recent finding has evidenced the significance of Hedgehog signaling in regulating self-renewal and the tumorigenic potential of gCSCs (53,54). These studies demonstrated that inhibition of the Hedgehog signaling pathway blocked the gCSC tumor growth and prevented viable neoplastic cells from propagating the tumor in vivo after cyclopamine treatment. Moreover, cyclopamine treatment has been shown to improve the effect of radiation on gCSCs (55).

These results indicated that the Hedgehog signaling pathway is critical for the maintenance of gCSCs and that targeting this pathway with a pharmacologic inhibitor may inhibit gCSC growth and improve the efficacy of conventional therapies.

Wnt Signaling

Wnt signaling, together with other signaling pathways, controls embryonic development and tissue homeostasis (56,57). Recent evidence has shown that Wnt/beta-catenin signaling may contribute to radioresistance in CSCs (58). Thus, it is possible that blockade of Wnt signaling may effectively and specifically target CSCs in GBM patients. Wnt/beta-catenin has also been implicated in mediating the radiation resistance of mouse mammary gland progenitor cells. Zhang et al. used isolated mammary CSCs from *p53*-null mice to show that their DNA damage response was more efficient, when compared to the bulk of the tumor (59). The use of Akt pharmacological inhibitors could inhibit the Wnt pathway as well as the ability to repair DNA in the CSC population, thereby sensitizing them to ionizing radiation treatment. In addition, Takahashi-Yanaga et al.

reported that ICG-001, a beta-catenin/CBP antagonist, was able to eradicate drug-resistant leukemic CSCs both in vitro and in vivo (60).

These results suggest that the mechanisms and signaling pathways that support stem cell renewal in normal and malignant tissues could become new targets for therapies designed to complement existing approaches and reduce tumor recurrence.

STAT3 Signaling

Signaling transducer and activator of transcription 3 (STAT3) is a crucial transcriptional regulator involved in a wide range of cellular activities in the development of the CNS as well as in immune responses, stem cell maintenance, and tumorigenesis. Constitutive activation of STAT3 has been observed in many human cancers, including breast, head and neck, prostate, thyroid, and melanoma (61). Recently, Sherry et al. reported that gCSCs express STAT3, which is phosphorylated on the activating tyrosine and serine residues (62). Inhibition of STAT3 in these cells by either small molecular inhibitors or RNAi resulted in the inhibition of growth and neurosphere formation. Cao et al. also found that inhibition of STAT3 with specific inhibitors, or targeting of STAT3 with specific shRNAs, disrupted proliferation and maintenance of gCSCs (63).

It has been shown that upstream pathways such as interleukin-6 (IL-6), erythropoietin, and Notch signaling can regulate STAT3 action. Targeting these upstream pathways will inhibit the STAT3 activation that in turn inhibits cell growth and self-renewal in gCSCs (64).

MICRORNAS REGULATE GLIOBLASTOMA STEM CELLS

MicroRNAs (miRNAs) control a wide array of physiological and pathological processes, including development, differentiation, cellular proliferation, programmed cell death, oncogenesis, and metastasis by modulating the expression of their cognate target genes through cleaving mRNA molecules or inhibiting their translation.

Self-renewal is a critical property and has been related to the tumorigenic properties of CSCs. Recently, Chan et al. demonstrated that miRNAs are critical in the regulation of cancer cell function in malignant gliomas (65). One of the potential explanations for such remarkable effects on glioma formation and expansion may be the identification of a network of regulatory miRNA, such as the cluster containing miRNAs-371/372/373, which epigenetically controls the levels of gene products involved in the maintenance of stem cell properties (66).

It is well documented that miRNA targeting must be sequence-specific instead of gene-specific. miRNA-21 is overexpressed in GBM tumors, while functional blockade of this miRNA induces apoptotic cell death (67). The levels of miR-124, miR-137, and miR-451 are significantly reduced in gCSCs when compared with non-stem tumor cells (68,69). Moreover, overexpression of these miRNAs in gCSCs suppresses proliferation and induces differentiation in gCSCs, suggesting that these miRNAs have important roles in maintaining gCSCs in vivo. These results indicate that critical miRNAs can be potentially used as molecular targets or therapeutic agents for gCSCs.

It is important to evaluate the effect of a specific miRNA-mediated therapy on a proteome-wide scale to prevent unwanted gene alteration. Potential delivery systems need to achieve high therapeutic efficiency. Thus, it is still a great challenge to deliver these miRNAs into gCSCs.

THE MECHANISM OF GLIOBLASTOMA CANCER STEM CELLS RESISTANT TO THE CURRENT CHEMOTHERAPY

Temozolomide (TMZ), an oral methylating chemotherapeutic agent, has been used in the management of gliomas. The pharmacological effect of TMZ is significantly cytotoxic to cancer cells, mainly by its methylation of the O6 position of guanine in DNA. The combination of TMZ with radiosensitization in GBM therapy has been most effective in improving survival (3). TMZ may slow GBM tumor growth and increase patients' survival by two years; however, long-term survivors are still rare due to drug resistance and tumor recurrence, indicating the presence of TMZ-resistant cancer cells in GBM (30).

Schatton et al. reported that a high expression of ABC (ATP binding cassette) drug transporters such as ABCG2 and ABCA3 in GBM cell lines may be one of the critical mechanisms that pump out chemotherapeutical agents and increase chemoresistance in CSCs (70). Moreover, Hirschmann-Jax et al. reported that a side population (SP) of CSCs derived from GBM cell lines express elevated levels of APC drug transporters, indicating that targeting of these drug transporters may be one strategy to reduce chemoresistance in gCSCs (71).

GLIOBLASTOMA STEM CELLS AND TUMOR ANGIOGENESIS

Malignant gliomas are vascular tumors that produce vascular endothelial growth factor (VEGF), which is an important mediator of angiogenesis.

Preclinical data indicate that angiogenesis is essential for the proliferation and survival of malignant glioma cells, which suggests that inhibition of angiogenesis may be an effective therapeutic strategy. One of the important roles of the CSC population in a tumor is to regulate tumor angiogenesis through VEGF signaling. Bao et al. demonstrated that gCSCs express high levels of VEGF and display great angiogenic potential in vitro and in vivo (72). gCSCs promote tumor angiogenesis partially through elevated expression of VEGF. The effect of gCSCs on tumor vascularization suggests that targeting gCSCs should involve the inhibition of tumor angiogenesis. Thus, targeting VEGF with bevacizumab specifically blocked the proangiogenic effects of gCSCs both in vitro and in vivo. More recently, Wang et al. demonstrated that blocking VEGF or silencing VEGFR2 inhibited the maturation of tumor endothelial progenitors into endothelium, but not the differentiation of CD133+ gCSCs into endothelial progenitors (73). Gamma-secretase inhibition or Notch silencing blocks the transition into endothelial progenitors when exposed to bevacizumab or gamma-secretase inhibitors.

HYPOXIA RESPONSES IN GLIOBLASTOMA STEM CELLS

In solid cancers, hypoxia is a well-recognized tumor microenvironmental condition that is linked to poor patient outcomes and resistance to therapies (74,75). A hypoxic condition had been thought to have a negative impact on tumor growth, including in GBM. However, hypoxia contributes to the progression of a variety of cancers by activating adaptive transcriptional programs that promote cell survival, motility, and tumor angiogenesis. Compelling evidences suggested that hypoxia actually promotes tumor angiogenesis, cancer invasion, and therapeutic resistance, such as radioresistance, in GBM (76).

Hypoxia-inducible factor (HIF), a heterodimeric transcription factor consisting of α and β subunits, regulates the expression of angiogenic factors, including VEGF. HIF stimulates the expansion and migration of endothelial cells into the tumor space, which allows new vessel growth from the existing vasculature structure surrounding the tumor. The formation of these vessels supplies the rapidly expanding tumor with nutrients and oxygen (77). Moreover, the cellular responses to hypoxia are mainly mediated through HIFs. As VEGF plays an important role in angiogenesis during tumor growth, the inhibition of VEGF-induced HIF is an attractive therapeutic target for tumor angiogenesis.

Recent results have demonstrated that overexpression of hypoxia-inducible factor-2α (HIF-2α) actually promotes the persistence of gCSCs (78). Thus, HIF-2 α represents a potential target specific for gCSCs. However, the role of HIF-2 α in other normal stem cells needs to be elucidated.

Although the importance of hypoxia and subsequent hypoxia-inducible factor-1α (HIF-1α) activation in tumor angiogenesis is well known, their role in the regulation of glioma-derived stem cells is unclear. It was reported that hypoxia (1% oxygen) promotes the self-renewal capacity of CD133+ human gCSCs. Propagation of glioma-derived CSCs in a hypoxic environment also led to the expansion of cells bearing CXCR4 (CD184), CD44 (low), and A2B5 surface markers. The enhanced self-renewal activity of the CD133$^+$ CSCs in hypoxia was preceded by upregulation of HIF-1α, suggesting that these signaling cascades may modulate the hypoxic response. These results suggest that CSCs, in response to hypoxia, involve the activation of HIF-1α, enhance the self-renewal activity of CD133$^-$ cells, and inhibit the induction of CSC differentiation (78).

Moreover, a recent work has demonstrated that HIF-2α and multiple HIF-regulated genes are preferentially expressed in gCSCs in comparison to non-stem tumor cells and normal neural progenitors. Targeting HIFs in gCSCs inhibits self-renewal, proliferation, and survival in vitro as well as attenuates the tumor initiation potential of gCSCs in vivo (79). Heddleston et al. indicated that the state of CSCs may be plastic and that microenvironmental conditions may promote the acquisition of a stem cell–like phenotype (80).

These studies suggest that the targeting of the microenvironment of CSCs such as hypoxia niches may provide a new avenue for the development of novel therapeutic approaches against gCSCs.

IMPLICATIONS FOR MOLECULAR TARGETED THERAPEUTICS

CSCs represent a subpopulation of cancer cells with extraordinary capacities to promote tumor angiogenesis, invasion, therapeutic resistance, and repopulation after treatment, making them a crucial cell population that should be targeted for anti-GBM therapies. Recent advances in this exciting research area have allowed us to gain remarkable insights into the molecular mechanisms or signaling pathways that are differentially present or regulated in gCSCs or non-stem tumor cells. Though most are still far from clinical applications, the anti-vascular niche treatment has shown promising results in clinical trials leading to FDA-approval for bevacizumab for the treatment of recurrent or progressive GBMs.

It is clear that the microenviroment is crucial to maintaining gCSC populations; gCSCs interact not only with the vascular niche but also with non-stem tumor cells, stromal elements, and immune cells. The emerging concepts and roles of CSCs are still rapidly evolving. For instance, recent studies demonstrate that the epithelial-mesenchymal transition (EMT) plays an important role in the acquisition of malignant and stem cell traits of cancer cells (81,82).

Molecular targeted therapy is a promising therapeutic strategy, in which the products of selectively expressed genes that contribute to the neoplastic phenotype are exploited as targets of antibodies, small molecules, or genetic constructs (83). Ideal targeted therapy should have a higher therapeutic index and be less toxic than current cytotoxic drugs. Although numerous challenges remain, a notable progress in the molecular characterization of GBM has paved the way for more rationally based treatment strategies that target specific genes and proteins.

Targeting Cancer Stem Cells Using Dendritic Cell-Based Immunotherapy

Immunotherapies harness the body's own immune system to counter tumor cells and potentially overcome difficulties in conventional treatments. Various strategies of immunotherapy have been reported, including active immunotherapy, passive immunotherapy, and cytokine therapy. Active immunotherapy (tumor vaccines), using dendritic cells (DCs) designed to generate vaccines, can stimulate the host's intrinsic immune response to the tumor and represents a promising therapeutic approach, though these efforts have only achieved limited clinical success. Major challenges include finding a means of overcoming inhibitory immune regulatory mechanisms and eliciting effective T-cell responses to antigens preferentially expressed by tumor cells.

Dendritic cells (DCs) are the most potent antigen-presenting cells (APCs) due to their superior capacity for acquiring and processing antigens for presentation to T-cells. The first DC vaccination study in cancer patients was published in 1996 (84). In this study, four patients with follicular B-cell lymphoma were treated with infusions of DCs isolated directly from the blood by leukapheresis and loaded with specific recombinant idiotype proteins ex vivo. Among these four patients, the measurable immune response and positive clinical effects obtained in three patients provided a considerable impetus to investigate this approach further. The primary advantages of DC-based active immunotherapy are its relative lack of side effects and its specificity against target tumor cells, as well as its capacity to generate a long-term memory response against tumor-specific antigens (85).

Human DCs are commonly generated from peripheral blood-derived monocytes, followed by a differentiation step using GM-CSF and IL-4 to produce immature DCs (iDCs). The iDCs undergo maturation and antigen loading steps to produce mature DCs. When DCs are pulsed with cancer antigens or tumor peptides, they induce an antigen-specific immune response with the potential to express high levels of co-stimulatory/co-inhibitory molecules that drive immune activation. Moreover, DCs have the capacity to modulate immune responses by instructing T-cell differentiation and polarization. Emerging evidence has shown that DC-mediated antigen presentation may be more effective than irradiated tumor cells, an early-stage active immunotherapy vaccine.

Accumulating evidence suggests that DC vaccination could increase tumor antigen presentation and elicit significant anti-tumor immune responses to successfully improve and prolong the survival of tumor-bearing experimental animals or patients (86). Clinical trials of antigen-pulsed DCs have been conducted in patients with various types of tumors, such as breast cancer, colorectal cancer, malignant melanoma, multiple myeloma, prostate cancer, renal cell carcinoma, and non-small-cell lung cancer (87). For glioma, immunotherapy with a DC vaccine, different tumor-associated antigens (TAAs), including specific tumor-associated peptides, tumor RNA and cDNA, tumor cell lysate and apoptotic tumor cells, have been tested in various studies (88). It has been reported that vaccination with DCs pulsed with acid-eluted glioblastoma peptides were well tolerated and could induce a systemic antigen-specific immunity in patients with recurrent GBM (89,90). An early phase I clinical study showed there were one or more tumor-associated antigen (TAA)-specific cytotoxic T-lymphocyte (CTL) clones against melanoma antigen-encoding gene-1(MAGE-1), gp100, and human epidermal growth factor receptor (HER)-2 in four out of nine patients based on a HLA-restricted tetramer staining assays (91). These promising results demonstrated the feasibility, safety, and clinical response of an autologous tumor lysate-pulsed DC vaccine for patients with malignant glioma.

The development of reproducible protocols for generating a large number of monocyte-derived and CD34+ precursor-derived DCs for clinical application has facilitated phase I and II clinical studies designed to analyze toxicity and clinical efficacy. To date, as much as 200 DC vaccine trials have been reported, with melanoma as the most frequent type of cancer treated with DC vaccines (92). These clinical trials have demonstrated the feasibility and safety of DC vaccines. However, these vaccines have not translated into meaningful therapeutic responses despite the induction of tumor-specific T-cell responses in many patients. Further understanding of immune tolerance and regulation may improve the immunogenicity of DC vaccines.

Recent studies have suggested that gCSCs may have implications for modifying GBM treatments, including DC vaccination–based immunotherapy (15,93,94). A critical consideration in the development of anti-gCSC immunity lies in presenting the immunogenic tumor antigens of gCSCs to T-cells in vivo. gCSCs-associated proteins may be used for cancer vaccination. SOX2 was regarded as a critical gene for self-renewal in both normal neural stem cells and brain cancer stem cells. The abundant and glioma-restricted overexpression of SOX2, and the generation of SOX2-specific peptides, may implicate this antigen as a target for T-cell–based immunotherapy of brain cancer stem cells (95). In one study, specific CTLs were induced against the HLA-A0201-restricted SOX2-derived peptide and were capable of lysing glioma cells. Recently, Pellegatta et al. demonstrated that DC targeting of mouse glioma GL261 neurosphere (GL261-NS) provided a more efficient protection against GL261 tumors than targeting of GL261 adherent cells (GL261-AC) (96). In this study, DC vaccination using CSC antigens lysed up to 80% of GL261 tumors, while DC vaccination using regular GL261 antigens did not lyse CSC-initiated tumors. This study also reported a robust tumor infiltration by CD8+ and CD4+ T-lymphocytes and highlighted the potential of gCSCs in inducing anti-tumor immune responses. Garcia-Hernandez et al. reported upon a CSC-based prostate cancer vaccine. In this study, mice having prostate cancer were vaccinated with prostate stem cell antigen. The results showed that the vaccine could induce MHC expression, cytokine production, lymphocyte infiltration, and long-term protection against prostate cancer (97). The results in murine models from both cancer vaccination studies supported the hypothesis that CSC-derived whole lysates or CSC-associated antigens may be superior to conventional tumor antigens in generating antigen-specific anti-tumor immune response. Due to the difference in cancer immunity between murine models and humans, it is important to explore how to translate and integrate CSC-targeting DC vaccination in murine models into human clinical trials. Recently, it has been demonstrated that GBM-derived CSCs expressed a range of TAAs and class I MHC molecules that are critical for immune recognition. In CSCs, the expression level of some TAAs was over 200 folds higher than that in differentiated daughter cells. Importantly, vaccination with DCs loaded with CSC antigens induced an antigen-specific Th1 immune response. In a 9L CSC brain tumor model, DC vaccination using 9L CSC tumor antigens achieved an antigen-specific anti-tumor T-cell immune response that provided a significant survival benefit (94).

To date, there are very few reports regarding CSC-targeted DC vaccination in animal models and patients. The success of such vaccines depends on the identification of appropriate tumor antigens, establishment of effective immunization strategies, and their capacity to circumvent inhibitory immune mechanisms. The challenge with vaccination strategies is to break tolerance so that the patient's immune system will recognize CSCs. Future vaccination therapies may be driven toward CSC lysates or specific tumor antigens of CSCs to improve and amplify the DC vaccine efficacy. Thus, activated immune systems could directly and specifically attack tumor CSCs. Importantly, CSC-targeted DC vaccination should not evoke an immune response specific to normal cells that may express common antigens. It has been demonstrated that there are very low levels of expression of cell surface MHC molecules in NSCs. Moreover, NSCs may also evade immune attacks due to decreased expression of co-stimulatory proteins (98). Cytotoxic chemotherapy may be integrated with DC vaccines using unique doses and schedules to break down barriers to cancer immunotherapy. New protocols combining chemotherapy with immunotherapy to achieve therapeutic synergy may benefit cancer therapy (99). It has been reported that sensitization of malignant gliomas to chemotherapy through DC vaccination provides a novel strategy to overcome the immune escape of CSCs by immunoediting (100,101).

Targeting Cancer Stem Cells Based on Mono-Antibody Therapy

Monoclonal antibodies (mAbs) have emerged as effective targeted therapies for the treatment of a number of human malignancies as they have target antigen specificity and generally minimal toxicity. One limitation of conventional antibody therapies is that they have limited efficacy against solid tumors. In a clinical setting, the toxin–monoclonal antibody complex may have utility as a topical or locally delivered chemotherapy for treating tumors at a very early stage that have the potential to develop into mature tumors.

The use of antibodies for cancer therapy has brought positive clinical outcomes and new options for targeting CSCs. The challenge now is how to segregate tumors most efficiently and effectively into treatment-relevant subgroups; this requires the development of necessary biomarkers. Thus, mAbs are well positioned as CSC-targeting therapies. One promising strategy for the development of mAbs targeting human CSCs involves first identifying cell surface antigens, expressed preferentially on CSCs compared with normal cells. In recent years, some cell surface markers specifically and frequently expressed by CSCs have been demonstrated (Table 15.1). The identification of cell surface molecules that are selectively or differentially expressed on acute myeloid leukemia (AML) stem cells relative to normal tissue suggests that antibody-based diagnostic or therapeutic opportunities may be forthcoming. For instance, CD44 has been identified as a cell surface marker in AML stem cells. Anti-CD44 antibody therapy represents a major approach called anti-CSC. In this leukaemic model, CSCs were discovered and characterized with six antibodies used to selectively induce differentiation or inhibit proliferation to eradicate them. Jin et al. reported that targeting AML CSCs in vivo resulted in lower engraftment, suggesting that anti-CD44 antibody treatment directly altered the fate of CSCs either by inducing differentiation or by inhibiting their repopulating ability (102). This study provided evidence that targeting CSCs using antibody could be effective.

Antibodies are typically used in combination with cytotoxic chemotherapy regimens. Such combinations have made a significant contribution to patient survival. Chemotherapy may, in fact, aid antibody functions such as penetration into the tumor and hence improving immunological performance. All colon cancer cells appear to express higher levels of IL-4 than normal colon tissues, suggesting a potential therapeutic index with anti-IL-4 therapy. Neutralizing antibodies targeting IL-4 or a dominant-negative IL-4 ligand increases the sensitivity of both colon cancer cells and colon CSCs. Todaro et al. reported that treatment with an IL-4α antagonist or an anti-IL-4 neutralizing antibody strongly enhanced the anti-tumor efficacy of a standard chemotherapeutic drug (fluorouracil) through selective sensitization of CD133$^+$ cells (103).

Targeting Signaling Pathways in Cancer Stem Cells

It is important to develop CSC-specific targeted therapies that avoid potential toxicity to NSCs, because CSCs and NSCs share common regulatory pathways and cell-surface markers. For instance, dimethylamino-parthenolide (DMAPT), a parthenolide analog, has been shown to be highly active in human acute myeloid leukemia (AML) stem cells but not in normal hematopoietic stem cells (HSCs). This potent inhibitor of NF-κB has been demonstrated to induce apoptosis of both AML and chronic myeloid leukemia (CML) blast crisis stem cells while sparing normal HSCs (104).

The utility of short-interfering RNAs (siRNAs) is a new approach to develop gene-oriented therapies. The ability of siRNAs to silence any gene in the genome makes it extremely promising as a potential targeted cancer therapy. Previous data have shown that the pleiotropic cytokine interleukin-6 (IL-6) contributes to malignant progression and apoptosis resistance of various cancer types (105). GBM samples have been shown to contain significantly higher levels of IL-6 protein compared to those of control brains (106), and higher IL-6 mRNA levels correlate with poor GBM patient survival (107). Recently, Wang et al. reported that targeting IL6Rα with shRNA, or IL-6 with siRNA or an antibody, increased tumor latency in mice that bear human glioma xenografts and significantly impaired their growth and survival in vitro (108). This finding suggests the importance of IL-6 autocrine signaling in maintaining CSCs. This result additionally suggests that IL-6 may be a novel therapeutic target directed at CSCs. Additionally, Sunayama et al. showed that targeted inactivation of both MEK/extracellular signal-regulated kinase (ERK) and PI3K/mTOR pathways in gCSCs using pharmacological inhibitors or siRNAs suppressed their self-renewal capacity and tumorigenicity (109).

CONCLUSIONS

The origin of gCSCs in GBM from different patients may vary and may thus also display different genetic and epigenic changes in complex tumor tissues. The next generation of treatment for GBM will rely on a unique combination of several targeted therapies based on cellular, molecular, genetic, and epigenic information from the specific tumors of individual patients.

Cellular and molecular analysis of tumor heterogeneity may accelerate biomarker development and the application of personalized medical therapy. However, great challenges lay ahead as gCSC populations are themselves also heterogeneous (110) and may evolve over time within GBM patients. It has been well known that primary tumors displaying a gene expression signature characteristic of the epithelial-mesenchymal transition are more likely to be associated with eventual distant metastasis and shorter periods of distant metastasis-free survival (111). Thus, aspects of the stem cell–like phenotype may contribute to tumor invasion and metastasis. These paradigms are exciting as they may provide new avenues for developing novel therapeutics to improve tumor treatment and reduce the tumor metastasis or recurrence that is the primary cause of most cancer deaths.

REFERENCES

1. Cohen MH, Shen YL, Keegan P, et al. FDA drug approval summary: bevacizumab (Avastin) as treatment of recurrent glioblastoma multiforme. Oncologist 2009; 14: 1131–8.
2. Paulino AC, Teh BS. Treatment of brain tumors. N Engl J Med 2005; 352: 2350–3.
3. Stupp R, Mason WP, van den Bent MJ, et al. Radiotherapy plus concomitant and adjuvant temozolomide for glioblastoma. N Engl J Med 2005; 352: 987–96.
4. Hegi ME, Diserens AC, Gorlia T, et al. MGMT gene silencing and benefit from temozolomide in glioblastoma. N Engl J Med 2005; 352: 997–1003.
5. Stupp R, Hegi ME, Mason WP, et al. Effects of radiotherapy with concomitant and adjuvant temozolomide versus radiotherapy alone on survival in glioblastoma in a randomised phase III study: 5-year analysis of the EORTC-NCIC trial. Lancet Oncol 2009; 10: 459–66.
6. Wicha MS, Liu S, Dontu G. Cancer stem cells: An old idea—A paradigm shift. Cancer Res 2006; 66: 1883–90.
7. Lapidot T, Sirard C, Vormoor J, et al. A cell initiating human acute myeloid leukaemia after transplantation into SCID mice. Nature 1994; 367: 645–8.
8. Bonnet D, Dick JE. Human acute myeloid leukemia is organized as a hierarchy that originates from a primitive hematopoietic cell. Nat Med 1997; 3: 730–7.
9. Al-Hajj M, Wicha SM, Benito-Hernandez A, et al. Prospective identification of tumorigenic breast cancer cells. Proc Natl Acad Sci USA 2003; 100: 3983–8.
10. Holyoake TL, Jiang X, Drummond MW, et al. Elucidating critical mechanisms of deregulated stem cell turnover in the chronic phase of chronic myeloid leukemia. Leukemia 2002; 16: 549–58.
11. Cox CV, Evely RS, Oakhill A, et al. Characterization of acute lymphoblastic leukemia progenitor cells. Blood 2004; 104: 2919–25.
12. Singh SK, Clarke ID, Terasaki M, et al. Identification of a cancer stem cell in human brain tumors. Cancer Res 2003; 63: 5821–8.
13. Galli R, Binda E, Orfanelli U, et al. Isolation and characterization of tumorigenic, stem-like neural precursors from human glioblastoma. Cancer Res 2004; 64: 7011–21.
14. Ignatova TN, Kukekov VG, Laywell ED, et al. Human cortical glial tumors contain neural stem-like cells expressing astroglial and neuronal markers in vitro. Glia 2002; 39: 193–206.
15. Yuan X, Curtin J, Xiong Y, et al. Isolation of cancer stem cells from adult glioblastoma multiforme. Oncogene 2004; 23: 9392–400.
16. Friel AM, Sergent PA, Patnaude C, et al. Functional analyses of the cancer stem cell-like properties of human endometrial tumor initiating cells. Cell Cycle 2008; 7: 242–9.
17. Pardal R, Clarke MF, Morrison SJ. Applying the principles of stem-cell biology to cancer. Nat Rev Cancer 2003; 3: 895–902.
18. Hermann PC, Huber SL, Herrler T, et al. Distinct populations of cancer stem cells determines tumor growth and metastatic activity in human pancreatic cancer. Cell Stem Cell 2007; 1: 313–23.
19. Li C, Heidt DG, Dalerba P, et al. Identification of pancreatic cancer stem cells. Cancer Res 2007; 67: 1030–7.
20. Ji J, Black KL, Yu JS. Glioma stem cell research for the development of immunotherapy. Neurosurg Clin N Am 2010; 21: 159–66.
21. O'Brien CA, Pollet A, Gallinger S, et al. A human colon caner cell capable of initiating tumour growth in immunodeficient mice. Nature 2007; 445: 106–10.
22. Collins AT, Berry PA, Hyde C, et al. Prospective identification of tumorigenic prostate cancer stem cells. Cancer Res 2005; 65: 10946–51.
23. Gudjonsson T, Villadsen R, Nielsen HL, et al. Isolation, immortalization, and characterization of a human breast epithelial cell line with stem cell properties. Genes Dev 2002; 16: 693–706.
24. Baumann P, Cremers N, Kroese F, et al. CD24 expression causes the acquisition of multiple cellular properties associated with tumor growth and metastasis. Cancer Res 2005; 65: 10783–93.
25. Gallacher L, Murdoch B, Wu DM, et al. Isolation and characterization of human CD34(-)Lin(-) and CD34(+)Lin(-) hematopoietic stem cells using cell surface markers AC133 and CD7. Blood 2000; 95: 2813–20.
26. Lang P, Bader P, Schumm M, et al. Transplantation of a combination of CD133+ and CD34+ selected progenitor cells from alternative donors. Br J Haematol 2004; 124: 72–9.
27. Mizrak D, Brittan M, Alison MR. CD133 : molecule of the moment. J Pathol 2008; 214: 3–9.
28. Singh SK, Hawkins C, Clarke ID, et al. Identification of human brain tumour initiating cells. Nature 2004; 432: 396–401.

29. Eramo A, Ricci-Vitiani L, Zeuner A, et al. Chemotherapy resistance of glioblastoma stem cells. Cell Death Differ 2006; 13: 1238–41.
30. Liu G, Yuan X, Zeng Z, et al. Analysis of gene expression and chemoresistance of CD133+ cancer stem cells in glioblastoma. Mol Cancer 2006; 5: 67.
31. Bao S, Wu Q, McLendon RE, et al. Glioma stem cells promote radioresistance by preferential activation of the DNA damage response. Nature 2006; 444: 756–60.
32. Lendahl U, Zimmerman LB, McKay RD. CNS stem cells express a new class of intermediate filament protein. Cell 1990; 60: 585–95.
33. Chou YH, Khuon S, Herrmann H, et al. Nestin promotes the phosphorylation-dependent disassembly of vimentin intermediate filaments during mitosis. Mol Biol Cell 2003; 14: 1468–78.
34. Hoffman RM. The potential of nestin-expressing hair follicle stem cells in regenerative medicine. Expert Opin Biol Ther 2007; 7: 289–291.
35. Almazán G, Vela JM, Molina-Holgado E, et al. Re-evaluation of nestin as a marker of oligodendrocyte lineage cells. Microsc Res Tech 2001; 52: 753–65.
36. Dahlstrand J, Collins VP, Lendahl U. Expression of the class VI intermediate filament nestin in human central nervous system tumors. Cancer Res 1992; 52: 5334–41.
37. Veselska R, Kuglik P, Cejpek P, et al. Nestin expression in the cell lines derived from glioblastoma multiforme. BMC Cancer 2006; 6: 32–43.
38. Thomas SK, Messam CA, Spengler BA, et al. Nestin is a potential mediator of malignancy in human neuroblastoma cells. J Biol Chem 2004; 279: 27994–9.
39. Ogden AT, Waziri AE, Lochhead RA, et al. Identification of A2B5+CD133- tumor-initiating cells in adult human gliomas. Neurosurgery 2008; 62: 505–14.
40. Nunes MC, Roy NS, Keyoung HM, et al. Identification and isolation of multipotential neural progenitor cells from the subcortical white matter of the adult human brain. Nat Med 2003; 9: 439–47.
41. Maric D, Maric I, Barker JL. Developmental changes in cell calcium homeostasis during neurogenesis of the embryonic rat cerebral cortex. Cereb Cortex 2000; 10: 561–73.
42. Tchoghandjian A, Baeza N, Colin C, et al. A2B5 cells from human glioblastoma have cancer stem cell properties. Brain Pathol 2010; 20: 211–21.
43. Maness PF, Schachner M. Neural recognition molecules of the immunoglobulin superfamily: signaling transducers of axon guidance and neuronal migration. Nat Neurosci 2007; 10: 19–26.
44. Bao S, Wu Q, Li Z, et al. Targeting cancer stem cells through L1CAM suppresses glioma growth. Cancer Res 2008; 68: 6043–8.
45. Reya T, Clevers H. Wnt signalling in stem cells and cancer. Nature 2005; 434: 843–50.
46. Artavanis-Tsakonas S, Rand MD, Lake RJ. Notch signaling: cell fate control and signal integration in development. Science 1999; 284: 770–6.
47. Fan X, Khaki L, Zhu TS, et al. NOTCH pathway blockade depletes CD133-positive glioblastoma cells and inhibits growth of tumor neurospheres and xenografts. Stem Cells 2010; 28: 5–16.
48. Wang J, Wakeman TP, Lathia JD, et al. Notch promotes radioresistance of glioma stem cells. Stem Cells 2010; 28: 17–28.
49. Hahn H, Wicking C, Zaphiropoulous PG, et al. Mutations of the human homolog of Drosophila patched in the nevoid basal cell carcinoma syndrome. Cell 1996; 85: 841–51.
50. Johnson RL, Rothman AL, Xie J, et al. Human homolog of patched, a candidate gene for the basal cell nevus syndrome. Science 1996; 272: 1668–71.
51. Yauch RL, Gould SE, Scales SJ, et al. A paracrine requirement for hedgehog signalling in cancer. Nature 2008; 455: 406–10.
52. Tian H, Callahan CA, DuPree KJ, et al. Hedgehog signaling is restricted to the stromal compartment during pancreatic carcinogenesis. Proc Natl Acad Sci USA 2009; 106: 4254–9.
53. Clement V, Sanchez P, de Tribolet N, et al. HEDGEHOG-GLI1 signaling regulates human glioma growth, cancer stem cell self-renewal, and tumorigenicity. Curr Biol 2007; 17: 165–72.
54. Ehtesham M, Sarangi A, Valadez JG, et al. Ligand-dependent activation of the hedgehog pathway in glioma progenitor cells. Oncogene 2007; 26: 5752–61.
55. Bar EE, Chaudhry A, Lin A, et al. Cyclopamine-mediated hedgehog pathway inhibition depletes stem-like cancer cells in glioblastoma. Stem Cells 2007; 25: 2524–33.
56. Clevers H. Wnt/beta-catenin signaling in development and disease. Cell 2006; 127: 469–80.
57. Klaus A, Birchmeier W. Wnt signalling and its impact on development and cancer. Nat Rev Cancer 2008; 8: 387–98.
58. Woodward WA, Chen MS, Behbod F, et al. WNT/beta-catenin mediates radiation resistance of mouse mammary progenitor cells. Proc Natl Acad Sci USA 2007; 104: 618–23.

59. Zhang M, Atkinson RL, Rosen JM. Selective targeting of radiation-resistant tumor-initiating cells. Proc Natl Acad Sci USA 2010; 107: 3522–7.
60. Takahashi-Yanaga F, Kahn M. Targeting Wnt signaling: can we safely eradicate cancer stem cells? Clin Cancer Res 2010; 16: 3153–62.
61. Bromberg J. Stat proteins and oncogenesis. J Clin Invest 2002; 109: 1139–42.
62. Sherry MM, Reeves A, Wu JK, et al. STAT3 is required for proliferation and maintenance of multipotency in glioblastoma stem cells. Stem Cells 2009; 27: 2383–92.
63. Cao Y, Lathia JD, Eyler CE, et al. Erythropoietin Receptor Signaling Through STAT3 Is Required For Glioma Stem Cell Maintenance. Genes Cancer 2010; 1: 50–61.
64. Wang H, Lathia JD, Wu Q, et al. Targeting interleukin 6 signaling suppresses glioma stem cell survival and tumor growth. Stem Cells 2009; 27: 2393–404.
65. Chan JA, Krichevsky AM, Kosik KS. MicroRNA-21 is an antiapoptotic factor in human glioblastoma cells. Cancer Res 2005; 65: 6029–33.
66. Suh MR, Lee Y, Kim JY, et al. Human embryonic stem cells express a unique set of microRNAs. Dev Biol 2004; 270: 488–98.
67. Conti A, Aguennouz M, La Torre D, et al. miR-21 and 221 upregulation and miR-181b downregulation in human grade II-IV astrocytic tumors. J Neurooncol 2009; 93: 325–32.
68. Silber J, Lim DA, Petritsch C, et al. miR-124 and miR-137 inhibit proliferation of glioblastoma multiforme cells and induce differentiation of brain tumor stem cells. BMC Med 2008; 6: 14.
69. Gal H, Pandi G, Kanner AA, et al. MIR-451 and Imatinib mesylate inhibit tumor growth of Glioblastoma stem cells. Biochem Biophys Res Commun 2008; 376: 86–90.
70. Schatton T, Murphy GF, Frank NY, et al. Identification of cells initiating human melanomas. Nature 2008; 451: 345–9.
71. Hirschmann-Jax C, Foster AE, Wulf GG, et al. A distinct "side population" of cells with high drug efflux capacity in human tumor cells. Proc Natl Acad Sci USA 2004; 101: 14228–33.
72. Bao S, Wu Q, Sathornsumetee S, et al. Stem cell-like glioma cells promote tumor angiogenesis through vascular endothelial growth factor. Cancer Res 2006; 66: 7843–8.
73. Wang R, Chadalavada K, Wilshire J, et al. Glioblastoma stem-like cells give rise to tumour endothelium. Nature 2010; 468: 829–33.
74. Teicher BA. Hypoxia and drug resistance. Cancer Metastasis Rev 1994; 13: 139–68.
75. Liang BC. Effects of hypoxia on drug resistance phenotype and genotype in human glioma cell lines. J Neurooncol 1996; 29: 149–55.
76. Jensen RL. Brain tumor hypoxia: tumorigenesis, angiogenesis, imaging, pseudoprogression, and as a therapeutic target. J Neurooncol 2009; 92: 317–3.
77. Baish JW, Jain RK. Cancer, angiogenesis and fractals. Nat Med 1998; 4: 984.
78. Heddleston JM, Li Z, McLendon RE, et al. The hypoxic microenvironment maintains glioblastoma stem cells and promotes reprogramming towards a cancer stem cell phenotype. Cell Cycle 2009; 8: 3274–84.
79. Soeda A, Park M, Lee D, et al. Hypoxia promotes expansion of the CD133-positive glioma stem cells through activation of HIF-1alpha. Oncogene 2009; 28: 3949–59.
80. Li Z, Bao S, Wu Q, et al. Hypoxia-inducible factors regulate tumorigenic capacity of glioma stem cells. Cancer Cell 2009; 15: 501–13.
81. Mani SA, Guo W, Liao MJ, et al. The epithelial-mesenchymal transition generates cells with properties of stem cells. Cell 2008; 133: 704–15.
82. Gupta PB, Chaffer CL, Weinberg RA. Cancer stem cells: mirage or reality? Nat Med 2009; 15: 1010–12.
83. Choi S, Myers JN. Molecular pathogenesis of oral squamous cell carcinoma: implications for therapy. J Dent Res 2008; 87: 14–32.
84. Hsu FJ, Benike C, Fagnoni F, et al. Vaccination of patients with B-cell lymphoma using autologous antigen-pulsed dendritic cells. Nat Med 1996; 2: 52–8.
85. Banchereau J, Steinman RM. Dendritic cells and the control of immunity. Nature 1998; 392: 245–52.
86. Fong L, Engleman EG. Dendritic cells in cancer immunotherapy. Annu Rev Immuno 2000; 18: 245–273.
87. Sabado RL, Bhardwaj N. Directing dendritic cell immunotherapy towards successful cancer treatment. Immunotherapy 2010; 2: 37–56.
88. Okada H, Kohanbash G, Zhu Xm, et al. Immunotherapeutic approaches for glioma. Crit Rev Immunol 2009; 29: 1–42.

89. Liau LM, Black KL, Martin NA, et al. Treatment of a patient by vaccination with autologous dendritic cells pulsed with allogeneic major histocompatibility complex class I-matched tumor peptides. Case Report. Neurosurg Focus 2000; 9: e8.

90. Yu JS, Wheeler CJ, Zeltzer PM, et al. Vaccination of malignant glioma patients with peptide-pulsed dendritic cells elicits systemic cytotoxicity and intracranial T-cell infiltration. Cancer Res 2001; 61: 842–7.

91. Yu JS, Liu G, Ying H, et al. Vaccination with tumor lysate-pulsed dendritic cells elicits antigen-specific, cytotoxic T-cells in patients with malignant glioma. Cancer Res 2004; 64: 4973–9.

92. Sabado RL, Bhardwaj N. Directing dendritic cell immunotherapy towards successful cancer treatment. Immunotherapy 2010; 2: 37–56.

93. Singh SK, Hawkins C, Clarke ID, et al. Identification of human brain tumour initiating cells. Nature 2004; 432: 396–401.

94. Xu Q, Liu G, Yuan X, et al. Antigen-specific T-cell response from dendritic cell vaccination using cancer stem-like cell-associated antigens. Stem Cells 2009; 27: 1734–40.

95. Schmitz M, Temme A, Senner V, et al. Identification of SOX2 as a novel glioma-associated antigen and potential target for T cell-based immunotherapy. Br J Cancer 2007; 96: 1293–301.

96. Pellegatta S, Poliani PL, Corno D, et al. Neurospheres enriched in cancer stem-like cells are highly effective in eliciting a dendritic cell-mediated immune response against malignant gliomas. Cancer Res 2006; 66: 10247–52.

97. Garcia-Hernandez Mde L, Gray A, Hubby B, et al. Prostate stem cell antigen vaccination induces a long-term protective immune response against prostate cancer in the absence of autoimmunity. Cancer Res 2008; 68: 861–9.

98. Odeberg J, Piao JH, Samuelsson EB, et al. Low immunogenicity of in vitro-expanded human neural cells despite high MHC expression. J Neuroimmunol 2005; 161: 1–11.

99. Emens LA, Jaffee EM. Leveraging the activity of tumor vaccines with cytotoxic chemotherapy. Cancer Res 2005; 65: 8059–64.

100. Liu G, Black KL, Yu JS. Sensitization of malignant glioma to chemotherapy through dendritic cell vaccination. Expert Rev Vaccines 2006; 5: 233–47.

101. Dunn GP, Bruce AT, Ikeda H, et al. Cancer immunoediting: from immunosurveillance to tumor escape. Nat Immunol 2002; 3: 991–8.

102. Jin L, Lee EM, Ramshaw HS, et al. Monoclonal antibody-mediated targeting of CD123, IL-3 receptor alpha chain, eliminates human acute myeloid leukemic stem cells. Cell Stem Cell 2009; 5: 31–42zsw.

103. Todaro M, Alea MP, Di Stefano AB, et al. Colon cancer stem cells dictate tumor growth and resist cell death by production of interleukin-4. Cell Stem Cell 2007; 1: 389–402.

104. Guzman ML, Rossi RM, Karnischky L, et al. The sesquiterpene lactone parthenolide induces apoptosis of human acute myelogenous leukemia stem and progenitor cells. Blood 2005; 105: 4163–9.

105. Weissenberger J, Loeffler S, Kappeler A, et al. IL-6 is required for glioma development in a mouse model. Oncogene 2004; 23: 3308–16.

106. Choi C, Gillespie GY, Van Wagoner NJ, et al. Fas engagement increases expression of interleukin-6 in human glioma cells. J Neurooncol 2002; 56: 13–19.

107. Tchirkov A, Khalil T, Chautard E, et al. Interleukin-6 gene amplification and shortened survival in glioblastoma patients. Br J Cancer 2007; 96: 474–6.

108. Wang H, Lathia JD, Wu Q, et al. Targeting interleukin 6 signaling suppresses glioma stem cell survival and tumor growth. Stem Cells 2009; 27: 2393–404.

109. Sunayama J, Matsuda K, Sato A, et al. Crosstalk between the PI3K/mTOR and MEK/ERK pathways involved in the maintenance of self-renewal and tumorigenicity of glioblastoma stem-like cells. Stem Cells 2010; 28: 1930–9.

110. Piccirillo SG, Binda E, Fiocco R, et al. Brain cancer stem cells. J Mol Med 2009; 87: 1087–95.

111. Kalluri R. EMT: when epithelial cells decide to become mesenchymal-like cells. J Clin Invest 2009; 119: 1417–19.

16 | RNA in cancer vaccine therapy

Smita Nair, David Boczkowski, Scott Pruitt, and Johannes Urban

INTRODUCTION

Immunotherapy is based on the concept of using the body's own immune system to fight disease. Cancer vaccines are a form of active immunotherapy with the goal to generate an endogenous and specific immune response to tumor antigens or tumor-associated antigens (TAAs) that can target and destroy cancer cells. Current vaccine strategies aim to induce not only a very robust and effective $CD8^+$ cytotoxic T-cell response but also $CD4^+$ T helper responses, B-cell responses, and natural killer (NK) cell activity. There are many ongoing phase III cancer vaccine trials nearing completion, and some of these are showing promise, an indication that cancer immunotherapy is here to stay. In 2010, sipuleucel-T (Provenge™, Dendreon Corporation, Seattle, WA), an autologous antigen-presenting cell- (APC) enriched vaccine preparation loaded with a prostatic acid phosphatase (PAP)–granulocyte-macrophage colony-stimulating factor (GM-CSF) fusion protein, was the first immunotherapy vaccine approved by the Food and Drug Administration for treatment of castration-resistant metastatic prostate cancer. As such, the future of immunotherapy will continue to evolve as these clinical trials shed light on tumor-specific immune mechanisms and will, without doubt, involve a multi-pronged approach that can translate to effective cancer vaccine therapies that have a sustained clinical benefit.

One component of the cancer vaccine is the tumor antigen itself, which can be either one antigen that is expressed by the tumor, or a complex mixture of TAAs (either known or unknown antigens). Since many tumor antigens are now known to be ineffective at stimulating robust immune responses, current research has widened to include approaches to make vaccination strategies more durable, including enhancing co-stimulation and blocking immune-suppression.

The role of RNA in immunity was first explored in studies demonstrating that extracts from the lymphoid tissues of animals injected with tumors could transfer specific immunity when incubated with splenocytes from nonimmunized animals (1,2). The transferred component that was responsible for the immunity was sensitive to degradation by RNase and could be isolated by the use of oligo-dT, suggesting that the activity was in the messenger RNA (mRNA) fraction, referred to as "immune RNA"(2).

In this chapter we focus on the use of RNA encoding tumor antigens to stimulate tumor immune responses and, additionally, highlight recent studies that use RNA to enhance immune responses. As outlined below, the current use of RNA in cancer vaccine therapy has been mostly pursued using two approaches: (*i*) RNA-transfected dendritic cells (DCs) (3–5) or (*ii*) direct injection of RNA in vivo (4,6).

ADVANTAGES OF RNA

The cancer vaccine field was reinvigorated by the identification of TAAs, proteins that are mutated and/or aberrantly overexpressed in tumors. These TAAs have been used in vaccine preparations in the form of peptide, protein, DNA, or RNA. So this raises the obvious question: Why use RNA encoding TAA?

Short peptides that bind specific human leukocyte antigen (HLA) molecules are an obvious choice for the induction of immune responses due to the simplicity of their use and ability to manufacture these peptides on a large scale. However, a significant drawback of using peptides is that for every TAA, one has to identify an immunogenic 8–9 amino acid fragment that binds a specific HLA molecule. The peptide, once identified, is limited for use in only patients expressing that specific HLA molecule. Unlike peptides, RNA vaccines as part of the cellular process will generate multiple peptides in the patient, some of which will bind to the patient's HLA molecules. Thus, the number of patients that can be treated with RNA-based vaccines is not limited by prior identification of the immunogenic peptides or knowledge of the patient's HLA type.

An alternative that can circumvent the problem associated with peptides is to use a TAA protein that allows the patient's cells to process the entire protein and to present all possible epitopes. This has the added appeal of producing epitopes that can bind not only to class I molecules, but also to MHC class II molecules, leading to the induction of CD8+ as well as CD4+ T-cell responses. Many reports have now documented the benefits of inducing CD4 and CD8 T cells for generating an effective and sustained immune response against tumors. Protein production and purification, however, is a cumbersome process, limiting its attractiveness as a source of antigen.

Another alternative is the use of DNA, which is not only easily produced in bulk but also overcomes the limitation of HLA specificity associated with peptide-based vaccines. However, DNA delivered to the cytoplasm of the cell must translocate to the nucleus to be transcribed into mRNA. The mRNA is next translated into a protein which is then subjected to the cell's class I processing mechanism to generate the relevant MHC-binding peptides. Although cells have been transfected with DNA by various methods, including cationic lipofection and electroporation, getting the DNA to the nucleus is not always efficient (7). In contrast, mRNA transferred to the cytoplasm is readily translated into proteins. A second potential problem associated with DNA use is that the DNA can integrate into the host-cell genome, a bigger concern if the transgene encodes a protein that is involved in the neoplastic process. This problem, although largely theoretical, is eliminated in RNA-based vaccines. Van Tendeloo et al. demonstrated another potential reason to choose mRNA over DNA by comparing CD34+ precursor-derived Langerhans cells (epidermal DCs), electroporated with Melan-A-encoding DNA or mRNA for their ability to stimulate interferon-γ (IFNγ) production from a Melan-A-specific CTL clone (7). Although both the mRNA-transfected and DNA-transfected cells stimulated the Melan-A CTL clone, cells electroporated with DNA encoding a protein other than Melan-A caused non-specific stimulation. Whereas, when mRNA was used, only cells electroporated with mRNA encoding Melan-A caused interferon-γ release from the CTL clone, highlighting the improved specificity of this approach. In another comparison it was found that human DCs transfected with mRNA encoding influenza matrix protein were superior to DCs lipofected with plasmid DNA in stimulating a CD8+ memory response (8).

When the TAA expressed by a particular cancer is known, producing large quantities of in vitro transcribed mRNA under good manufacturing practice is a straightforward and inexpensive process that involves a one-time cloning of the appropriate cDNA into a vector that encodes a bacteriophage promoter and a poly(A) tail. For mRNA generation, the cDNA-containing plasmid is linearized by restriction digestion and used as a template for in vitro transcription in a reaction that contains buffers, ribonucleotide triphosphates, and bacteriophage RNA polymerase. After transcription, the plasmid template is digested with DNase and the mRNA is cleaned up for subsequent use.

USING mRNA ENCODING A DEFINED TAA VERSUS RNA ISOLATED FROM TUMOR CELLS

Vaccination with defined TAA has some advantages over the use of total RNAs derived from tumors. First, there is no requirement for the growth of tumor cells or the isolation of antigen for each patient. Secondly, the antigen preparation is of high purity and a majority of the loaded DCs present the same epitope(s) in the context of MHC on their surface. Thirdly, the risk of autoimmunity induced by the inclusion of nonmutated, normally expressed proteins is reduced or eliminated. However, there are some limitations to using a defined TAA for vaccination. The primary one is that TAAs for many tumors remain unknown, although the identification of novel TAAs is a field of active research. Another drawback is that not all TAAs identified are necessarily the best antigens for inducing an anti-tumor immune response. Finally, there is always the potential of developing tumor escape mutants that will downregulate the expression of the cognate protein under selective pressure from an activated immune system.

An alternative to using defined tumor antigen is to use complex antigen mixtures that have been derived from the patient's tumor in the form of RNA. This eliminates the need to identify antigens expressed by the patient's tumor, thus significantly enhancing the number of cancers that can be treated with this approach. In addition, because the entire spectrum of antigenic determinants will be displayed, the immune system can use those that are most effective and simultaneously reduce the risk of escape mutants. There are drawbacks to vaccinating with total tumor-derived material though, with a major disadvantage being the large amount of tumor required to isolate tumor antigen, thus excluding patients with low tumor burden from such a vaccination protocol. Secondly, unfractionated tumor-derived antigen will contain non-tumor-specific self proteins, which can potentially induce autoimmunity. Another potential problem is that many tumors express immunosuppressive molecules such as transforming growth factor beta (TGF-β) and/or interleukin-10 (IL-10). Transfecting DCs with tumor-derived RNA can also result in the translation of these suppressive mRNAs and thereby suppress immune responses.

Based on the discussion above, there are legitimate reasons for choosing either a defined antigen or unfractionated, tumor-derived antigen for vaccine preparation. In certain scenarios where the only option is total tumor-derived RNA, there is still the possibility of having insufficient amount of tumor for isolation of antigen and, even if there is enough material, the theoretical concern of autoimmunity still exits. These concerns can be addressed by using mRNA that has been amplified from the tumor as the antigen source. We have shown that RNA extracted from tumors and amplified via RT-PCR or cDNA library construction can be used to elicit immune responses in mice (9). In addition, DCs pulsed with mRNA amplified from microdissected frozen sections of human carcinoembryonic antigen (CEA) positive colorectal tumor were capable of stimulating an in vitro cytotoxic T lymphocyte (CTL) response against CEA (9). Heiser et al. have shown that human monocyte-derived DCs generated from prostate cancer patients and transfected with mRNA that was amplified from microdissected frozen tumor sections stimulated a polyclonal T-cell response that recognized the patient's tumor cells as well as prostate-specific antigen (PSA) and telomerase reverse transcriptase (TERT)-expressing target cells (10). Grunebach et al. demonstrated that DCs transfected with amplified mRNA from a green fluorescent protein (GFP)-expressing renal cancer cell line expressed GFP protein and stimulated CTL responses comparable to responses generated by DCs transfected with non-amplified RNA (11). In addition, this technique allows not only for an unlimited amount of tumor antigen but also may lessen autoimmunity-related issues.

EX VIVO MODIFICATION OF CELLS WITH RNA

The concept of using DCs transfected with RNA to induce anti-tumor immunity has now been shown in multiple labs and has also been the subject of many comprehensive reviews. Our laboratory pioneered this concept by demonstrating that mice vaccinated with DCs pulsed with RNA from tumor expressing chicken ovalbumin (OVA) or with in vitro transcribed OVA mRNA could be protected from tumor challenge (12). In a stringent model, mice that had a primary melanoma tumor removed had significantly fewer lung metastases if they were vaccinated with DCs transfected with melanoma RNA than DCs transfected with an unrelated RNA (12). By using human DCs from healthy volunteers and a cancer patient, we demonstrated that DCs transfected with total RNA from CEA+ tumor cells could elicit a CTL response comparable to DCs transfected with CEA mRNA (13). Notably, DCs from a patient with CEA+ adenocarcinoma loaded with CEA mRNA stimulated an in vitro CEA-specific CTL response (13).

The notion of vaccinating against an antigen that is expressed in all tumors is appealing. The catalytic subunit of TERT is an attractive candidate because it is silent in normal tissues but reactivated in more than 85% of cancers. We, and others, have demonstrated induction of TERT-specific CTLs that are capable of lysing target cells transfected with hTERT mRNA, as well as tumor cells (14,15). Zeis et al. showed that vaccination of mice with survivin mRNA-transfected DCs induced resistance to challenge by a survivin-expressing lymphoma (16) and demonstrated that survivin, a member of the inhibitor of apoptosis protein family, has the potential to act as a tumor rejection antigen. CTL responses and tumor immunity can be induced by immunization against angiogenesis-associated products such as vascular endothelial growth factor (VEGF), VEGF receptor-2, or Tie2 (17). Notably, combined immunotherapy against angiogenic targets and TAA exerted a synergistic antitumor effect. We have also demonstrated that fibroblast activation protein, a product that is preferentially expressed in the tumor-associated fibroblasts, could function as a tumor rejection antigen in a range of cancers (18).

In 2001, Van Tendeloo et al. published the first study that used electroporation to load DCs with RNA (7). Most importantly, electroporated DCs were more effective stimulators than DCs that were passively loaded with RNA. In addition to transfecting DCs with RNA that encodes TAA, many laboratories are now focusing on ways to enhance the function and potency of these DC-RNA vaccines. The use of RNA to enhance the function of DCs has now taken center stage and was covered in depth in a recent review by Boczkowski and Nair (3). As an alternative approach, many groups are also using siRNA that target negative immune response modifiers as a way to enhance DC function. Due to space concerns, and because genetic modification of DCs is the subject of another chapter, we will not discuss siRNA-mediated modulation of DC function here.

Critical parameters that can enhance the function of DCs transfected with TAA-encoding mRNA include (*i*) the number of immunizations, (*ii*) the route of immunization to facilitate DC migration to the lymph node, (*iii*) the maturational state of the DCs (mature DCs have now been shown to be more effective at stimulating immune responses), (*iv*) RNA modifications to improve translation or antigen presentation, (*v*) efficient RNA loading into DCs (electroporation is now the method of choice in many clinical trials), and (*vi*) co-transfecting DCs with mRNA encoding immune stimulatory molecules.

Table 16.1 shows some of the studies that have harnessed RNA co-transfection with TAA-encoding mRNA and mRNA that encodes molecules that can enhance DC function.

CLINICAL TRIALS WITH RNA-TRANSFECTED CELLS

Based on compelling data from in vitro studies and preclinical immunotherapy models, many phase I clinical trials were initiated in patients with cancer to test the safety and efficacy of RNA-transfected DCs as vaccines (Table 16.2). In the first report (29), Rains et al. isolated DCs from 15 colorectal cancer patients and pulsed them with autologous tumor RNA and keyhole limpet hemocyanin. The study demonstrates that the approach is feasible and the vaccines were well tolerated. The serum levels of CEA, a surrogate marker of anti-tumor response, were decreased in 7 of the 13 patients (29).

In a study by Heiser et al., prostate cancer patients were vaccinated with DCs transfected with PSA mRNA (30). Feasibility and safety were demonstrated, as was the induction of PSA-specific immunity. A PSA-specific T-cell response was consistently detected in all patients and the log slope of PSA levels decreased significantly in six of seven patients. Moreover, a transient clearance of PSA tumor cells from the circulation was confirmed by real-time RT-PCR in all tested patients (n = 3) (30).

A phase I clinical trial was performed in patients with advanced CEA-expressing malignancies using immature DCs transfected with CEA mRNA as vaccine (32,33). The immunizations were well tolerated and no toxicities were observed. Of the 24 evaluable patients, there was 1 complete response, 2 minor responses, 3 with stable disease, and 18 patients with progressive disease (33).

In another clinical trial, renal cell carcinoma (RCC) patients were immunized with immature DCs transfected with tumor RNA isolated from autologous tumors, and no evidence of dose-limiting toxicity or vaccine-related adverse effects, including autoimmunity, were observed (34). Notably, immunization stimulated polyclonal T-cell responses that were directed

Table 16.1 Enhancing Dendritic Cell (DC) Function Using RNA

Objective	RNA Used	Results	Reference
Enhancing DC migration	E/L selectin	Human DCs were successfully electroporated with E/L selectin RNA and TAA RNADCs were capable of presenting antigen and E/L selectin expressing DCs could roll on sialyl-Lewisx coated slides	Dorrie et al. (19)
Enhancing DC function using immune-stimulating molecules	IL-12	Human DCs transfected with IL-12 RNA-stimulated lymphocytes by shifting them from a Th1 phenotype to a Th2 phenotype	Minkis et al. (20)
	Chimeric RNA encoding ubiquitin, MART, and IL-12	Human DCs transfected with chimeric RNA that also includes IL-12 were more effective at stimulating MART-specific T cells	Bontkes et al. (21)
	CD40-ligand (L)	Human DCs transfected with truncated CD40-L matured and produced more IL-12	Tcherepanova et al. (22)
	Constitutively active (ca)TLR4	Human DCs transfected with caTLR4 were superior at secreting IL-12 and TNF-α	Cisco et al. (23)
		DCs transfected with caTLR4 RNA and MART RNA were superior at T-cell activation	Abdel-Wahab et al. (24)
	CD40-L, caTLR4 and CD70 (also referred to as TriMix)	CD40-L and caTLR4 transfected human DCs showed increased IL-12 secretion	Bonehill et al. (25)
		Addition of CD70 RNA to the mix also enhanced the percentage and absolute numbers of T cells generated	
		TriMix RNA and tumor antigen encoding RNA transfected into DCs together simplified the clinical generation of antigen-loaded and matured DCs	
	OX40-L	Human DCs transfected with OX40-L enhanced CD4 T-cell responses and CD8 CTL response	Dannull et al. (26)
		Murine DCs transfected with OX40-L and tumor antigen RNA demonstrated improved anti-tumor response	
	4-1BB-L	Human DCs co-transfected with 4-1BB-L RNA and HER2/neu RNA induced increased levels of antigen-specific CTL	Grunebach et al. (27)
Engineering DCs to secrete immune-modulating proteins	Anti-GITR antibody (murine) Anti-CTLA-4 antibody (murine and human) Soluble GITR-L (murine and human)	Co-injection of murine DCs transfected with anti-GITR or anti-CTLA-4 with TAA RNA-transfected DCs enhanced anti-tumor immunity	Boczkowski et al. (28) Pruitt et al. (to be published, clinical trials. gov NCT01216436)
		Co-stimulation of T cells with human TAA RNA-transfected DCs in conjunction with CTLA-4- or soluble GITR-L-secreting DCs enhances the induction of antigen-specific T cells	

Abbreviations: CTLA, cytotoxic T lymphocyte antigen; GITR, glucocorticoid-induced tumor necrosis factor receptor (TNFR)-related protein; IL-12, interleukin-12; MART, melanoma antigen recognized by T-cells; (ca)TLR, constitutively active Toll-like receptor; TAA, tumor-associated antigen; TNF-α, tumor necrosis factor α.

Table 16.2 Summary of Clinical Trials Using Dendritic Cells Transfected with RNA as Vaccines

Type of Cancer	RNA Source/ Target Antigen	Vaccination Schedule	# of Patients	Immunological Response	Clinical Response	Reference
Colorectal	Total autologous tumor	10^6 DCs pulsed with 25 µg RNA and KLH IV 4 times at monthly intervals	15	NA	NA Decreased CEA Short follow-up	Rains et al. (29)
Prostate	PSA	10^7–5×10^7 DCs transfected with 1.5 µg RNA/10^6 DCs given IV 3 times biweekly with escalating dose and 10^7 given ID Feasibility and safety phase I study	16	9/9	NA	Heiser et al. (30)
Lung adeno-carcinoma	Total autologous tumor	3×10^7 DCs transfected with 300 µg RNA given IV, followed by 10^6 DCs transfected with 25 µg RNA given ID 4 times at monthly intervals	1	1/1	NA	Nair et al. (31)
Pancreatic	CEA	10^7 DCs transfected with 20 µg RNA given ID 6 times at monthly intervals Feasibility and safety phase I study	3	NA	NA	Morse et al. (32)
CEA-express-ing cancers	CEA	Phase I: 10^7–10^8 DCs transfected with 2 µg RNA/10^6 DC given IV and 0–10^6 DC given ID 4 times biweekly Phase I: dose-escalation phase (29 patients, 24 evaluable) Phase II: 3×10^7 DCs IV and 10^6 DCs ID every 2 wks for 4 doses Phase II: 13 patients	42	NA	Phase I: 1 response based on tumor marker 2 minor response 3 stable disease 18 progression Phase II: 9/13 relapsed (median 122 days)	Morse et al. (33)
Renal cell	Total autologous tumor	10^7–5×10^7 DCs given IV 3 times biweekly RNA/10^7 DCs given IV 3 times biweekly with escalating dose and 10^7 given ID Feasibility and safety phase I study	10	6/7 evaluable	8/10 underwent secondary therapy 1/10 progression 1/10 SD (22 months)	Su et al. (34)
Brain	Total autologous tumor	0.5–5×10^7 DC/m^2 transfected with 5 µg RNA/10^6 DCs given IV and 0.5×10^7 DC/m^2 given ID, 3 times biweekly with escalating dose, 3 times at 3-mo intervals	9	NA	2/7 stable disease	Caruso et al. (35)
Neuroblastoma	Total autologous tumor	0.5–5×10^7 DC/m^2 transfected with 5 µg RNA/10^6 DCs given IV and 0.5×10^7 DC/m^2 given ID, 3 times biweekly with escalating dose, 3 times at 3-mo intervals	11	NA	1/7 stable disease	Caruso et al. (36)

Cancer	RNA/Antigen	Protocol	Number	Immune response	Clinical response	Reference
Renal (RCC), ovarian (OVA)	Total RNA from tumor tissue classified as clear cell carcinoma	Arm 1: 10^7 DCs electroporated with 5 µg RNA/10^6 DCs given ID 3 times biweekly, 18 µg/kg DAB389IL-2 (ONTAK) given prior to vaccination. Arm 2: 10^7 DCs electroporated with 5 µg RNA/10^6 DCs given ID 3 times biweekly	11 Arm 1:7 Arm 2:4 RCC: 10 OVA: 1	10/11 Arm 1: 7/7 Arm 2: 3/4 Increased immune response in Arm 1	NA	Dannull et al. (37)
Prostate	hTERT, hTERT-LAMP	Arm 1: 10^7 DCs electroporated with 1 µg hTERT RNA/10^6 DCs given ID, 3 times (6 patients) or 6 times (5 patients) weekly Arm 2: 10^7 DCs electroporated with 1 µg hTERT-LAMP RNA/10^6 DCs given ID, 3 times (6 patients) or 6 times (3 patients) weekly	20 Arm 1: 11 Arm 2: 9	17/18 Enhanced immune response detected in the Arm 2	12/18 evaluated by serum PSA levels No objective clinical response	Su et al. (38)
Prostate	Total RNA from cell lines DU145, LNCaP, PC-3	2×10^7 DCs electroporated with total allo-tumor RNA from 5×10^7 tumor cells per vaccination given IN or ID, at least 4 times weekly	19	12/19	11/19 SD (by serum PSA levels)	Mu et al. (39)
Melanoma	Total autologous tumor	Arm 1: 2×10^7 electroporated DCs ID 4 times weekly Arm 2: 2×10^7 electroporated DCs IN 4 times weekly	22 Arm 1:10 Arm 2: 12	9/19 T-cell assays 8/18 DTH reaction	2/22 SD 18/22 progression 2/22 not evaluable (no tumor post-surgery)	Kyte et al. (40)
Metastatic ovarian cancer	Folate receptor-alpha (FR-α)	10 injections of electroporated DCs at 4-week intervals IN into unaffected inguinal lymph nodes. First 2 doses 2×10^6 DCs followed by 17-25.2×10^6 DCs. First vaccination with fresh DCs subsequent with cryopreserved	1	1/1	PR Cancer antigen (CA)-125 levels decreased	Hernando et al. (41)
Melanoma	MAGE-A3, MAGE-C2, tyrosinase, gp100	1.25×10^7 electroporated TriMix DCs given ID, 4 times biweekly TriMix DCs: DCs electroporated with mRNA encoding CD40L, CD70 and caTLR4	3	2/2	NA	Bonehill et al. (42)
Melanoma	gp100 or tyrosinase	12×10^6 DCs grown in presence of KLH were electroporated with 20 µg RNA. DCs were labeled with SPIO prior to electroporation. 4 IN vaccinations at day 0 (fresh), 14, 28 and 42 (frozen/thawed)	11	6/8 KLH antibody 11/11 KLH-specific T-cell proliferation 7/11 tetramer+ CD8 T-cell responses from DTH sites	NA	Schuurhuis et al. (43)

(Continued)

Table 16.2 (*Continued*) Summary of Clinical Trials Using Dendritic Cells Transfected with RNA as Vaccines

Type of Cancer	RNA Source/ Target Antigen	Vaccination Schedule	# of Patients	Immunological Response	Clinical Response	Reference
AML	Wilm's tumor gene 1 (WT1)	5–20 × 10⁶ WT1 RNA electroporated DCs injected ID 4 times biweekly to patients in hematological remission First vaccination with fresh DCs subsequent with cryopreserved	10	2/5 evaluable patients had increased (>1.5-fold) frequencies of WT-1 specific tetramer + CD8 cells	2/10 CR	Van Tendeloo et al. (44)
End-stage endometrial carcinoma	WT1	4 weekly injections of WT1-RNA-electroporated DCs (6–8.8 × 10⁶ DCs) given ID in imiquimod pretreated skin	1	2.5-fold increase in WT1-specific T cells	1/1 SD CA-125 decreased after 2 injections	Coosemans et al. (45)
Melanoma	Amplified autologous tumor RNA	4 SC injections of 5 × 106 electroporated DCs once every 3 weeks Note: DCs were cultured in maturation medium for 2 days following EP prior to being frozen	6	0/6	0/6	Markovic et al. (46)

Abbreviations: CR, complete response; DCs, dendritic cells; DTH, delayed-type hypersensitivity; ID, intradermally; IN, intranodally; IV, intravenously; KLH, keyhole limpet hemocyanin; NA, not applicable; PR, partial response; SC, subcutaneously; SD, stable disease; TERT, telomerase reverse transcriptase.

toward TERT, RCC-associated antigen G250, and oncofetal antigen (OFA), but not against cellular proteins expressed by normal renal tissue. Tumor-related mortality was low in 3 out of 10 patients dying from the disease after a mean follow-up of 20 months. The clinical efficacy of this vaccination protocol was not evaluable because patients underwent secondary therapies after vaccination (34).

In a recent clinical study, Dannull et al. investigated whether elimination of CD4+CD25+ regulatory T cells (T_{REGS}) using the recombinant IL-2-diphtheria toxin conjugate, denileukin diftitox (ONTAK™, Eisai Co., Ltd., Tokyo), is capable of enhancing the immune responses elicited by RCC tumor, RNA-transfected DCs (37). T_{REG} depletion significantly improved the stimulation of tumor-specific T-cell responses in RCC patients when compared with vaccination alone.

Bonehill et al. demonstrated that DCs can be electroporated with constitutively active (ca) TLR4, CD40-L, and CD70 mRNAs (referred to as "TriMix") (42) in combination with mRNA encoding antigen, yielding a simplified, one-step antigen-loading and maturation procedure. The antigens were Mage-A3, Mage-C2, tyrosinase, and gp100. DCs from two HLA-A2+, stage III or IV melanoma patients were electroporated with the TriMix mRNAs along with one of the antigen-encoding mRNAs and were then mixed so that DCs expressing all of the antigens were combined. Patients were given four biweekly intradermal injections; two weeks after the final vaccination, CD8+ T cells from their peripheral blood were analyzed for increases in antigen-specific cells. Although reactivity against known HLA-A2-restricted peptides for the antigens could not be detected by tetramer staining, a strong vaccine-induced response was observed when tested for lytic activity/stimulation using a CD107a/CD137 assay and intracellular staining for IFNγ and tumor necrosis factor α (TNFα) (42). This effect could be attributed to unknown immunogenic epitopes that were present in the full-length RNA-encoded TAA protein, further illustrating the advantage of using RNA over peptides as antigens.

The clinical trials summarized in Table 16.2 list the different DC-RNA vaccines that have been tested thus far. Several new strategies including combination therapies to optimize DC-RNA immunotherapy protocols are currently under investigation.

IN VIVO INJECTION OF RNA

In a seminal study, Wolff et al. demonstrated that unformulated "naked" mRNA gets locally expressed after intramuscular injection in mice (47). This study highlights the fact that naked RNA injection in vivo results in uptake by cells and translation into protein, an important prerequisite for inducing immune responses. Subsequent studies have focused on the optimization of mRNA and its delivery for in vivo gene vaccination.

OPTIMIZATION OF mRNA FOR DIRECT INJECTION IN VIVO

The intrinsic instability of RNA and the presence of nucleases on the skin and in body fluids have long discouraged researchers to exploit mRNA as a vehicle for gene transfer in vivo. However, both historic and recent findings have brought new attention to mRNA-based gene therapy, and a strategic optimization aiming at improved mRNA stability and prolonged in vivo expression has been conducted. Essentially all features of mature mRNAs, such as 5′cap structure, untranslated regions (UTRs), coding region, poly (A) tail, and the overall RNA chemistry have successfully been altered in the course of these studies.

The 5′cap structure of eukaryotic mRNAs is essential for recognition by the translational machinery and required for efficient protein production. Unfortunately, bacteriophage polymerases used to incorporate common m^7GpppG cap analogs co-transcriptionally into in vitro transcribed mRNA also utilize the 3′OH of the 7-methylguanosine moiety, thereby producing about 50% translation-incompetent mRNA with the cap in the wrong orientation. "Anti-reverse" cap analogs (ARCAs) such as $m_2^{7,3'-O}GpppG$, in which the 3′OH is eliminated to ensure incorporation in the correct orientation, have been designed and result in mRNA with increased translation efficacy (48). The beneficial effect of ARCA-modified mRNA as compared with m^7GpppG-capped species is highlighted by a 25-, 12-, and 2-fold higher translational output upon transfection into the murine DC line JAWSII, immature human DCs, and mature human DCs, respectively (49). In the near future, novel phosphorothioate cap analogs, such as $m_2^{7,2'-O}Gpp_spG$ (β-S-ARCA), might challenge the status of unmodified ARCA as the gold standard in RNA-based immunotherapy approaches. In β-S-ARCA, a non-bridging oxygen in the β-phosphate moiety is substituted by sulfur which results in reduced susceptibility to 5'-3' decay of the mRNA in vivo, without compromising recognition by the translational machinery. Accordingly, β-S-ARCA mRNAs have a longer half-life and yield more protein upon electroporation into immature human DCs as compared to conventional ARCA mRNA (50). In line with this finding, direct injection of naked β-S-ARCA mRNA into the inguinal lymph nodes of C57Bl/6 mice leads to increased and prolonged protein expression in vivo and more efficient de novo priming of naive T cells (50).

By optimizing the 3'untranslated region (3'UTR) in vitro transcribed mRNA can be further improved. The substitution of the natural 3'UTR of mRNA of interest by a heterologous 3'UTR, derived from an mRNA with exceptional stability, is generally believed to prolong its half-life. Holtkamp and colleagues report an enhanced RNA stability and translational yield of mRNAs equipped with two tandem human β-globin 3'UTRs cloned in head to tail orientation (51). Moreover, protein yields improve with increasing length of the 3'-poly(A) tail, and mRNAs harboring a free-ending poly(A) tail composed of 120 adenosine residues show a higher stability and protein output compared with non-optimized mRNAs.

Another option that remains to be proven in immunotherapy studies is to enhance the translational capacity of mRNA by incorporating modified nucleotides during in vitro transcription. A recent study demonstrated that substitutions of uridine by pseudouridine (ψ) and cytidine by 5-methylcytidine (5mC) enhanced the protein yield of reporter mRNAs by 5 and 2 folds, respectively, upon transfection into precursor-derived murine DCs (52).

In summary, mRNA optimizations act additively to enhance protein production which translates into increased and prolonged expression of antigen-specific peptide–MHC complexes and superior T-cell expansion, a prerequisite in RNA-based immunotherapy.

Delivery of mRNA In Vivo

The ex vivo manipulation of DCs with TAA-encoding mRNA is an effective, but also a laborious and costly means to induce anti-tumor immunity. An alternative is the direct injection of mRNA in vivo to elicit an immune response. The efficacy of the immune response primed by directly injected mRNA is not only strongly influenced by the site chosen for delivery, but also by the formulation of the mRNA. Preclinical studies so far describe the induction of anti-tumor immunity using unformulated mRNA (either needle injection of "naked" RNA in solution or gene gun-mediated delivery after coating onto gold particles) or formulated mRNA that has been complexed with liposomes or protamine.

In a pilot study, intramuscular injection of naked mRNA encoding CEA as an immunogen induced a CEA-specific antibody response after challenge with syngeneic CEA-expressing tumor cells (53). Intradermal injection of naked total RNA isolated from tumor cells, but not from control cells, significantly delayed the tumor growth in a murine challenge model in the absence of an adjuvant (54). Following these early observations, a more thorough characterization of the induced immune response in mice indicates that antigen-specific CTL and IgG antibodies are readily generated after injection of antigen-encoding unprotected mRNA into the ear pinna (55). This route of vaccination primarily triggers a Th2 immune response, characterized by induction of IgG1 antibodies and moderate CTL activation, which can be shifted toward a Th1 response with an increased CTL activation by injecting GM-CSF one day after immunization (56). A systematic comparison of different administration routes revealed an increased potency of antigen-specific T-cell immunity upon intranodal injection of antigen-encoding mRNA, compared with intradermal or subcutaneous administrations (57). Intranodal injection leads to not only a selective uptake of the mRNA into lymph node-resident DCs followed by efficient translation and antigen processing, but also a TLR-mediated upregulation of

Table 16.3 Clinical Trials Using RNA Injected In Vivo

Type of Cancer	Rna Source/Target Antigen	Vaccination Schedule	# of Patient	Immunological Response	Clinical Response	Reference
Melanoma	Amplified autologous tumor RNA	200 µg injected ID, 4 vaccinations every 2 weeks followed by 6 monthly injections. Each vaccination was followed 24 h later by 150 µg GM-CSF SC. Feasibility and safety phase I study	15	NA	2/13 MR 3/13 NED	Weide et al. (62)
Melanoma	Melan-A, tyrosinase, gp100, Mage-A1, Mage-A3, survivin	Arm 1: 3.2–80 µg RNA per antigen + 128 µg protamine injected ID on days 1, 3, 5, weeks 2, 3, 4, 5, 6, 7, 11, 15 and 19. Each vaccination was followed 24 h later by 200 µg GM-CSF SCArm 2: 3.2-80 µg RNA per antigen + 128 µg protamine + 4 mg KLH injected ID on days 1, 3, 5, weeks 2, 3, 4, 5, 6, 7, 11, 15 and 19. Each vaccination was followed 24 h later by 200 µg GM-CSF SC	21 Arm 1: 11 Arm 2: 10	2/4 vaccine-directed T cells (intracellular IFN-γ analysis)	Arm 1: 1/11 CR 4/11 NED Arm 2: 1/10 NED	Weide et al. (63)
Renal cell carcinoma	MUC1, CEA, Her-2/ Neu, telomerase, survivin, MAGE-1	Arm 1: 20 µg naked RNA per antigen injected ID on days 0, 14, 28, 42, followed by monthly injections Each vaccination was followed 24 h later by 100 µg/m2 GM-CSF SC Arm 2: 50 µg naked RNA per antigen injected ID on days 0-3, 7-10, 28, 42 followed by monthly injections. Each vaccination was followed 24 h later by 250 µg/m2 GM-CSF SC	30 Arm 1: 14 Arm 2: 16	ELISpot: 3/7 CD4+ T cells 8/9 CD8+ T cells Chromium-release assay: 7/11 CD8+ CTL	Arm 1: 1/14 PR 6/14 SD Arm 2: 9/16 SD	Rittig et al. (64)

Abbreviations: CR, complete response; GM-CSF, granulocyte-macrophage colony-stimulating factor; ID, intradermally; IN, intranodally; KLH, keyhole limpet hemocyanin; MR, mixed response; NED, no evidence of disease; NA, not applicable; PR, partial response; SC, subcutaneous; SD, stable disease.

co-stimulatory molecules and proinflammatory cytokines. The induced immune response protects 90% of vaccinated mice from subsequent tumor challenge and leads to complete regression of established tumors in 60% of the treated animals.

An alternative to unformulated mRNA administration via needle injection is the particle-mediated epidermal delivery of mRNA using a gene gun. Herein, the mRNA is precipitated onto microscopic gold particles which are forced to penetrate the skin by a high-pressure helium flow, and readily deliver the mRNA to the cytosol and nuclei of epidermal cells, including resident APCs. mRNA delivered by gene gun bombardment gets efficiently translated and induces both specific humoral and cellular immunity against the encoded protein (58). Moreover, mice immunized with mRNA encoding the melanoma self antigen TRP-2 fused to enhanced green fluorescent protein are protected against experimentally induced B16 melanoma lung metastasis (58). Although most immunotherapeutic studies thus far focused on gene gun-mediated delivery of antigen-encoding plasmid DNA, mRNA-based vaccination is a viable alternative. It is likely that a number of optimization methods that have been successfully integrated into particle-mediated DNA-based vaccination regimes will be adapted to improve the efficacy of gene gun-mediated mRNA immunizations in the near future.

Besides naked mRNA immunizations, mRNA has been complexed with cationic liposomes or cationic polymers to increase the stability of the nucleic acid and induce an immune response. Mice immunized with OVA mRNA entrapped in liposomes are protected from challenge with OVA-expressing murine melanoma cells. In addition, as little as 1 µg of liposome-encapsulated mRNA is sufficient to induce detectable CTL and can be further increased by co-encapsulation of GM-CSF-encoding mRNA (59). Cationic polymers, such as the arginine-rich protein protamine, form stable complexes with RNA and have been used to protect antigen-encoding mRNA from degradation by serum nucleases (55). Immunization of mice with either protamine-complexed mRNA alone or mRNA encapsulated into liposomes leads to the induction of antigen-specific CTL and reactive IgG antibodies. The use of the mRNA–protamine complex has two opposing effects on the efficacy of the induced immune response. First, the complexed mRNA is protected from nuclease-mediated degradation and acts as a potent danger signal via recognition by TLR7 upon uptake into endosomal compartments of the cell. TLR7 signaling leads to mRNA sequence-independent activation of innate immunity, which is characterized by the activation of several blood cells including APCs and the secretion of proinflammatory cytokines. Second, even though the stimulation of innate immunity acts as a potent adjuvant, the translation efficacy of protamine-complexed mRNA is strongly reduced, thereby impairing the antigen-specificity of the vaccine (60). Recent work solved this problem by vaccination with a mixture of protamine-complexed mRNA and uncomplexed mRNA to ensure both unspecific mRNA-mediated activation of the innate immunity and induction of a potent humoral and cellular immunity specific to the mRNA-encoded antigen (61). This dual vaccine showed promising results in a preclinical tumor model that evaluated both prophylactic and therapeutic murine tumor challenge and may provide a basis for future clinic trials in humans.

To date, a few clinical trials have been carried out with RNA injected in vivo and they are summarized in Table 16.3. These studies demonstrated some immune response induction, but clinical responses were not observed. One of the factors attributed to the lack of clinical response was the role of immunosuppressive cells. On the other hand, some of the studies described above have demonstrated a significant therapeutic effect in murine tumor models and, therefore, these improvised strategies, combined with immune-stimulating mechanisms and inhibition of immune-suppressive mechanisms, would be a critical next step in the advancement of RNA vaccine clinical trials.

SUMMARY

The objective for which the RNA vaccine research is moving forward is clear: identify a vaccine that translates to clinical benefit. As our understanding of immune response mechanisms and the counteracting immune suppression continues to evolve, so will vaccine design efforts.

In clinical trials, new paradigms are constantly being tested to determine if there is any improvement in clinical benefit. A number of clinical trials currently underway are utilizing a multi-pronged vaccine approach, such as modulating T_{REG} function or eliminating T_{REGS} to enhance vaccine-mediated immunity, based on compelling evidence in pre-clinical animal models. One remains hopeful that these strategies, combined with RNA vaccination, will ultimately result in a successful vaccine for cancer.

REFERENCES

1. Fishman M, Adler FL. Antibody formation initiated in vitro. II. Antibody synthesis in x-irradiated recipients of diffusion chambers containing nucleic acid derived from macrophages incubated with antigen. J Exp Med 1963; 117: 595–602.
2. Pilch YH, Ramming KP. Transfer of tumor immunity with ribonucleic acid. Cancer 1970; 26: 630–7.
3. Boczkowski D, Nair S. RNA as performance-enhancers for dendritic cells. Expert Opin Biol Ther 2010; 10: 563–74.
4. Bringmann A, Held SA, Heine A, Brossart P. RNA vaccines in cancer treatment. J Biomed Biotechnol 2010; 2010: 623687. Published online June 1 2010.
5. Gilboa E, Vieweg J. Cancer immunotherapy with mRNA-transfected dendritic cells. Immunol Rev 2004; 199: 251–63.
6. Pascolo S. Vaccination with messenger RNA (mRNA). Handb Exp Pharmacol 2008; 183: 221–35.
7. Van Tendeloo VF, Ponsaerts P, Lardon F, et al. Highly efficient gene delivery by mRNA electroporation in human hematopoietic cells: superiority to lipofection and passive pulsing of mRNA and to electroporation of plasmid cDNA for tumor antigen loading of dendritic cells. Blood 2001; 98: 49–56.
8. Strobel I, Berchtold S, Gotze A, et al. Human dendritic cells transfected with either RNA or DNA encoding influenza matrix protein M1 differ in their ability to stimulate cytotoxic T lymphocytes. Gene Ther 2000; 7: 2028–35.
9. Boczkowski D, Nair SK, Nam JH, Lyerly HK, Gilboa E. Induction of tumor immunity and cytotoxic T lymphocyte responses using dendritic cells transfected with messenger RNA amplified from tumor cells. Cancer Res 2000; 60: 1028–34.
10. Heiser A, Maurice MA, Yancey DR, et al. Induction of polyclonal prostate cancer-specific CTL using dendritic cells transfected with amplified tumor RNA. J Immunol 2001; 166: 2953–60.
11. Grunebach F, Muller MR, Nencioni A, Brossart P. Delivery of tumor-derived RNA for the induction of cytotoxic T-lymphocytes. Gene Ther 2003; 10: 367–74.
12. Boczkowski D, Nair SK, Snyder D, Gilboa E. Dendritic cells pulsed with RNA are potent antigen-presenting cells in vitro and in vivo. J Exp Med 1996; 184: 465–72.
13. Nair SK, Boczkowski D, Morse M, et al. Induction of primary carcinoembryonic antigen (CEA)-specific cytotoxic T lymphocytes in vitro using human dendritic cells transfected with RNA. Nat Biotechnol 1998; 16: 364–9.
14. Heiser A, Maurice MA, Yancey DR, et al. Human dendritic cells transfected with renal tumor RNA stimulate polyclonal T-cell responses against antigens expressed by primary and metastatic tumors. Cancer Res 2001; 61: 3388–93.
15. Nair SK, Heiser A, Boczkowski D, et al. Induction of cytotoxic T cell responses and tumor immunity against unrelated tumors using telomerase reverse transcriptase RNA transfected dendritic cells. Nat Med 2000; 6: 1011–17.
16. Zeis M, Siegel S, Wagner A, et al. Generation of cytotoxic responses in mice and human individuals against hematological malignancies using survivin-RNA-transfected dendritic cells. J Immunol 2003; 170: 5391–7.
17. Nair S, Boczkowski D, Moeller B, et al. Synergy between tumor immunotherapy and antiangiogenic therapy. Blood 2003; 102: 964–71.
18. Lee J, Fassnacht M, Nair S, Boczkowski D, Gilboa E. Tumor immunotherapy targeting fibroblast activation protein, a product expressed in tumor-associated fibroblasts. Cancer Res 2005; 65: 11156–63.
19. Dorrie J, Schaft N, Muller I, et al. Introduction of functional chimeric E/L-selectin by RNA electroporation to target dendritic cells from blood to lymph nodes. Cancer Immunol Immunother 2008; 57: 467–77.
20. Minkis K, Kavanagh DG, Alter G, et al. Type 2 Bias of T cells expanded from the blood of melanoma patients switched to type 1 by IL-12p70 mRNA-transfected dendritic cells. Cancer Res 2008; 68: 9441–50.

21. Bontkes HJ, Kramer D, Ruizendaal JJ, Meijer CJ, Hooijberg E. Tumor associated antigen and interleukin-12 mRNA transfected dendritic cells enhance effector function of natural killer cells and antigen specific T-cells. Clin Immunol 2008; 127: 375–84.

22. Tcherepanova IY, Adams MD, Feng X, et al. Ectopic expression of a truncated CD40L protein from synthetic post-transcriptionally capped RNA in dendritic cells induces high levels of IL-12 secretion. BMC Mol Biol 2008; 9: 90. Published online 17 October 2008.

23. Cisco RM, Abdel-Wahab Z, Dannull J, et al. Induction of human dendritic cell maturation using transfection with RNA encoding a dominant positive toll-like receptor 4. J Immunol 2004; 172: 7162–8.

24. Abdel-Wahab Z, Cisco R, Dannull J, et al. Cotransfection of DC with TLR4 and MART-1 RNA induces MART-1-specific responses. J Surg Res 2005; 124: 264–73.

25. Bonehill A, Tuyaerts S, Van Nuffel AM, et al. Enhancing the T-cell stimulatory capacity of human dendritic cells by co-electroporation with CD40L, CD70 and constitutively active TLR4 encoding mRNA. Mol Ther 2008; 16: 1170–80.

26. Dannull J, Nair S, Su Z, et al. Enhancing the immunostimulatory function of dendritic cells by transfection with mRNA encoding OX40 ligand. Blood 2005; 105: 3206–13.

27. Grunebach F, Kayser K, Weck MM, et al. Cotransfection of dendritic cells with RNA coding for HER-2/neu and 4-1BBL increases the induction of tumor antigen specific cytotoxic T lymphocytes. Cancer Gene Ther 2005; 12: 749–56.

28. Boczkowski D, Lee J, Pruitt S, Nair S. Dendritic cells engineered to secrete anti-GITR antibodies are effective adjuvants to dendritic cell-based immunotherapy. Cancer Gene Ther 2009; 16: 900–11.

29. Rains N, Cannan RJ, Chen W, Stubbs RS. Development of a dendritic cell (DC)-based vaccine for patients with advanced colorectal cancer. Hepatogastroenterology 2001; 48: 347–51.

30. Heiser A, Coleman D, Dannull J, et al. Autologous dendritic cells transfected with prostate-specific antigen RNA stimulate CTL responses against metastatic prostate tumors. J Clin Invest 2002; 109: 409–17.

31. Nair SK, Morse M, Boczkowski D, et al. Induction of tumor-specific cytotoxic T lymphocytes in cancer patients by autologous tumor RNA-transfected dendritic cells. Ann Surg 2002; 235: 540–9.

32. Morse MA, Nair SK, Boczkowski D, et al. The feasibility and safety of immunotherapy with dendritic cells loaded with CEA mRNA following neoadjuvant chemoradiotherapy and resection of pancreatic cancer. Int J Gastrointest Cancer 2002; 32: 1–6.

33. Morse MA, Nair SK, Mosca PJ, et al. Immunotherapy with autologous, human dendritic cells transfected with carcinoembryonic antigen mRNA. Cancer Invest 2003; 21: 341–9.

34. Su Z, Dannull J, Heiser A, et al. Immunological and clinical responses in metastatic renal cancer patients vaccinated with tumor RNA-transfected dendritic cells. Cancer Res 2003; 63: 2127–33.

35. Caruso DA, Orme LM, Neale AM, et al. Results of a phase 1 study utilizing monocyte-derived dendritic cells pulsed with tumor RNA in children and young adults with brain cancer. Neuro Oncol 2004; 6: 236–46.

36. Caruso DA, Orme LM, Amor GM, et al. Results of a Phase I study utilizing monocyte-derived dendritic cells pulsed with tumor RNA in children with Stage 4 neuroblastoma. Cancer 2005; 103: 1280–91.

37. Dannull J, Su Z, Rizzieri D, et al. Enhancement of vaccine-mediated antitumor immunity in cancer patients after depletion of regulatory T cells. J Clin Invest 2005; 115: 3623–33.

38. Su Z, Dannull J, Yang BK, et al. Telomerase mRNA-transfected dendritic cells stimulate antigen-specific CD8+ and CD4+ T cell responses in patients with metastatic prostate cancer. J Immunol 2005; 174: 3798–807.

39. Mu LJ, Kyte JA, Kvalheim G, et al. Immunotherapy with allotumour mRNA-transfected dendritic cells in androgen-resistant prostate cancer patients. Br J Cancer 2005; 93: 749–56.

40. Kyte JA, Kvalheim G, Aamdal S, Saeboe-Larssen S, Gaudernack G. Preclinical full-scale evaluation of dendritic cells transfected with autologous tumor-mRNA for melanoma vaccination. Cancer Gene Ther 2005; 12: 579–91.

41. Hernando JJ, Park TW, Fischer HP, et al. Vaccination with dendritic cells transfected with mRNA-encoded folate-receptor-alpha for relapsed metastatic ovarian cancer. Lancet Oncol 2007; 8: 451–4.

42. Bonehill A, Van Nuffel AM, Corthals J, et al. Single-step antigen loading and activation of dendritic cells by mRNA electroporation for the purpose of therapeutic vaccination in melanoma patients. Clin Cancer Res 2009; 15: 3366–75.

43. Schuurhuis DH, Verdijk P, Schreibelt G, et al. In situ expression of tumor antigens by messenger RNA-electroporated dendritic cells in lymph nodes of melanoma patients. Cancer Res 2009; 69: 2927–34.

44. Van Tendeloo VF, Van de Velde A, Van Driessche A, et al. Induction of complete and molecular remissions in acute myeloid leukemia by Wilms' tumor 1 antigen-targeted dendritic cell vaccination. Proc Natl Acad Sci USA 2010; 107: 13824–9.

45. Coosemans A, Wolfl M, Berneman ZN, et al. Immunological response after therapeutic vaccination with WT1 mRNA-loaded dendritic cells in end-stage endometrial carcinoma. Anticancer Res 2010; 30: 3709–14.
46. Markovic SN, Dietz AB, Greiner CW, et al. Preparing clinical-grade myeloid dendritic cells by electroporation-mediated transfection of in vitro amplified tumor-derived mRNA and safety testing in stage IV malignant melanoma. J Transl Med 2006; 4: 35. Published online 15 August 2006.
47. Wolff JA, Malone RW, Williams P, et al. Direct gene transfer into mouse muscle in vivo. Science 1990; 247: 1465–8.
48. Stepinski J, Waddell C, Stolarski R, Darzynkiewicz E, Rhoads RE. Synthesis and properties of mRNAs containing the novel "anti-reverse" cap analogs 7-methyl(3'-O-methyl)GpppG and 7-methyl (3'-deoxy)GpppG. RNA 2001; 7: 1486–95.
49. Mockey M, Goncalves C, Dupuy FP, et al. mRNA transfection of dendritic cells: synergistic effect of ARCA mRNA capping with Poly(A) chains in cis and in trans for a high protein expression level. Biochem Biophys Res Commun 2006; 340: 1062–8.
50. Kuhn AN, Diken M, Kreiter S, et al. Phosphorothioate cap analogs increase stability and translational efficiency of RNA vaccines in immature dendritic cells and induce superior immune responses in vivo. Gene Ther 2010; 17: 961–71.
51. Holtkamp S, Kreiter S, Selmi A, et al. Modification of antigen-encoding RNA increases stability, translational efficacy, and T-cell stimulatory capacity of dendritic cells. Blood 2006; 108: 4009–17.
52. Kariko K, Muramatsu H, Welsh FA, et al. Incorporation of pseudouridine into mRNA yields superior nonimmunogenic vector with increased translational capacity and biological stability. Mol Ther 2008; 16: 1833–40.
53. Conry RM, LoBuglio AF, Wright M, et al. Characterization of a messenger RNA polynucleotide vaccine vector. Cancer Res 1995; 55: 1397–400.
54. Granstein RD, Ding W, Ozawa H. Induction of anti-tumor immunity with epidermal cells pulsed with tumor-derived RNA or intradermal administration of RNA. J Invest Dermatol 2000; 114: 632–6.
55. Hoerr I, Obst R, Rammensee HG, Jung G. In vivo application of RNA leads to induction of specific cytotoxic T lymphocytes and antibodies. Eur J Immunol 2000; 30: 1–7.
56. Carralot JP, Probst J, Hoerr I, et al. Polarization of immunity induced by direct injection of naked sequence-stabilized mRNA vaccines. Cell Mol Life Sci 2004; 61: 2418–24.
57. Kreiter S, Selmi A, Diken M, et al. Intranodal vaccination with naked antigen-encoding RNA elicits potent prophylactic and therapeutic antitumoral immunity. Cancer Res 2010; 70: 9031–40.
58. Steitz J, Britten CM, Wolfel T, Tuting T. Effective induction of anti-melanoma immunity following genetic vaccination with synthetic mRNA coding for the fusion protein EGFP.TRP2. Cancer Immunol Immunother 2006; 55: 246–53.
59. Hess PR, Boczkowski D, Nair SK, Snyder D, Gilboa E. Vaccination with mRNAs encoding tumor-associated antigens and granulocyte-macrophage colony-stimulating factor efficiently primes CTL responses, but is insufficient to overcome tolerance to a model tumor/self antigen. Cancer Immunol Immunother 2006; 55: 672–83.
60. Scheel B, Braedel S, Probst J, et al. Immunostimulating capacities of stabilized RNA molecules. Eur J Immunol 2004; 34: 537–47.
61. Fotin-Mleczek M, Duchardt KM, Lorenz C, et al. Messenger RNA-based vaccines with dual activity induce balanced TLR-7 dependent adaptive immune responses and provide antitumor activity. J Immunother 2011; 34: 1–15.
62. Weide B, Carralot JP, Reese A, et al. Results of the first phase I/II clinical vaccination trial with direct injection of mRNA. J Immunother 2008; 31: 180–8.
63. Weide B, Pascolo S, Scheel B, et al. Direct injection of protamine-protected mRNA: results of a phase 1/2 vaccination trial in metastatic melanoma patients. J Immunother 2009; 32: 498–507.
64. Rittig SM, Haentschel M, Weimer KJ, et al. Intradermal vaccinations with RNA coding for TAA generate CD8(+) and CD4(+) immune responses and induce clinical benefit in vaccinated patients. Mol Ther 2010. [Epub ahead of print].

17 | Induction of innate immunity by nucleic acids: A potential adjuvant for cancer vaccines?

Bo Jin and Anthony E. T. Yeo

SIGNIFICANT EFFECTS OF ADJUVANTS IN VACCINE IMMUNIZATION

A vaccine adjuvant should boost the potency and/or the longevity of specific immune response to antigens as seen by a reduction in the antigen dosage used and/or the number of immunizations. An adjuvant also should be associated with minimal or no toxicity (1). In attenuated live vaccines where adjuvants are not used, foreign antigens using pathogen-associated molecular patterns activate pattern recognition receptors (PRRs) inducing both innate immunity and adaptive immunity. With newer vaccines that use highly characterized recombinant antigens, a diminished ability to induce immune protection is present unless an adjuvant is used (2). For certain diseases such as cancer, the immune response induced by protein- or peptide-based vaccine (i.e., the type-2 T helper (Th2) cell response) needs to be complemented by a Th1-biased, antigen-specific cytotoxic T lymphocyte (CTL) response. Hence, an adjuvant should induce both antigen-specific Th1 and CTL responses (2,3) (Fig. 17.1).

Adaptive immunity significantly depends on the innate immunity that arises through the activation of dendritic cells (DCs), that is, antigen-presenting cells (APCs). DCs, through germ-line encoded PRRs, recognize molecular patterns present in microorganisms, and can direct a response which includes determining the magnitude, duration, polarity of the response for example toward Th1-, Th2-, or Th17-biased response, and the production of long-term memory (4). Therefore, PRR agonists can be used as adjuvants. One canonical family of PRRs is toll-like receptors (TLRs) (4,5).

THE TLR FAMILY

TLRs can be classified as cell surface TLRs or intracellular TLRs. The TLRs and the corresponding ligands are summarized in Table 17.1. TLRs on cell surface mainly recognize molecules on the surface of the pathogenic microorganisms while those localized intracellularly sense nucleic acids which are released by intracellular degradation of the invading pathogen (11).

Intracellular TLRs can only be activated after being transported from the endoplasmic reticulum (ER) to endolysosomes (11). UNC93B1 is specifically involved in the complex trafficking of nucleotide-sensing TLRs (12). Upon binding ligands, TLRs form homodimer or heterodimer units and recruit adaptor molecules. Four adaptor molecules have been characterized: myeloid differentiation protein 88 (MyD88) (13), Toll/IL-1 receptor (TIR) domain-containing adapter protein (TIRAP)/MyD88-adapter-like (Mal) (14), TIR domain-containing adaptor inducing interferon-β (TRIF)/TIR domain containing adaptor molecule-1 (TICAM-1) (15), and TRIF-related adaptor molecule (16). MyD88 is the essential adaptor for all the TLRs except TLR3. Upon ligand recognition, TLR recruits MyD88 to its cytoplasmic TIR domain by its association with the TIR domain of the adaptor molecule (Fig. 17.2A). Through a series of signals, translocation of the nuclear factor-κB (NF-κB) to the nucleus induces the transcription of proinflammatory cytokines.

TRIF is the sole adaptor of TLR3 and adjunctive adaptor of TLR4 (Fig. 17.2B). After sensing double-stranded RNA (dsRNA), the TIR domain of TLR3 associates TRIF TIR and then TRIF interacts with receptor-interacting protein 1 (RIP1) through the RIP homotypic interaction motif. The tumor necrosis factor (TNF) associated factor-6 (TRAF6) is also recruited to the N-terminal domain of TRIF and through a series of various signals stimulates proinflammatory cytokine production (6). TRIF also associates its adaptor protein NF-κB activating kinase (NAK)-associated protein 1 (NAP1) to activate TRAF family member-associated NF-κB activator-binding kinase 1 (TBK1) and IκB kinase-related kinase ε (IKKε) resulting in the phosphorylation and nuclear translocation of interferon regulatory factor 3 (IRF3), which induces

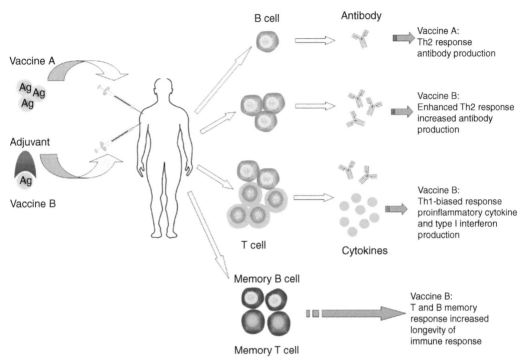

Figure 17.1 Effects of vaccine adjuvant. Protein or polypeptide antigen in Vaccine A can induce a Th2- biased response and antibody production. Using an adjuvant (Vaccine B) can improve the efficacy by reducing the antigen dosage and/or the number of immunizations and/or increase antibody production. An adjuvant can also promote long memory in B and/or T cells. Some adjuvants can qualitatively alter the induction mix of Th1-biased and antigen-specific cytotoxic T lymphocyte responses. *Abbreviation*: Th, T helper cell.

the expression of interferon beta (IFN–β) (17). TRAF3 combines with the TBK1/IKKε complex and is also involved in the TRIF-mediated IRF3 activation (18). TRIF also interacts with Fas-associated cell death domain (FADD) protein through RIP1 which in turn activates procaspase-8 to initiate the cell apoptosis (19). Recently, a TIR-less splice variant of TRIF (designated as TRIS) was found capable of activating IRF3 through the interaction with TBK1 and stimulates NF-κB via RIP1 (20).

PARADIGMS REGARDING THE ADJUVANTICITY OF NUCLEIC ACIDS FOR CANCER VACCINES

Cross-priming is the process whereby DCs and macrophages, using PRRs, sense malignantly transformed cells to activate Th1 and/or CTL cells. Cancer cells express antigens that are not expressed or are found only in trace amounts in healthy hosts and are referred to as tumor-associated antigens (TAAs). In order to immunologically control such cells, adaptive immunity is essential (21). Indeed, the prognosis of cancer patients is largely determined by the recruitment of tumor infiltrating lymphocytes, especially CD8[+] T cells (22,23). In the usual clinical situation, host immunity is weak or anergic due to either the weak antigenicity of TAAs or due to the presence of immune suppression. Therefore, enhancing the TAA-specific CTL response and overcoming immune suppression by targeting TLRs, has attracted a significant amount of research (24).

Application of TLR agonists in cancer therapy dates back to 1891 when patients with cancer were treated with Streptococci. Later the mixture was altered to heat-killed *Streptococcus pyogenes*

Table 17.1 TLR Ligands and Potential Vaccine Adjuvant Candidates (1,6,7–10)

Receptor	Exogenous Ligands	Endogenous Ligands	Vaccine Adjuvant Candidate	Location	Type of Immune Response
TLR1/TLR2	Triacyl lipopeptide	–	Pam₃Cys	Cell surface	Th1, antibody, NK
TLR2	Peptidoglycan Lipoprotein/Lipopeptide Lipoteichoic acid Glycoinositol phospholipids Atypical lipopolysaccharides Porins Zymosan	Gp96 Hsp60, 70, 96 Hyaluronic acid HMGB1	–	Cell surface	Th1, antibody, NK
TLR2/TLR6	Diacryl lipopeptide Peptidoglycan Zymosan Lipoproteins	–	Pam₂Cys MALP-2	Cell surface	Th1, antibody, NK
TLR3	dsRNA	Self dsRNA Stathmin	Poly(I:C) Poly(ICLC) Poly(I:C12U) PIKA Poly(A:U)	Endosome	NK, Th1, CTL, antibody
TLR4	Lipopolysaccharide Zymosan Viral fusion protein Viral envelope protein Pertussis toxin Toxol Hyphae Glycoinositolphospholipids	GP96 Hsp22, 60, 70, 96 Hyaluronic acid Heparan sulfate Fibrinogen Fibronectin Surfactant-protein A, D HMGB1β-defensin α-A Crystallin	MPLA (MPL®) AS02 (MPL+saponin QS-21) AS04 (MPL+alum) RC-529 (MPL derivative)	Cell surface	Strong Th1, antibody

TLR	Ligand	Endogenous ligand	Agonist	Location	Response
TLR5	Flagellin	–	Flagellin	Cell surface	Th1, CTL, antibody
TLR7	ssRNA	Endogenous RNA	ssRNA, Imidazoquinolines (e.g., resiquimod, imiquimod), Bropyrimine, Adenosine derivatives, Guanosine derivatives (e.g., loxoribine), Poly(A:U)	Endosome	Strong Th1, CTL
TLR8	ssRNA	Endogenous RNA	ssRNA, Imidazoquinolines (e.g. Resiquimod), Adenosine derivatives, Guanosine derivatives	Endosome	Strong Th1, CTL
TLR9	CpG DNA, Hemozoin	Endogenous DNA, Chromatin immune complex	CpG-ODN	Endosome	Strong Th1, CTL, antibody, NK
TLR10	Pam$_3$CSK$_4$? PamCysPamSK4?	–	–	Cell surface	–
TLR11	Uropathogenic bacteria, Protozoan profilin	–	–	Cell surface	Th1

Abbreviations: AS, Adjuvant System® (GlaxoSmithKline Biologicals, Rixensart, Belgium), a biological tool comprising more than one adjuvant, developed by GSK Biologicals; CpG, unmethylated cytosine-phosphate-guanine motif; CTL, cytotoxic T lymphocyte; dsRNA, double-stranded RNA; HMGB1, high mobility group box 1; Hsp, heat shock protein; MALP-2, macrophage-activating lipoprotein-2; MPL, Corixa Corporation, Hamilton, MT), monophosphoryl lipid A; NK, natural killer cell; ODN, oligodeoxynucleotide; PIKA, a stabilized dsRNA; poly(A:U), polyadenylic:polyuridylic acid; poly(I:C), polyriboinosinic:polyribocytidylic acid; poly(I:C12U), polyriboinosinic:polyribocytidylic acid; poly(I:C12U), cytosine replaced by uracil at every 13th cytosine of poly(I:C); poly(ICLC), poly(I:C) with poly-L-lysine and carboxymethylcellulose; ssRNA, single-stranded RNA; Th1, type-1 T helper cell; TLR, Toll-like receptor.

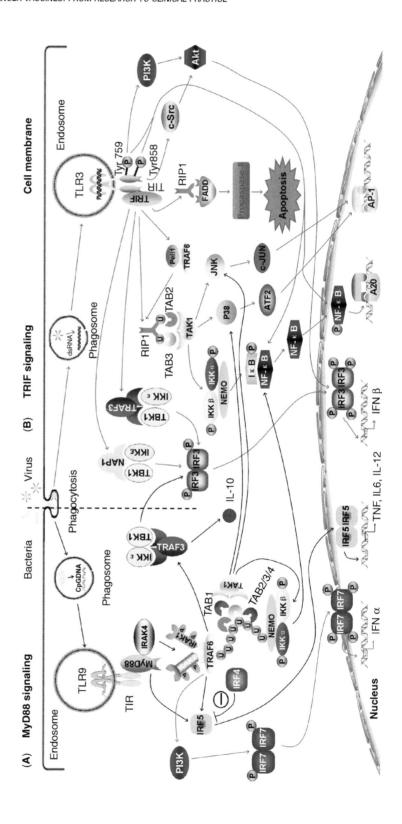

Figure 17.2 Intracellular TLR signal pathway. Conventional murine dendritic cells take up viruses or bacteria into cytoplasm by phagocytosis. The phagosomes fuse with late endosomes or lysosomes where the viruses or bacteria are broken down to release viral dsRNA or bacterial CpG DNA that are recognized by intracellular TLR3 or TLR9 respectively. (**A**): CpG DNA signaling through TLR9. TLR9 recognizes bacterial CpG DNA or synthetic unmethylated CpG-ODN and recruits MyD88 via its cytoplasmic TIR domain. MyD88 associates IRAK4 through the interaction of their DD. Then IRAK4 phosphorylates IRAK1 and IRAK2 and activates TRAF6. TRAF6 induces the synthesis of polyubiquitin chains that link TRAF6, NEMO, IRAK1, TAB2, TAB3, and TAB4. The ubiquitination of TAB2/3/4 in association with TAB1 activates TAK1. This induces phosphorylation of IKK complex resulting in the dissociation of IκB and NF-κB. NF-κB then translocates into nucleus to induce the transcription of proinflammatory cytokines. The TAK1 also activates JNK and p38 which induces AP1 activation. MyD88 and TRAF6 both activate IRF5 and induce proinflammatory cytokines. This activation is inhibited by IRF4. TRAF6 also interacts with TRAF3 and then recruits TBK1 to activate IRF3 and IFNβ production. TRAF3 alternatively induces the anti-inflammatory cytokine IL-10. In humans, TLR9 is present in plasmacytoid dendritic cells and absent in myeloid dendritic cells. A signaling pathway through MyD88 activates PI3K promoting the nuclear translocation of IRF7 and induces a significant IFNα production (indicated by pink arrow). (**B**): dsRNA signaling through TLR3. dsRNA that is internalized in endosome binds to TLR3. TLR3 possesses two dsRNA binding sites near the N-terminus and C-terminus, respectively. When combined with dsRNA, a sole dsRNA molecule associates two TLR3 molecules through four dsRNA binding sites in an "m" shape. TLR3 TIR domain combines with the TIR domain of TRIF. The interaction of TRIF with RIP1 or TRAF6 and Peli1 results in polyubiquitination of RIP1, the latter binds ubiquitin receptors TAB2 and TAB3 which activates TAK1. Activated TAK1 induces phosphorylation of IKK complex composed of IKKα, IKKβ, and NEMO, leading to phosphorylation and degradation of IκB. This results in the release and nuclear translocation of NF-κB to activate the specific gene promoter A20. TAK1 also acts with JNK and p38 which activates c-JUN and ATF2. This triggers the AP-1 transcription factors' family. TRIF acting through NAP1 also activates TBK1 and IKKε. This induces phosphorylation and nuclear translocation of IRF3 culminating in IFNβ production. TRAF3 binds with the TBK1–IKKε complex inducing IRF3 activation. Combination of TRIF results in the phosphorylation of Tyr759 and Tyr858 in the TLR3 TIR domain which subsequently induces the phosphorylation of, and degradation of IκB leading to NF-κB release. Phosphorylated Tyr759 recruits PI3K and activates kinase Akt for full phosphorylation and activation of IRF3 in the nucleus. Tyrosine kinase c-Src also plays a role in Akt activation. A unique feature of TRIF signaling is that it interacts with FADD through RIP1 and activates procaspase-8 to initiate cell apoptosis. *Abbreviations:* AP-1, activator protein-1; ATF2, activating transcription factor 2; CpG, unmethylated cytosine-phosphate-guanine motif; DD, death domain; dsRNA, double-stranded RNA; FADD, Fas-associated cell death domain; IFN, interferon; IKK, IκB kinase-related kinase; IRAK, interleukin-1 receptor-associated kinase; IRF, interferon regulatory factor; JNK, c-Jun N-terminal kinase; MyD88, myeloid differentiation protein 88; NAP, NF-κB activating kinase-associated protein; NEMO, NF-κB essential modulator; NF-κB, nuclear factor-κB; PI3K, phosphatidylinositol 3-kinase; RIP, receptor-interacting protein; TAB, TAK1-binding protein; TAK, transforming growth factor α-activated kinase; TBK, TRAF family member-associated NF-κB activator-binding kinase; TIR, Toll/IL-1 receptor; TLR, Toll-like receptor; TRAF, tumor necrosis factor receptor associated factor; TRIF, TIR domain-containing adaptor inducing interferon-β.

and *Serratia marcescens* with the main components of lipopolysaccharides and bacterial DNA products. When TLRs were finally discovered in the 1990s, the mechanism of action being mediated by TLR4 and TLR9 signaling was elucidated. Induction of the TLR4 and TLR9 signaling pathways leads to cytokine production and activation of natural killer (NK) and CTL cells (25).

Endosomal nucleic acid-sensing TLRs, such as TLR3, TLR7, TLR8, and TLR9, are specific for cancer (25). Activation of TLR3 on cancer cells by dsRNA elicits either an IFN-mediated response or a cellular apoptosis (25,26). Apoptosis releases copious amounts of TAAs that can be processed by DCs. These are then presented to Th1 cells and CTLs by DCs with the help of cytokines from the TRIF signaling pathway resulting in a long-term immune response. The classical dsRNA analog, polyriboinosinic:polyribocytidylic acid [poly(I:C)], an IFN inducer, has been clinically tested and systemic toxicity restricts its clinical utility (27). Poly(I:C12U) is derived from poly(I:C) with substitution of every 13th cytosine (C) with uracil (U). It is more easily degraded and demonstrates less toxicity than poly(I:C). Poly(I:C12U) is capable of inducing the maturation of monocyte-derived DCs and the production of proinflammatory cytokines in animal models. Even in the presence of immunosuppressive cytokines in cancer patients, a response is still elicited (28). $CD8^+$ T cells from the ascites of ovarian cancer can lyse autologous cancer cells when co-cultured with DCs primed with tumor lysate and stimulated with poly(I:C12U) (29). Poly(ICLC) is poly(I:C) complexed with poly-L-lysine and carboxymethyl cellulose and is more stable against hydrolysis by ribonucleotidase (30). In a murine glioma model, subcutaneous injections of synthetic peptides encoding CTL epitopes with intramuscular injections of poly(ICLC) induced a robust transcription of C-X-C motif chemokine 10 (CXCL10) in the tumor and efficient targeting of brain sites by antigen-specific type-1 CTL. This activity can be abrogated by a monoclonal antibody against CXCL10, the absence of IFNα receptor 1, or the absence of IFNγ (31). In a phase I/II clinical trial of patients with recurrent malignant gliomas using α-1 polarized DCs loaded with synthetic peptides for glioma associated antigen epitopes, co-administered with poly(ICLC), 58% of patients had positive responses. A sustained complete response was seen in one patient, while 12-months progression-free survival was achieved in 41% of patients (32). It was also shown to improve efficacy of radiotherapy or chemo-radiotherapy in patients with gliomas (33). Polyadenylic:polyuridylic acid [poly(A:U)], another type of synthetic dsRNA analog, engages human TLR3 but not retinoic acid-inducible gene-I (RIG-I)-like receptors (RLRs) and therefore is less efficient in NK cell activation (34). Additionally, it can induce type-I IFN through TLR7 in plasmacytoid DCs (pDCs). Poly(A:U) induces Th1 cell generation and antibody production in mice when co-administered with protein antigen (35). In vivo targeted delivery of tumor-associated epitope to APCs in conjunction with poly(A:U) results in control of tumor growth, establishment of immune memory, and protection against antigenic variants (36).

TLR7 and TLR8 that can sense viral single-stranded RNA (ssRNA) activates NF-κB through the MyD88 signal pathway in myeloid DCs (mDCs) and IRF7 to produce IFNα in pDCs. The adjuvanticity of TLR7 agonists to induce Th1 and CTL responses is mediated by the IFNα produced by pDCs (37). Natural ssRNA and small molecular imidazoquinolines are ligands of TLR7/8 and have been studied extensively. Imiquimod and gardiquimod are human and murine TLR7 ligands respectively and resiquimod is the ligand of human TLR7/8 and murine TLR7. Imiquimod is also capable of triggering Bcl-2- and caspase-dependent proapoptotic activity against tumor cells at higher concentrations of 25–50 μg/ml, 5–10 fold higher than those required for TLR-mediated cytokine induction in DCs (38). TLR7/8 agonists can decrease the regulatory T-cell activity and increase the tumor antigen-specific CTL response simultaneously. Topical resiquimod can enhance the cross-priming of subcutaneously administered protein antigen in mice eliciting an antigen-specific CTL response. Induced CTLs mediate antigen-specific killing in vivo and are effective in vivo against antigen-bearing tumor challenge (39). Imiquimod cream at a 5% concentration (Aldara®, 3M Pharmaceuticals, St. Paul, MN) has been approved for the treatment of a variety of conditions including superficial basal cell cancer and a non-melanotic skin cancer (38). Recent research suggests that mRNA vaccines work by expression of encoded TAA and activation of TLR7 signaling by mRNA, a type of ssRNA (40). This produces TAA-induced antigen-specific Th1 and CTL responses. However, the activation of TLR7/8 in lung cancer cells induces cell survival and chemoresistance. Hence, even though TLR7 or TLR8 agonists are considered adjuvants, the expression of these TLRs in tumor cells should be noted (41).

TLR9 is mainly expressed in human B lymphocytes and pDCs and activated by unmethylated cytosine-phosphate-guanine (CpG) motif-containing microbial DNA or synthetic oligodeoxynucleotides (ODNs) (42). These act on NF-κB to induce production of cytokines or co-stimulatory molecules in human B cells and pDCs. Recruitment of MyD88 is the central event of TLR9 signaling (42). MyD88 is also involved in the production of IFNα in pDCs by activation of IRF7 (Fig. 17.2A) (42,43). The different signaling methods of TLR9 depends on the location of the intracellular compartment where triggering takes place. When TLR9 is triggered in early endosomes, IRF7 is activated to induce IFNα production, while in late endosomes, TLR9 preferentially activates NF-κB to induce maturation of pDCs and to produce proinflammatory cytokines (44). Artificial TLR9 ligands are synthetic CpG-ODNs that have a nuclease-resistant phosphorothioate (PS) backbone for improved stability. This can be divided into three classes. A-class CpG-ODN (also known as D type) is defined by G runs with PS linkages at the 5'- and 3'-ends surrounding a phosphodiester palindromic CpG containing sequence and capable of inducing strong pDC IFNα production. However, its effect on pDC maturation and B cell proliferation is weak (45). B-class CpG-ODN (also known as K type), the most commonly used CpG-ODN in human oncology contains 6-mer CpG motifs with the general formula "purine-pyrimidine-C-G-pyrimidine-pyrimidine" induces strong B-cell response with maturation of human pDC and monocytes (45). C-class CpG-ODN combines the characteristics of the A- and B-classes, induces strong B-cell responses and IFNα production from pDC (46,47). Although TLR9 is not expressed in resting T cells, in mature DCs it can create a Th1-like cytokine milieu resulting in a strong Th1 response (46).

In a study of 19 vaccine adjuvants used with the tumor antigens, MUC1 peptide and GD3 ganglioside, CpG-ODN induced the most Th1-biased immune responses with the highest levels of IFNγ secretion in mice (48). CpG-ODN is also synergistic with other anti-cancer treatments in murine models, for example, with surgery, radiotherapy, chemotherapy, and monoclonal anti-tumor antibodies (46). Unfortunately, human clinical trials have been disappointing (49). In a phase II trial for non-small-cell lung cancer, CpG-ODN showed an increased response rate and improved survival in combination with chemotherapy (50). Yet, in the following phase III trials, no improvement in overall survival or progression-free survival was observed and further studies were discontinued (46). However, a recent phase I trial using a CpG-ODN, IMO-2125, in combination with ribavirin to treat patients with hepatitis C virus infection, revealed a good tolerability to antiviral activity comparable to that obtained from the standard hepatitis C virus therapy (51). Another pilot trial of 15 patients with B-cell lymphoma who received low-dose radiotherapy and CpG-ODN injection at the same site had a single case of a complete response and three partial responses (52). As B-cell lymphoma is TLR9 positive, further research into tumors bearing TLR9 seems logical.

IMMUNOMODULATORY PATHWAYS OF DOUBLE-STRANDED RNA THROUGH TLR3

TLR3 activation recruits TRIF to induce NF-κB activation and IFNβ production. This unique property distinguishes it from other TLR pathways. This target may be valuable as an adjunct to multiple immunotherapy strategies (53).

TLRs are involved in the functioning of DCs. Putatively, upon sensing invading microorganisms, DCs, with the participation of ER, phagocytose the invader. The neutral pH and low proteolytic activity of the early endosome/early phagosome allows the ingested antigen to escape from the endosomal/phagosomal hydrolysis and translocated into cytosol where it is degraded by the cytosolic proteasome. The processed peptides are either imported into the ER through a transporter associated with antigen processing (TAP), trimmed by ER aminopeptidase (ERAP), loaded onto class-I MHC (MHC-I) molecules and then transported extracellularly through Golgi complex for cross-presentation to CD8$^+$ T cells (the cytosolic pathway); or re-imported to endosomes by TAP recruited upon phagocytosis, trimmed by insulin-regulated aminopeptidase, assembled with recycling MHC-I molecules and exported out of DCs for cross-presentation (the vacuolar pathway) (54). Furthermore, a third complementary proteasome-independent vacuolar pathway may exist (55). (Fig. 17.3)

Mature DCs, characterized by enhanced antigen presentation capacity and referred to as APCs, migrate to draining lymph nodes and interact with T and/or B lymphocytes. The

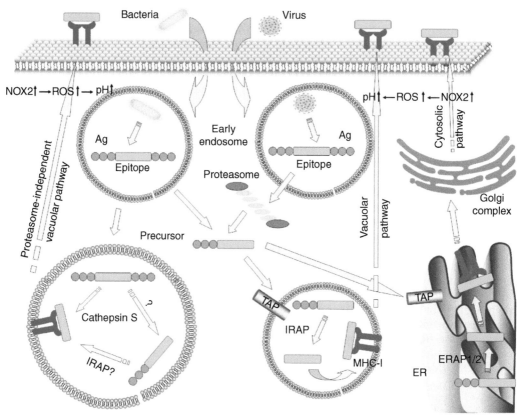

Figure 17.3 Cross-presentation pathway. Activated DCs take up the invading pathogen by phagocytosis into early phagosome. NOX2 is recruited to the early phagosome and endosome inducing generation of reactive oxygen species and H$^+$ consumption. This causes alkalinization of the compartment resulting in a neutral pH in the early phagosome/endosome and thereby establishing a role for a low hydrolysis of antigens and a high pH. In addition, DCs express lower levels of most lysosomal proteases than macrophages. Low proteolysis and high pH prevent the degradation of incoming antigen and MHC-I- restricted epitopes, and possibly load the peptides onto MHC-I molecules in endosome more efficiently. The ingested antigens are then transferred into cytosol to undergo proteolysis by cytosol proteasome. The resulting peptides can be translocated into ER or re-imported into endosome via TAP. The peptides taken into ER are further trimmed by ERAP1/2 turning into mature epitopes with 8–10 residues, loaded on the MHC-I molecules synthesized in the ER and transported to the cell surface through Golgi complex for cross-presentation (the cytosolic pathway). The peptides reimported into an endosome are trimmed by IRAP, assembled with recycling MHC-I molecules and exported out of DCs for cross-presentation (the vacuolar pathway). It is expected that cross-presentation of bacterial antigen is via endosomal pathway and of viral or tumor antigen is through cytosolic pathway. Cathepsin S plays an important role in the generation of epitopes for MHC-I binding in the proteasome-independent vacuolar pathway. The involvement of other proteases like IRAP is possible. *Abbreviations*: DC, dendritic cell; ER, endoplasmic reticulum; ERAP, ER aminopeptidase; IRAP, insulin-regulated aminopeptidase; NOX2, NADPH oxidase; TAP, transporter associated with antigen processing.

lymphocytes are activated by pathogen-derived peptides along with MHC-I molecules (cross-presentation), co-stimulatory molecules including CD80 and CD86, and the instructional signals, interleukin 12p70 (IL-12p70) for Th1, IL-4 for Th2, and IL-6 and IL-23 for Th17 by cross-priming (56) (Fig. 17.3). TLR3 signals affect DC maturation and cross-presentation at different levels. Poly(I:C) is able to induce autophagy in macrophages and this can be inhibited by TRIF short hairpin RNA (57). In poly(I:C) pretreated DCs, the ability of antigen uptake was impaired, suggesting that once the propagation of an endosomal TRIF-dependent signal has been recorded, DCs would ensure the antigen capture has occurred and terminate the subsequent antigen uptake (58). An enhanced efficiency of cross-presentation and of cross-priming was observed when antigen was taken up concurrently with poly(I:C) (59) and TRIF deficiency reduced cross-presentation up to 40% (60). Type-I IFN produced via TLR3 signal pathway plays a major role in the cross-priming of CD8+ T cells by promoting the expression of co-stimulatory molecules of DCs. Upon stimulation by TLR3, mDCs express a TRIF-inducing membrane protein named IRF-3-dependent NK-activating molecule, functional in both mDCs and NK cells and facilitates NK-cell activation (61). Another report suggested that poly(I:C) activates mDCs by co-triggering TLR3 and RLRs, and activates NK cells through RLRs (34). Human DCs stimulated by poly(I:C) terminate the ubiquitination of the MHC-II complex and protect the MHC-II complex from degradation resulting in an increase in MHC-II complex and CD86 (62). However, poly(I:C) with different molecular weights has differential effects on the maturation of DCs (63).

Cross-priming occurs when activated mDCs present antigen epitopes with MHC-II molecules (for CD4+ T cells) or MHC-I molecules (for CD8+ T cells), co-stimulatory molecules and other co-factors to naïve CD4+ or CD8+ T cells. Newly primed CD4+ T cells are programmed by various cytokines and other factors from DCs to differentiate into Th1, Th2, Th17, follicular helper T (Tfh) effector cells, or regulatory T cells (T_{REG}) (64). IL-12 produced from mDCs is the instructional signal that induces expression of the molecules: signal transducer and activator of transcription (STAT) 4, STAT1, and T box expressed in T cells (T-bet) resulting in Th1-cell differentiation. Upon activation, Th1 cells secrete IL-2 and IFNγ that are essential for the proliferation and function of CD8+ CTLs and feedback activation of mDCs (65). Th1 activation is a critical element against intracellular pathogens. IL-4 by activating STAT5 and GATA-binding protein 3 (GATA3) directs naïve CD4+ T cells to differentiate into Th2 cells. IL-4 is also involved in B cell differentiation and antibody production to eliminate extracellular parasites (66). Transforming growth factor (TGF) β stimulates naïve CD4+ T cells to cause Th17 transcription factor retinoic acid receptor related orphan receptor-γt (ROR-γt or ROR-c for human) in the presence of IL-6. Transcription of the IL-17 gene induces Th17 cells to control extracellular bacteria and mediate autoimmunity. Alternatively, TGF-β promoting forkhead box P3 (FoxP3) expression induces T_{REG} (iT_{REG}) cells in the presence of IL-2 (or IL-1β in human) to cause immunosuppression (67). An inappropriate regulation of Th17 activities is associated with chronic inflammation and autoimmunity (68). Primed CD4+ T cells in the presence of IL-6 (mouse) or IL-12 (human) expressing IL-21 and transcriptional repressor B-cell lymphoma 6 (Bcl-6) are able to differentiate into Tfh cells. Tfh cells then promote B cells to differentiate into long-lived plasma cells or memory B cells (69). IL-21 by feedback can cause further Tfh differentiation. When activated DCs cross-present antigen epitope with MHC-I to CD8+ T cells, activated Th1 cells in the presence of TLR ligands secrete IL-2, CC-chemokine ligand 3 (CCL3), CCL4 and CCL5 to recruit DCs for cross-priming by the CD40 ligand (CD40L)-CD40 interaction (70). Antigen-specific CTLs are indispensable in the immunity against intracellular pathogens and cancer. (Fig. 17.4)

dsRNA is capable of inducing robust IL-12p70 production which reduces the threshold of Th1 response and promotes Th1-biased adaptive immunity through the TLR3 and c-Jun N-terminal kinase pathways. Furthermore, the induction of robust type-I IFN production can elicit a Th1 response. This occurs owing to the upregulation of MHC-I and MHC-II, CD40, CD80, CD86, and CD83, which then results in increased chemokine receptor CCR7 expression and thus sensitizes and activates mDCs to CCL19 and CCL21. Consequently, migration of mDCs from peripheral tissues into lymphoid organs occurs (71). Other proinflammatory

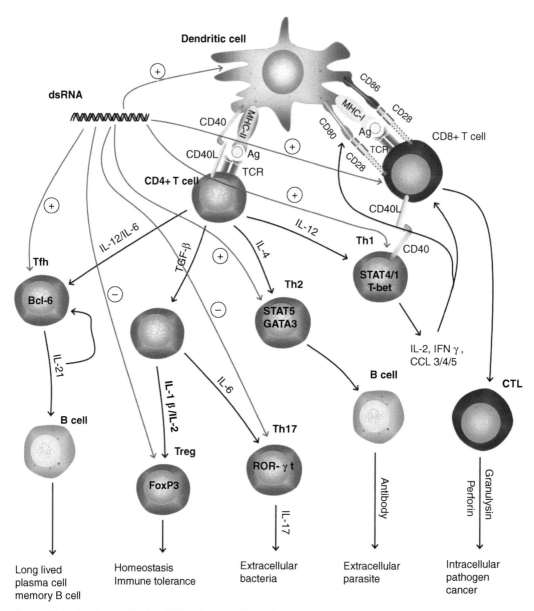

Figure 17.4 Dendritic cell-primed T lymphocytic differentiation. For complete activation of naïve T cells to occur, at least 2 signals need to be present. The first signal would be antigen in a peptide-MHC complex that is presented by APCs. Recognition of this complex would allow TCR to mount a specific response. The second one, the co-stimulatory signal, is also provided by the APCs. This signal engages T cells as well and is a vital part of the development of adaptive immunity. This T-cell co-stimulation is necessary for T-cell proliferation, differentiation, and survival. In the absence of co-stimulation T-cell anergy, deletion or the development of immune tolerance may occur. DCs take up the invading microbes by phagocytosis, process the protein antigen into epitopes, and present to CD4+ T cells on MHC-II molecules or to CD8+ T cells on MHC-I molecules along with co-stimulatory molecules, for example, CD80, CD86, or CD40. CD28 interacts with co-stimulatory molecules CD80 and CD86 located on APCs. The interaction of CD80 and CD86 with CD28, in the context of TCR signaling, expands the population of antigen-stimulated T cells to differentiate into effector and memory cells. Under the instruction from IL-12, the primed CD4+ T cell differentiates into Th1 cell to express STAT4 and STAT 1 and T-bet. In the presence of TLR ligands, the activated Th1 cell secretes IL-2, CCL3, CCL4, and CCL5 which license DCs to cross-prime via CD40L-CD40 interactions. The activated Th1 cell also secrets IFNγ to promote co-stimulatory molecules of DCs. (*Continued*)

cytokines like TNF-α and IL-18 also play important roles in the induction of Th1 response by dsRNA. dsRNA at low concentration (0.1–1 μg/ml) can induce human lymphocytes to express prototypic Th2 cytokine IL-4 (72). In addition, co-administration of dsRNA and protein antigen induces robust Th1-biased immunity and enhanced Th2 immune responses (10). Poly(I:C) through TLR3 can activate mDCs to produce IL-12p70 and IL-27. IL-12p70 activates Th1 cells to produce IFNγ which can inhibit Th17 cell generation and IL-27 inhibits Th17 cell differentiation in a STAT1-dependent manner. Thus, TLR3 agonist induces Th1 responses and dampens Th17 responses whereas TLR2 or dectin stimulation enhances Th17 responses (68,73). Moreover, activation of naïve Th cells with poly(I:C) in vitro drives differentiation toward an IL-21 but not IL-17-producing phenotype (74) suggesting that poly(I:C) may directly stimulate naïve Th cells to differentiate into Th1 or Tfh rather than Th17. A recent study suggested that c-Rel, a member of NF-κB family, plays an important role in the expression of IL-21 in T cells and subsequently in IL-21-dependent Tfh cell development (75). As activation of NF-κB is an important signal in TLR signaling, these results implicate TLRs in Tfh cell differentiation. Further evidence to support this can be seen in the response to antigen combined with poly(I:C) where type-I IFN signaling in DCs selectively stimulates Tfh cell development. In addition, the ability of DCs to produce IL-6 and the antibody affinity maturation are reduced without the type-I IFN signaling. CXCR5+ Tfh cells are also preferentially generated under strong immunogenic stimulations (76) and T_{REG} cells are responsible for homeostasis (77) and induction of immune tolerance toward cancer. Type-I IFN induced by TLR3 agonist can activate NK cells which are capable of suppressing the development of T_{REG} cells (78). The suppressive function of T_{REG} cells can also be blocked by the activation of melanoma differentiation-associated gene 5 (MDA-5) expressed in T_{REG} cells (79). MDA-5 belongs to RLRs and is the cytosolic adaptor of dsRNA, and thus dsRNA signaling might suppress the regulatory function of T_{REG} cells. Furthermore, an early study found that IL-6 is critical for overcoming T_{REG} suppression (80). When stimulated by dsRNA along with a specific antigen, activated DCs are able to induce the activation of antigen-specific CD8+ CTLs through cross-presentation and cross-priming mechanisms (56). Type-I IFN produced through dsRNA triggered signaling enhances the cross-priming ability of mDCs possibly via augmenting their capacity to deliver co-stimulatory signals or by directly stimulating CD8+ T cells (81). Upregulation of the co-stimulatory molecule CD40L in DCs directly promotes optimal priming of CTLs in the absence of CD4+ T-cell stimulation (82). For effective CTL priming, a cognate linkage between TLR3 and MHC-I molecules on the same DC cell is required (83). However, human DCs that capture dead cells containing the TLR3 agonist poly(I:C) fail to elicit CTL responses. This inhibition is specific for MHC-I restricted cross-presentation of dead cells bearing viral or poly(I:C) stimulus signals (84). This would therefore inhibit cross-presentation and hence prevent activation of self antigen–specific CTLs in viral infections. This suggests that caution should be exercised when using whole dead tumor cells as antigens in any developmental cancer vaccine. Nevertheless, live tumor cells combined with poly(I:C) can induce tumor-specific CD8+ and CD4+ T-cell responses, increase the clonal burst of tumor-specific CD8+ T-cells, and enhance the capacity of tumor-specific CD8+ T-cell expansion

Figure 17.4 (*Continued*) The antigen-specific CTL plays a critical role in fighting intracellular microorganisms and cancer cells. With the help of IL-4, the primed CD4+ T cell differentiates into Th2 cell to express STAT5 and GATA3 which boost antibody production. Stimulated by TGF-β, the primed CD4+ T cell differentiates into two reciprocal subtypes. In the presence of IL-6, this cell differentiates into IL-17-producing Th17 cell to play a role in eliminating extracellular bacteria. The other subtype differentiated from the TGF-β stimulated CD4+ T cell is T_{REG}. T_{REG} expresses FoxP3 when stimulated by IL-1β or IL-2. IL-6 or IL-12 can cause CD4+ T cells to differentiate into Tfh cell to express IL-21 and Bcl-6. Tfh cell is involved in the maintenance of long-lived plasma cells and memory B cells. dsRNA can promote DC maturation and Th1, Th2, CTLs and probably Tfh, and inhibit T_{REG} and perhaps Th17 cells. *Abbreviations*: CCL, CC-chemokine ligand; CD40L, CD40 ligand; CTL, cytotoxic T lymphocyte; DC, dendritic cell; FoxP3, forkhead box P3; GATA3, GATA-binding protein 3; IFN, interferon; IL, interleukin; STAT, signal transducer and activator of transcription; T-bet, T box expressed in T cell; TCR, T-cell receptor; Tfh, follicular helper T cell; TGF, transforming growth factor; Th, T helper cell; TLR, Toll-like receptor; Treg, regulatory T cell.

following restimulation with tumor antigens (85). Thus, dsRNA is able to promote Th1, Th2, CTL, and probably Tfh, and can inhibit T_{REG} and perhaps Th17 cells (Fig. 17.4).

EFFECTS OF DOUBLE-STRANDED RNA IN ANTI-CANCER IMMUNIZATION: A FRIEND OR A FOE?

Chronic inflammation is related to carcinogenesis (86) and the activation of TLRs can induce the production of proinflammatory cytokines through a signaling molecule cascade that can induce inflammation. This raises the questions: What is the relationship between activated TLRs and inflammation-associated tumorigenesis (87) considering that TLRs are expressed on DCs, other immune cells, and cancer cells? Can the activation of TLRs enhance the activity of T_{REG} cells or promote the growth of cancer cells (88,89)? The fact that viral infection is closely related with carcinogenesis and approximately 20% of all cancers are associated with infectious agents brings the third concern that dsRNA may act as a viral replication intermediate involved in carcinogenesis (6).

TLR4 is overexpressed in primary human colon cancer arising from chronic ulcerative colitis which is consistent with results from murine models when azoxymethane is used. In this model, mice genetically deficient in TLR4 are protected from inflammation-induced carcinogenesis. This TLR4-dependent tumorigenesis is associated with activation of epidermal growth factor receptor signaling and induction of cyclooxygenase-2 expression (90). The expression of other TLRs, like TLR7-TLR10 for example, is also upregulated in human colorectal cancer samples (91). The TLR2–TLR6 heterodimer can be activated by versican, an extracellular matrix proteoglycan, to induce TNF-α production and generate an inflammatory microenvironment to favor metastasis of Lewis lung carcinoma (92). Besides the proinflammatory mechanism, MyD88 can activate and amplify the canonical RAS pathway to induce murine and human cell transformation (87).

T_{REG} cells have been shown to suppress cytotoxic immunity against cancer (93) and the activation of TLR2, TLR4, and TLR5 on T cells can enhance the suppressive function of T_{REG} cells. Interestingly, naturally occurring T_{REG} cells express higher levels of TLR2, TLR4, TLR5, TLR7/8, and TLR10 than effector $CD4^+CD25^-$ T cells. iT_{REG} can be induced by 1α, 25-dihydroxyvitamin D3, the active form of vitamin D3, in vitro or in vivo, to express IL-10, and these iT_{REG} cells highly express TLR9. Pretreatment of the iT_{REG} cells with CpG-ODN resulted in decreased IL-10 and IFNγ synthesis and a concurrent loss of regulatory function (94). A recent study demonstrated that poly(I:C) induced peripheral expansion of functional T_{REG} in a TRIF- and IL-6-dependent manner in vivo. The property of poly(I:C) to induce expansion of naturally occurring T_{REG} is mediated indirectly through IL-6 produced from DCs and this is inhibited by IFNα from poly(I:C)-stimulated DCs. This suggests that the balance of IL-6 and IFNα produced via the signaling pathway triggered by poly(I:C) critically affects the number of peripheral T_{REG}. TLR agonists thus possess anti-inflammatory and regulatory properties to control excessive inflammation (89).

The involvement of TLRs in tumorigenesis and metastasis primarily affects TLRs that are MyD88 dependent rather than TLR3 which is TRIF dependent. This unique property of TLR3 in the TLR family is that it may have particular effects on immune response against cancer (53). The growth of murine-implanted syngeneic tumor was retarded by a subcutaneous injection of poly(I:C) that activated NK activation. This growth suppression was absent in TRIF(-/-) mice and present in MyD88(-/-) animals (95).

Synthetic dsRNA analogs have been used in cancer treatment (96). A randomized trial conducted 30 years ago using poly(A:U) as an adjuvant in the treatment of operable breast cancer suggested a beneficial trend in patients with auxiliary lymph node involvement (97). A later study focusing on TLR3 expression in patients with auxiliary lymph node metastasis, discovered that the 20-year overall survival was 88% in those with strong TLR3 expression on cancer cells and poly(A:U) treatment. In stark contrast, the survival rate was 41% in those with the same treatment but without TLR3 expression on tumor cells (98). The body of evidence suggests that activation of TLR3 elicits an immune response against cancer and also triggers the apoptosis (99). The growth of implanted transgenic adenocarcinoma of the mouse prostate tumor was significantly increased in TLR3$^{-/-}$ mice compared to TLR3$^{+/+}$ mice. Treatment with poly(I:C) strongly suppresses both implanted tumors and orthotopic prostate cancers in transgenic mice (78). Human DCs activated by dsRNA compared to DCs activated by other TLR ligands, produce a stronger Th1-polarized immune responses.

TLR3 expressed in tumor cells or T lymphocytes would induce biological effects different from those in DCs. TLR3 mRNA expression can be upregulated and poly(I:C)-induced apoptosis can be increased in colorectal cancer cell line by treating with 5-fluorouracil and/or IFNα. Melanoma cells treated with poly(I:C) conjugated with polyethyleneimine are induced to apoptosis through the activation of MDA-5 (99). Activation of TLR3 in HepG2 cell line by poly(I:C) results in a biased response toward the induction of an apoptosis with no production of proinflammatory factors. TLR3 was found to be expressed both membranously and cytoplasmically in hepatocellular carcinoma cells, and only cytoplasmic activation of TLR3 with transfected poly(I:C) significantly induced the apoptosis. Thus, it seems that dsRNA directly causes the cancer cell apoptosis (100). Activation of TLR3 in nasopharyngeal carcinoma cells can inhibit cell migration by downregulation of chemokine receptor CXCR4 and reduce the capacity of these cells to form metastasis when injected into athymic mice. All these results suggest an anti-metastatic activity of endogenous human TLR3 expression.

TLR3 is found to be expressed in both CD4$^+$ T cell and CD8$^+$ T cell but not in naturally occurring T$_{REG}$ cell. In human CD8$^+$ T cell, TLR3 is expressed in effector and effector memory subtypes but not in naïve and central memory subtypes (101). Addition of poly(I:C) significantly increased the quantity of IFNγ released by phytohemagglutinin-activated effector and/or effector memory CD8$^+$ T cells. However, poly(I:C) by itself cannot induce detectable IFNγ release by CD8$^+$ T cell, suggesting the co-stimulatory property of poly(I:C). Poly(I:C) also has no influence on the activity of CTLs or the cytolytic activity of antigen-specific cloned CD8$^+$ T cells (101). In murine models, a brief conditioning of purified naïve T-cell receptor (TCR) transgenic OT-1 (CD8$^+$) T cells in vitro with poly(I:C) induced activation of these cells in the absence of antigen stimulation. When these in vitro poly(I:C)-conditioned OT-1 cells were transferred into naïve recipients and vaccinated by peptide, recipients showed superior expansion and activation to their naïve counterparts which suggests that murine CD8$^+$ T-cells can be activated by triggering their TLR3 (102).

In summary, dsRNA through its enhanced cross-presentation and cross-priming ability can augment Th1 response and CTL response against cancer. It can also induce the cell apoptosis by endogenous TLR3 activation. It is involved in the activation of CD8$^+$ T cells through co-stimulatory mechanism. dsRNA can thus be regarded as being host protective (friendly).

PERSPECTIVES

TAA-specific CTL immunity is the major mechanism by which the host eliminates cancer cells. An adjuvant plays a significant role in enhancing the TAA-specific Th1-biased CTL-dominated response. TLR3 agonist appears to be an important adjuvant (53) with promising results from animal models (103). Unfortunately, clinical trials using TLR3 agonist-adjuvanted vaccines have not achieved sufficient positive results. Nevertheless, it is possible that the effect of TLR3 expression on cancer cells could play an important role in any dsRNA-adjuvanted cancer vaccine. In situ administration of such a vaccine may be more effective than systemic application (52,104). And in addition to TLR3 agonist, incorporation of other immunostimulating adjuvants could synergistically enhance the TAA-specific immune response (2,3,105).

ACKNOWLEDGMENTS

The authors thank Dr. James W. Shih, PhD, National Institute of Vaccine and Diagnostics, P.R.China for his advice.

This work is supported by the 11th Five-year Project for Medical Research from Chinese PLA (grant no. 06H003).

REFERENCES

1. Reed SG, Bertholet S, Coler RN, et al. New horizons in adjuvants for vaccine development. Trends Immunol 2009; 30: 23–32.
2. Mbow ML, De Gregorio E, Valiante NM, et al. New adjuvants for human vaccines. Curr Opin Immunol 2010; 22: 411–16.
3. Coffman RL, Sher A, Seder RA. Vaccine adjuvants: putting innate immunity to work. Immunity 2010; 33: 492–503.
4. Palm NW, Medzhitov R. Pattern recognition receptors and control of adaptive immunity. Immunol Rev 2009; 227: 221–33.
5. Pasare C, Medzhitov R. Control of B-cell responses by Toll-like receptors. Nature 2005; 438: 364–8.
6. Jin B, Sun T, Yu XH, et al. Immunomodulatory effects of dsRNA and its potential as vaccine adjuvant. J Biomed Biotechnol 2010; 2010: 690438.
7. Bauer S, Muller T, Hamm S. Pattern recognition by Toll-like receptors. Adv Exp Med Biol 2009; 653: 15–34.
8. Dubensky TW, Jr, Reed SG. Adjuvants for cancer vaccines. Semin Immunol 2010; 22: 155–61.
9. Chang ZL. Important aspects of Toll-like receptors, ligands and their signaling pathways. Inflamm Res 2010; 59: 791–808.
10. Jin B, Wang RY, Qiu Q, et al. Induction of potent cellular immune response in mice by hepatitis C virus NS3 protein with double-stranded RNA. Immunology 2007; 122: 15–27.
11. McGettrick AF, O'Neill LA. Localisation and trafficking of Toll-like receptors: an important mode of regulation. Curr Opin Immunol 2010; 22: 20–7.
12. Kim YM, Brinkmann MM, Paquet ME, et al. UNC93B1 delivers nucleotide-sensing toll-like receptors to endolysosomes. Nature 2008; 452: 234–8.
13. Wesche H, Henzel WJ, Shillinglaw W, et al. MyD88: an adapter that recruits IRAK to the IL-1 receptor complex. Immunity 1997; 7: 837–47.
14. Fitzgerald KA, Palsson-McDermott EM, Bowie AG, et al. Mal (MyD88-adapter-like) is required for Toll-like receptor-4 signal transduction. Nature 2001; 413: 78–83.
15. Oshiumi H, Matsumoto M, Funami K, et al. TICAM-1, an adaptor molecule that participates in Toll-like receptor 3-mediated interferon-beta induction. Nat Immunol 2003; 4: 161–7.
16. Yamamoto M, Sato S, Hemmi H, et al. TRAM is specifically involved in the Toll-like receptor 4-mediated MyD88-independent signaling pathway. Nat Immunol 2003; 4: 1144–50.
17. Sasai M, Oshiumi H, Matsumoto M, et al. Cutting edge: NF-kappaB-activating kinase-associated protein 1 participates in TLR3/Toll-IL-1 homology domain-containing adapter molecule-1-mediated IFN regulatory factor 3 activation. J Immunol 2005; 174: 27–30.
18. Hacker H, Redecke V, Blagoev B, et al. Specificity in Toll-like receptor signalling through distinct effector functions of TRAF3 and TRAF6. Nature 2006; 439: 204–7.
19. Kaiser WJ, Offermann MK. Apoptosis induced by the toll-like receptor adaptor TRIF is dependent on its receptor interacting protein homotypic interaction motif. J Immunol 2005; 174: 4942–52.
20. Han KJ, Yang Y, Xu LG, et al. Analysis of a TIR-less splice variant of TRIF reveals an unexpected mechanism of TLR3-mediated signaling. J Biol Chem 2010; 285: 12543–50.
21. Wang RF, Miyahara Y, Wang HY. Toll-like receptors and immune regulation: implications for cancer therapy. Oncogene 2008; 27: 181–9.
22. Galon J, Costes A, Sanchez-Cabo F, et al. Type, density, and location of immune cells within human colorectal tumors predict clinical outcome. Science 2006; 313: 1960–4.
23. Laghi L, Bianchi P, Miranda E, et al. CD3+ cells at the invasive margin of deeply invading (pT3-T4) colorectal cancer and risk of post-surgical metastasis: a longitudinal study. Lancet Oncol 2009; 10: 877–84.
24. Rakoff-Nahoum S, Medzhitov R. Toll-like receptors and cancer. Nat Rev Cancer 2009; 9: 57–63.
25. Hennessy EJ, Parker AE, O'Neill LA. Targeting Toll-like receptors: emerging therapeutics? Nat Rev Drug Discov 2010; 9: 293–307.
26. Salaun B, Coste I, Rissoan MC, et al. TLR3 can directly trigger apoptosis in human cancer cells. J Immunol 2006; 176: 4894–901.
27. Field AK, Tytell AA, Lampson GP, et al. Inducers of interferon and host resistance. II. Multistranded synthetic polynucleotide complexes. Proc Natl Acad Sci USA 1967; 58: 1004–10.
28. Navabi H, Jasani B, Reece A, et al. A clinical grade poly I:C-analogue (Ampligen) promotes optimal DC maturation and Th1-type T cell responses of healthy donors and cancer patients in vitro. Vaccine 2009; 27: 107–15.
29. Jasani B, Navabi H, Adams M. Ampligen: a potential toll-like 3 receptor adjuvant for immunotherapy of cancer. Vaccine 2009; 27: 3401–4.

30. Levy HB, Baer G, Baron S, et al. A modified polyriboinosinic-polyribocytidylic acid complex that induces interferon in primates. J Infect Dis 1975; 132: 434–9.
31. Zhu X, Fallert-Junecko BA, Fujita M, et al. Poly-ICLC promotes the infiltration of effector T cells into intracranial gliomas via induction of CXCL10 in IFN-alpha and IFN-gamma dependent manners. Cancer Immunol Immunother 2010; 59: 1401–9.
32. Okada H, Kalinski P, Ueda R, et al. Induction of CD8+ T-cell responses against novel glioma-associated antigen peptides and clinical activity by vaccinations with {alpha}-type 1 polarized dendritic cells and polyinosinic-polycytidylic acid stabilized by lysine and carboxymethylcellulose in patients with recurrent malignant glioma. J Clin Oncol 2011; 29: 330–6.
33. Rosenfeld MR, Chamberlain MC, Grossman SA, et al. A multi-institution phase II study of poly-ICLC and radiotherapy with concurrent and adjuvant temozolomide in adults with newly diagnosed glioblastoma. Neuro Oncol 2010; 12: 1071–7.
34. Perrot I, Deauvieau F, Massacrier C, et al. TLR3 and Rig-like receptor on myeloid dendritic cells and Rig-like receptor on human NK cells are both mandatory for production of IFN-gamma in response to double-stranded RNA. J Immunol 2010; 185: 2080–8.
35. Wang L, Smith D, Bot S, et al. Noncoding RNA danger motifs bridge innate and adaptive immunity and are potent adjuvants for vaccination. J Clin Invest 2002; 110: 1175–84.
36. Bot A, Smith D, Phillips B, et al. Immunologic control of tumors by in vivo Fc gamma receptor-targeted antigen loading in conjunction with double-stranded RNA-mediated immune modulation. J Immunol 2006; 176: 1363–74.
37. Rajagopal D, Paturel C, Morel Y, et al. Plasmacytoid dendritic cell-derived type I interferon is crucial for the adjuvant activity of Toll-like receptor 7 agonists. Blood 2010; 115: 1949–57.
38. Schon MP, Schon M. TLR7 and TLR8 as targets in cancer therapy. Oncogene 2008; 27: 190–9.
39. Chang BA, Cross JL, Najar HM, et al. Topical resiquimod promotes priming of CTL to parenteral antigens. Vaccine 2009; 27: 5791–9.
40. Fotin-Mleczek M, Duchardt KM, Lorenz C, et al. Messenger RNA-based vaccines with dual activity induce balanced TLR-7 dependent adaptive immune responses and provide antitumor activity. J Immunother 2011; 34: 1–15.
41. Cherfils-Vicini J, Platonova S, Gillard M, et al. Triggering of TLR7 and TLR8 expressed by human lung cancer cells induces cell survival and chemoresistance. J Clin Invest 2010; 120: 1285–97.
42. Bauer S, Kirschning CJ, Hacker H, et al. Human TLR9 confers responsiveness to bacterial DNA via species-specific CpG motif recognition. Proc Natl Acad Sci USA 2001; 98: 9237–42.
43. Kawai T, Sato S, Ishii KJ, et al. Interferon-alpha induction through Toll-like receptors involves a direct interaction of IRF7 with MyD88 and TRAF6. Nat Immunol 2004; 5: 1061–8.
44. Schreibelt G, Tel J, Sliepen KH, et al. Toll-like receptor expression and function in human dendritic cell subsets: implications for dendritic cell-based anti-cancer immunotherapy. Cancer Immunol Immunother 2010; 59: 1573–82.
45. Vollmer J, Weeratna R, Payette P, et al. Characterization of three CpG oligodeoxynucleotide classes with distinct immunostimulatory activities. Eur J Immunol 2004; 34: 251–62.
46. Vollmer J, Krieg AM. Immunotherapeutic applications of CpG oligodeoxynucleotide TLR9 agonists. Adv Drug Deliv Rev 2009; 61: 195–204.
47. Krieg AM. Development of TLR9 agonists for cancer therapy. J Clin Invest 2007; 117: 1184–94.
48. Kim SK, Ragupathi G, Musselli C, et al. Comparison of the effect of different immunological adjuvants on the antibody and T-cell response to immunization with MUC1-KLH and GD3-KLH conjugate cancer vaccines. Vaccine 1999; 18: 597–603.
49. Stevenson FK, Johnson PW. Harnessing innate immunity to suppress lymphoma. J Clin Oncol 2010; 28: 4295–6.
50. Manegold C, Gravenor D, Woytowitz D, et al. Randomized phase II trial of a toll-like receptor 9 agonist oligodeoxynucleotide, PF-3512676, in combination with first-line taxane plus platinum chemotherapy for advanced-stage non-small-cell lung cancer. J Clin Oncol 2008; 26: 3979–86.
51. Idera P. Idera Pharmaceuticals Announces Preliminary Data from Phase 1 Clinical Trial of IMO-2125 in Treatment-Naive Genotype 1 HCV Patients. News; [Available from: http://ir.iderapharma.com/ phoenix.zhtml?c=208904&p=irol-newsArticle&ID=1509338&highlight 2010].
52. Brody JD, Ai WZ, Czerwinski DK, et al. In situ vaccination with a TLR9 agonist induces systemic lymphoma regression: a phase I/II study. J Clin Oncol 2010; 28: 4324–32.
53. Nicodemus CF, Berek JS. TLR3 agonists as immunotherapeutic agents. Immunotherapy 2010; 2: 137–40.
54. Saveanu L, Carroll O, Weimershaus M, et al. IRAP identifies an endosomal compartment required for MHC class I cross-presentation. Science 2009; 325: 213–17.

55. Rock KL, Farfan-Arribas DJ, Shen L. Proteases in MHC class I presentation and cross-presentation. J Immunol 2010; 184: 9–15.
56. Joffre O, Nolte MA, Sporri R, et al. Inflammatory signals in dendritic cell activation and the induction of adaptive immunity. Immunol Rev 2009; 227: 234–47.
57. Shi CS, Kehrl JH. MyD88 and Trif target Beclin 1 to trigger autophagy in macrophages. J Biol Chem 2008; 283: 33175–82.
58. Watts C, West MA, Zaru R. TLR signalling regulated antigen presentation in dendritic cells. Curr Opin Immunol 2010; 22: 124–30.
59. Schlosser E, Mueller M, Fischer S, et al. TLR ligands and antigen need to be coencapsulated into the same biodegradable microsphere for the generation of potent cytotoxic T lymphocyte responses. Vaccine 2008; 26: 1626–37.
60. Burgdorf S, Scholz C, Kautz A, et al. Spatial and mechanistic separation of cross-presentation and endogenous antigen presentation. Nat Immunol 2008; 9: 558–66.
61. Ebihara T, Azuma M, Oshiumi H, et al. Identification of a polyI:C-inducible membrane protein that participates in dendritic cell-mediated natural killer cell activation. J Exp Med 2010; 207: 2675–87.
62. Walseng E, Furuta K, Goldszmid RS, et al. Dendritic cell activation prevents MHC class II ubiquitination and promotes MHC class II survival regardless of the activation stimulus. J Biol Chem 2010; 285: 41749–54.
63. Avril T, de Tayrac M, Leberre C, et al. Not all polyriboinosinic-polyribocytidylic acids (Poly I:C) are equivalent for inducing maturation of dendritic cells: implication for alpha-type-1 polarized DCs. J Immunother 2009; 32: 353–62.
64. Manicassamy S, Pulendran B. Modulation of adaptive immunity with Toll-like receptors. Semin Immunol 2009; 21: 185–93.
65. Smith-Garvin JE, Koretzky GA, Jordan MS. T cell activation. Annu Rev Immunol 2009; 27: 591–619.
66. Paul WE. What determines Th2 differentiation, in vitro and in vivo? Immunol Cell Biol 2010; 88: 236–9.
67. Flavell RA, Sanjabi S, Wrzesinski SH, et al. The polarization of immune cells in the tumour environment by TGFbeta. Nat Rev Immunol 2010; 10: 554–67.
68. Korn T, Bettelli E, Oukka M, et al. IL-17 and Th17 Cells. Annu Rev Immunol 2009; 27: 485–517.
69. Dienz O, Eaton SM, Bond JP, et al. The induction of antibody production by IL-6 is indirectly mediated by IL-21 produced by CD4+ T cells. J Exp Med 2009; 206: 69–78.
70. Kurts C, Robinson BW, Knolle PA. Cross-priming in health and disease. Nat Rev Immunol 2010; 10: 403–14.
71. Longhi MP, Trumpfheller C, Idoyaga J, et al. Dendritic cells require a systemic type I interferon response to mature and induce CD4+ Th1 immunity with poly IC as adjuvant. J Exp Med 2009; 206: 1589–602.
72. Kehoe KE, Brown MA, Imani F. Double-stranded RNA regulates IL-4 expression. J Immunol 2001; 167: 2496–501.
73. Duraisingham SS, Hornig J, Gotch F, et al. TLR-stimulated CD34 stem cell-derived human skin-like and monocyte-derived dendritic cells fail to induce Th17 polarization of naive T cells but do stimulate Th1 and Th17 memory responses. J Immunol 2009; 183: 2242–51.
74. Holm CK, Petersen CC, Hvid M, et al. TLR3 ligand polyinosinic:polycytidylic acid induces IL-17A and IL-21 synthesis in human Th cells. J Immunol 2009; 183: 4422–31.
75. Chen G, Hardy K, Bunting K, et al. Regulation of the IL-21 gene by the NF-kappaB transcription factor c-Rel. J Immunol 2010; 185: 2350–9.
76. Cucak H, Yrlid U, Reizis B, et al. Type I interferon signaling in dendritic cells stimulates the development of lymph-node-resident T follicular helper cells. Immunity 2009; 31: 491–501.
77. Waldmann H, Cobbold S. Regulatory T cells: context matters. Immunity 2009; 30: 613–15.
78. Chin AI, Miyahira AK, Covarrubias A, et al. Toll-like receptor 3-mediated suppression of TRAMP prostate cancer shows the critical role of type I interferons in tumor immune surveillance. Cancer Res 2010; 70: 2595–603.
79. Anz D, Koelzer VH, Moder S, et al. Immunostimulatory RNA blocks suppression by regulatory T cells. J Immunol 2010; 184: 939–46.
80. Pasare C, Medzhitov R. Toll pathway-dependent blockade of CD4+CD25+ T cell-mediated suppression by dendritic cells. Science 2003; 299: 1033–6.
81. Le Bon A, Tough DF. Type I interferon as a stimulus for cross-priming. Cytokine Growth Factor Rev 2008; 19: 33–40.

82. Johnson S, Zhan Y, Sutherland RM, et al. Selected Toll-like receptor ligands and viruses promote helper-independent cytotoxic T cell priming by upregulating CD40L on dendritic cells. Immunity 2009; 30: 218–27.
83. Davey GM, Wojtasiak M, Proietto AI, et al. Cutting edge: priming of CD8 T cell immunity to herpes simplex virus type 1 requires cognate TLR3 expression in vivo. J Immunol 2010; 184: 2243–6.
84. Frleta D, Yu CI, Klechevsky E, et al. Influenza virus and poly(I:C) inhibit MHC class I-restricted presentation of cell-associated antigens derived from infected dead cells captured by human dendritic cells. J Immunol 2009; 182: 2766–76.
85. McBride S, Hoebe K, Georgel P, et al. Cell-associated double-stranded RNA enhances antitumor activity through the production of type I IFN. J Immunol 2006; 177: 6122–8.
86. Kluwe J, Mencin A, Schwabe RF. Toll-like receptors, wound healing, and carcinogenesis. J Mol Med 2009; 87: 125–38.
87. Coste I, LeCorf K, Kfoury A, et al. Dual function of MyD88 in RAS signaling and inflammation, leading to mouse and human cell transformation. J Clin Invest 2010; 120: 3663–7.
88. Huang B, Zhao J, Unkeless JC, et al. TLR signaling by tumor and immune cells: a double-edged sword. Oncogene 2008; 27: 218–24.
89. Conroy H, Marshall NA, Mills KH. TLR ligand suppression or enhancement of Treg cells? A double-edged sword in immunity to tumours. Oncogene 2008; 27: 168–80.
90. Fukata M, Chen A, Vamadevan AS, et al. Toll-like receptor-4 promotes the development of colitis-associated colorectal tumors. Gastroenterology 2007; 133: 1869–81.
91. Grimm M, Kim M, Rosenwald A, et al. Toll-like receptor (TLR) 7 and TLR8 expression on CD133+ cells in colorectal cancer points to a specific role for inflammation-induced TLRs in tumourigenesis and tumour progression. Eur J Cancer 2010; 46: 2849–57.
92. Kim S, Takahashi H, Lin WW, et al. Carcinoma-produced factors activate myeloid cells through TLR2 to stimulate metastasis. Nature 2009; 457: 102–6.
93. Nishikawa H, Sakaguchi S. Regulatory T cells in tumor immunity. Int J Cancer 2010; 127: 759–67.
94. Urry Z, Xystrakis E, Richards DF, et al. Ligation of TLR9 induced on human IL-10-secreting Tregs by 1alpha,25-dihydroxyvitamin D3 abrogates regulatory function. J Clin Invest 2009; 119: 387–98.
95. Akazawa T, Ebihara T, Okuno M, et al. Antitumor NK activation induced by the Toll-like receptor 3-TICAM-1 (TRIF) pathway in myeloid dendritic cells. Proc Natl Acad Sci USA 2007; 104: 252–7.
96. Levine AS, Levy HB. Phase I-II trials of poly IC stabilized with poly-L-lysine. Cancer Treat Rep 1978; 62: 1907–12.
97. Lacour J, Lacour F, Ducot B, et al. Polyadenylic-polyuridylic acid as adjuvant in the treatment of operable breast cancer: recent results. Eur J Surg Oncol 1988; 14: 311–16.
98. Andre F, Zitvogel L, Sabourin JC. Treatment of cancer using TLR3 agonists. US Patent 7378249; [Available from: http://patft.uspto.gov/netacgi/nph-Parser?Sect1=PTO1&Sect2=HITOFF&d=PALL&p=1&u=%2Fnetahtml%2FPTO%2Fsrchnum.htm&r=1&f=G&l=50&s1=7378249.PN.&OS=PN/7378249&RS=PN/7378249 2008].
99. Alonso-Curbelo D, Soengas MS. Self-killing of melanoma cells by cytosolic delivery of dsRNA: wiring innate immunity for a coordinated mobilization of endosomes, autophagosomes and the apoptotic machinery in tumor cells. Autophagy 2010; 6: 148–50.
100. Matijevic T, Pavelic J. Toll-like receptors: cost or benefit for cancer? Curr Pharm Des 2010; 16: 1081–90.
101. Tabiasco J, Devevre E, Rufer N, et al. Human effector CD8+ T lymphocytes express TLR3 as a functional coreceptor. J Immunol 2006; 177: 8708–13.
102. Salem ML, Diaz-Montero CM, El-Naggar SA, et al. The TLR3 agonist poly(I:C) targets CD8+ T cells and augments their antigen-specific responses upon their adoptive transfer into naive recipient mice. Vaccine 2009; 27: 549–57.
103. Trumpfheller C, Caskey M, Nchinda G, et al. The microbial mimic poly IC induces durable and protective CD4+ T cell immunity together with a dendritic cell targeted vaccine. Proc Natl Acad Sci USA 2008; 105: 2574–9.
104. Scarlett UK, Cubillos-Ruiz JR, Nesbeth YC, et al. In situ stimulation of CD40 and Toll-like receptor 3 transforms ovarian cancer-infiltrating dendritic cells from immunosuppressive to immunostimulatory cells. Cancer Res 2009; 69: 7329–37.
105. Zhu Q, Egelston C, Vivekanandhan A, et al. Toll-like receptor ligands synergize through distinct dendritic cell pathways to induce T cell responses: implications for vaccines. Proc Natl Acad Sci USA 2008; 105: 16260–5.

18 | Passive immunotherapy by T cell–engaging bispecific antibodies

Patrick A. Baeuerle and Benno Rattel

INTRODUCTION

Cytotoxic T cells are unique in their capability to eliminate cancer cells whether these are proliferating or temporarily non-dividing, and whether they are cancer stem cells or their progeny. Moreover, T cells are found and can act in almost all compartments of the body with limited activity only in immunoprivileged sites such as the brain or testes. In mouse models, numerous approaches have shown that T cells can—as a monotherapy—eradicate large established tumors (1–4). The capacity of T cells to completely eradicate target cells is also evident from their key role in fighting viral diseases by eliminating virus-infected cells. It is therefore highly attractive to find a means of mounting T-cell responses against malignant cells for cancer therapy. However, given the enormous cytotoxic potential of T cells, the specificity of target recognition and a tight control of their activity are important for the therapeutic use of T cells in cancer treatment. The induction of various kinds of autoimmune reactions by anti- cytotoxic T lymphocyte-associated antigen 4 antibody ipilimumab concurrent with its anti-tumor activity (5) demonstrates the difficulty of mounting T-cell responses that are specific for tumor cells.

The ultimate goal of therapeutic vaccination of cancer patients is to mount an effective mono- or oligoclonal, cytotoxic, tumor-specific T-cell response that is curative by eradicating tumor and clearing of the disseminated cancer cells, followed by long-term protection of patients from a relapse. Even if the T-cell response can only establish equilibrium between cancer cell proliferation and ongoing lysis, thereby stabilizing tumors, this may translate into increased survival time for patients. This latter scenario could explain the intriguing observations that patients with T cell–infiltrated tumors live much longer than patients with tumors containing few or no T cells. This has been reported for ovarian cancer (6), colorectal cancer (7), and non-Hodgkin lymphoma (NHL) patients (8). The number of CD8+ effector memory T cells appeared to be mostly responsible for the highly significant correlation between survival and the degree of T-cell infiltration of tumors (7).

Analogous to anti-viral T-cell responses, anti-tumor T-cell responses have the potential to establish a long-term memory, which becomes relevant once tumor cells grow back years or decades after the primary disease. However, as with viruses, cancer cells selected under T-cell pressure will have acquired new mutations that may require the generation of T-cell clones with novel specificities. Apart from losing the target antigen, tumor cells can become selected for multiple evasion mechanisms allowing their escape from regular T-cell recognition (9). Prominent mechanisms include loss or lowered expression of major histocompatibility complex (MHC) class I molecules, β2-microglobulin, or of transporters associated with antigen processing. Antigen presentation by tumor cells can likewise be hampered by changes in proteasome subunits that will prevent the generation of certain peptide antigens. An alternative defense strategy of tumor cells is interference with the differentiation of cytotoxic T cells by secretion of immunosuppressive cytokines such as interleukin (IL) 10, IL-4, or transforming growth factor beta. Tumor cells can functionally impair T cells by expressing ligands that find negative regulatory or death receptors on T cells, such as B7-H1/PD-L1, or Fas ligand. They can also silence T cells by expressing indoleamine-pyrrole 2,3 dioxygenase, which can tolerize or even kill T cells by local tryptophane degradation and resulting metabolites. Furthermore, tumor cells have the potential to create an immune suppressive microenvironment by attracting regulatory T cells and a host of other negative regulatory immune cells. Hence, it is conceivable that tumors have accumulated in late-stage disease a multitude of escape mechanisms, which in their combination, can very effectively intercept immunosurveillance at various levels, thereby allowing for a deadly disease progression.

Table 18.1 T Cell-Engaging Antibodies and Fusion Proteins in Clinical Development

T Cell-Engaging Antibody	Targets	Format	Development Stage (2010)	Indication	Co-treatment	Institution
Removab® Rexomun® Lymphomun®	EpCAM and CD3 HER2 and CD3 CD20 and CD3	Triomab (ttifunctional Mab)	Market Phase II Phase I	Malignant ascites Solid tumors B-NHL	All monotherapies	Trion Pharma/ Fresenius Biotech AG
ANYARA®	5T4 and TCR/3	Superantigen/Fab fragment fusion	Pivotal	Renal cell cancer	+Interferon-alpha	Active Biotech AB
Blinatumomab MT110 MEDI-565/MT111	CD19 and CD3 EpCAM and CD3 CEA and CD3 TCR-beta	Bispecific T-cell engager (tandem ScFvs)	Pivotal Phase I Phase I	B-ALL, B-NHL Solid tumors Solid tumors	All monotherapies	Micromet. Inc. Micromet. Inc./ MedImmune/AZ
Her2Bi	HER2 and CD3	Chemically cross-linked commercial MAbs	Phase II	Breast cancer	+GM-CSF +IL2	Barbara Karmanos Cancer Center
IMCgp100	gp100 peptide-HLA-A2 complex and CD3	Soluble T-cell receptor/anti-CD3 scFv fusion	Phase I	Melanoma	Monotherapy	Immunocore, Ltd

Abbreviations: ALL, acute lymphoblastic leukemia; GM-CSF, granulocyte-macrophage colony stimulating factor; NHL, non-Hodgkin lymphoma.

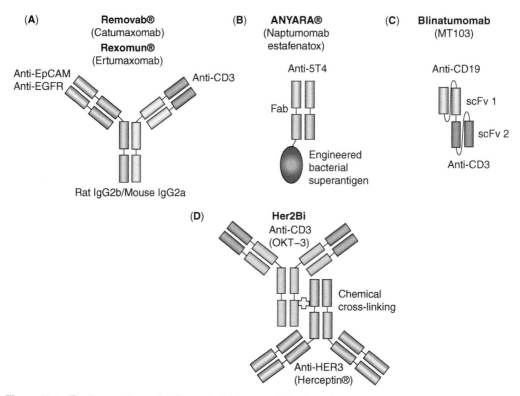

Figure 18.1 T cell–engaging antibodies and a fusion protein in phase II or pivotal clinical testing. The structural features of proteins are shown and drawn at the same scale. Red and green colours depict the two binding specificities of molecules. *Abbreviations*: EGFR, epidermal growth factor receptor; IgG, immunoglobulin.

More than 20 years ago, cell culture studies showed that T cells when forced into close proximity with cancer cells by bispecific antibodies can exert redirected lysis irrespective of their T-cell receptor (TCR) specificity (10). This indicated that the killing program inherent to cytotoxic T cells can be unleashed independently from the interaction of TCRs with the MHC class I/peptide complex and, furthermore, that any by-standing or circulating cytotoxic T cell can potentially be recruited for redirected lysis of cancer cells. The attractiveness of T cell–engaging antibodies has not faded since then resulting in multiple technical solutions for engagement of polyclonal T cells by using antibodies and antibody fragments (11). Apart from deciphering the optimal bispecific design for T-cell engagement, the key challenges of such bispecific antibodies have been to safely mount a polyclonal T-cell response, to activate unstimulated T cells, to support serial lysis by activated T cells, to avoid T-cell anergy, and to produce in sufficient amounts stable antibodies or antibody-based constructs that comply with the ever increasing quality criteria for therapeutic biological products.

We will in the following text focus on those bispecific T cell–engaging biologics that are currently most advanced in pharmaceutical development, that is, those that have reached the stage of formal clinical safety and efficacy testing (Table 18.1). The structural features of all proteins discussed are depicted in Figures 18.1 and 18.2.

TRIFUNCTIONAL ANTIBODIES

More than 20 years of bispecific antibody development has culminated in 2009 with the market approval in the EU of Removab® (catumaxomab) (Fresenius Biotech, Munich, Germany) for the treatment of malignant ascites in patients with EpCAM-expressing carcinoma (12).

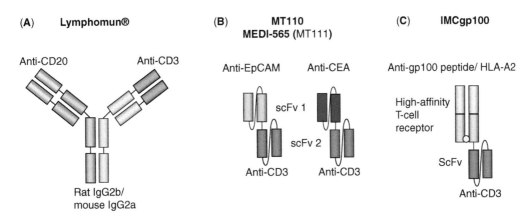

Figure 18.2 T cell–engaging antibodies and a fusion protein in phase I clinical testing. The structural features of proteins are shown and drawn at the same scale. Red and green colours depict the two binding specificities of molecules. *Abbreviations*: CEA, carcinoembryonic antigen; HLA, human leukocyte antigen; IgG, immunoglobulin.

Treatment with this EpCAM/CD3-bispecific antibody resulted in a highly significant prolongation of paracentesis intervals, and in a subgroup of patients, a trend toward an increased survival, which is being further explored in ongoing clinical studies. Serial analyses of ascites samples from patients treated with the drug showed that catumaxomab induced in the ascites of essentially every patient a fast and potent elimination of cancer cells as well as a proliferation and activation of T cells, including a respective release of cytokines. The antibody is intraperitoneally administered every other day at escalating doses of 10, 20, 50, and 150 µg resulting in a local mean dose level of ca.10 ng/ml in ascites, and systemic Cmax values of 0.4 ng/ml with a mean serum half-life of 2.13 days (13). Due to its murine/rat origin, catumaxomab elicits a strong neutralizing antibody response in all patients at the end of infusion, which can prevent re-treatment.

Catumaxomab and related antibodies are asymmetric by design in that one heavy chain is derived from rat IgG2b and the other from mouse IgG2a (Figs. 18.1A and 18.2A). They are produced as secreted proteins by quadroma cell lines derived by fusion of two hybridoma cell lines of rat and mouse origin, respectively. A particular advantage of using murine immunoglobulin G (IgG)2a and rat IgG2b antibodies is that rat and mouse heavy chains heterodimerize with high preference while at the same time light chains will dimerize with their respective heavy chains of the same species (14). This guarantees that a high yield of properly arranged antibody is formed.

Catumaxomab is frequently referred to as "trifunctional", or as a Triomab. This relates to its Fcγ part, which represents a third binding domain in addition to its two distinct binding domains for EpCAM and the CD3ε subunit of the TCR complex. The Fcγ part binds with various affinities to several Fcγ receptors, which are expressed on a great variety of immune and endothelial cells. The Fcγ part of trifunctional antibodies is capable of mediating antibody-dependent cellular cytotoxicity and complement-dependent cytotoxicity, which are thought to amplify the cytotoxicity mediated by redirected lysis via T cells. Moreover, the Fcγ part of trifunctional antibodies can bind Fcγ receptors on APCs and the neonatal receptor FcRn on endothelial cells, which mediates the long serum half-life of antibodies. A recent non-clinical study supports the assumption that the Fcγ part is essential for the anti-tumor activity of catumaxomab (15).

However, the Fcγ part may likewise contribute to the low systemic tolerability of catumaxomab. In a study with lung cancer patients, the maximum tolerated dose of intravenously infused antibody was found to be 5 µg per patient and required co-administration of steroids (16). Side effects appeared to be related to overt cytokine release and transaminitis. In support of a negative impact of the Fcγ part of catumaxomab on systemic tolerability is the observation that the

EpCAM/CD3-bispecific Bispecific T-cell engager (BiTE) antibody MT110 (Fig. 18.2B), which is lacking an Fcγ part, has thus far been well tolerated up to 24 µg per patient per day following continuous i.v. infusion for 4–8 weeks (17). The difference in tolerability is further highlighted by the higher systemic exposure achieved by continuous i.v. infusion of MT110 compared with the repeated intraperitoneal short-term administration of the short-lived trispecific antibody. Intriguingly, an HER-2-specific trifunctional antibody called ertumaxomab (Rexomun®) (Fig. 18.2A), which shares the anti-CD3 arm with catumaxomab, has shown a much higher systemic tolerability with a maximum tolerated i.v. dose of 100 µg per patient (18), indicating that the targeted tumor antigen and its accessibility may also significantly contribute to the safety profile of this class of antibodies.

So far, a total of three TriomAbs have been investigated in patients. Apart from the EpCAM and HER-2-specific antibodies Removab and Rexomun, also the CD20-specific TriomAb Lymphomun® (Fig. 18.2A) was tested in a small trial with chronic lymphocytic leukemia patients (19). In all three cases, biological activity and anti-tumor activity were evident at very low doses of antibodies. However, a future challenge of this T cell–engaging antibody format will be to improve their risk/benefit profile after systemic administration allowing a sufficiently high exposure for a clinically significant impact on disease progression and survival, and to manage their high immunogenic potential, which severely limits a prolonged or repeated treatment. A particular promise of trifunctional antibodies is that patients treated with catumaxomab developed anti-tumor immunity (20), a feature that has not yet been reported for other T cell–engaging antibodies. A vaccination effect of catumaxomab may add efficacy to antibody-dependent cellular cytotoxicity and redirected T-cell lysis.

BACTERIAL SUPERANTIGEN/ANTIBODY FUSION PROTEIN

Superantigens (SAgs) can be considered naturally occurring, T cell–engaging bispecific proteins released by microbes as a defense against the host's immune system (21). While a specific T-cell response activates only 0.001–0.0001% of all T cells, SAgs can in a polyclonal fashion activate up to 20% of all T cells by direct binding to a variable region of the TCR-β chain. The second binding domain of certain SAgs recognizes MHC class II, which is expressed on a variety of immune cells. At extremely low concentrations, a simultaneous binding of SAgs to T cells and MHC class II-expressing cells triggers T-cell mitosis, overt cytokine release, and redirected lysis of target cells. Acute clinical manifestations of these events can be rashes, fever, hypotension, multi-organ failure, toxic shock syndrome, coma, and death. Prolonged exposure to SAgs leads to T-cell anergy by multiple mechanisms.

Of the great variety of bacterial and viral SAgs, the staphylococcal enterotoxin A (SEA) has been selected for crafting a T cell–engaging antibody called ANYARA® (naptumomab estafenatox; ABR- or PNU-214936) (22). As a target antigen for binding to cancer cells, the oncofetal antigen 5T4 has been selected, which is frequently found expressed on human cancers but only at low levels on normal tissues. As shown in Figure 18.1B, ANYARA uses the Fab fragment of an anti-5T4 murine mAb to which SEA is C-terminally fused by a recombinant DNA technology. Binding of the SEA moiety to MHC class II has been largely abrogated by mutating Asp 227 to Ala while retaining binding to the TCR β-chain. In cell culture assays, a redirected lysis of 5T4-expressing cancer cells by T cells required only 10^{-10} M ANYARA, while it took a 1000-fold higher concentration to trigger lysis of MHC class II-expressing cells (23).

ANYARA has completed a phase III trial with more than 500 renal cell carcinoma (RCC) patients with final results expected for 2012. Results from phase I dose escalation studies in 78 RCC patients (24), 39 non-small-cell lung cancer (NSCLC) patients as monotherapy, and 17 NSCLC patients in combination with docetaxel (25), and a phase II study in 43 RCC patients (26) have been reported. In these studies, the dose levels of ANYARA had to be individually adjusted in order to titrate the patients' pre-existing anti-SEA antibody levels from previous bacterial infections. This resulted in a wide dose range of ANYARA from as low as 44 ng/kg to 22 µg/kg which has been tested in the various trials. Patients received

4–5 consecutive daily 3-hour infusions, and a second cycle 4–6 weeks later. The terminal serum half-life of ANYARA was rather short, lasting only 0.9–1.38 hours, likely resulting in very low systemic drug exposure.

The phase I study by Cheng et al. (24) revealed 5 minor responses in 66 evaluable RCC patients (7.6%) persisting 4 weeks or longer, and 25 patients (38%) had stable disease by day 28 of cycle 1. All other patients in the trial showed progress. In the docetaxel combo phase 1 study with non-small-cell lung cancer (NSCLC) patients (25), 14/39 monotherapy patients (36%) had stable disease on day 56 in the monotherapy arm. In the combination therapy arm with 17 patients, 2 patients (15%) had a partial response, and 5 patients (38%) had stable disease on day 56. In the RCC study (26), 1/40 (2.5%) evaluable patients had a partial response and 16 patients (40%) were diagnosed with stable disease 4 months after starting the treatment. Patients receiving a higher dose resulting in higher drug exposure lived almost twice as long as those with low drug exposure. Retrospective analyses suggested that the IL2 levels induced by ANYARA on day 2 correlated with an increased survival.

The most frequent clinical adverse events of ANYARA were as expected for a polyclonal T cell–engaging agent and included fever, hypotension, nausea, vomiting, chills, rigors, fatigue, diarrhea, and lymphocytopenia. Incidences of grade 3 and 4 events (i.e., hypotension, rigors, and nausea) were highest in response to the first treatment cycle consistent with an adaptive response of T cells. In one study, the dose-limiting toxicity was reached at 22 μg/kg (plus docetaxel), which caused one event of a lethal neutropenic sepsis.

The most significant challenges of ANYARA are its high immunogenicity requiring dose adaptation for pre-existing anti-SEA serum titers, its residual binding to MHC class II-expressing cells, which may contribute to the adverse event profile, and its very short serum half-life. The first two issues have been addressed by the construction of a novel version of naptumomab estafenatox called 5T4FabV18-SEA/E-120 or ABR-217620 (27). It is less sensitive to high anti-SEA titers, has a 10-fold increased cytoxic activity in vitro and high activity in mouse models, and is now 10,000 folds less active in lysing MHC class II-expressing immune cells. This new version of ANYARA has already been tested in a phase I trial (25). Superantigen fusion proteins with other target specificities have been constructed and characterized but have not entered clinical testing.

BITE

BiTE antibodies have a minimalistic design for T-cell engagement (Figs. 18.1C and 18.2B). They link two single-chain antibodies (scFvs), which represent the minimal antigen-binding domains of two monoclonal antibodies (mAbs). By use of three non-immunogenic linker sequences, a single polypeptide chain of 55–60 kDa is created, which is lacking an Fcγ domain, and can be produced by eukaryotic cell cultures (28,29). One BiTE arm is binding to the CD3ε invariable chain of the TCR complex and the other arm to a surface target antigen. Through the forced approximation of a cytotoxic T cell to a target cell, a cytolytic synapse is formed allowing for comprehensive T-cell activation (30–33). As a consequence, exactly the same process is induced that specific T cells use to lyse target cells after connecting via their TCR to MHC class I–peptide complexes. This process involves discharge of cytotoxic granules, insertion of perforin pores, and delivery of granzymes into the cytoplasm of target cells leading to membrane leakage, induction of apoptosis, and disintegration of the target cell by membrane blebbing (33).

In cell culture assays, BiTE antibodies mediate target cell lysis at half maximal concentrations between low pg/ml (10^{-13} M) (34) and low ng/ml (10^{-10} M) (35) largely depending on the nature of the target antigen, its surface density, and the binding affinity of the BiTE antibody for the respective target. Unstimulated peripheral blood mononuclear cells or purified CD8+ or CD4+ T cells can all be used as effector cells, whereby effector memory T cells (CD8+ or CD4+, CD45RO, CCR7-) show the highest activity with BiTE antibodies (36). Of note, BiTE antibodies have been shown to support serial lysis of T cells at very low effector-to-target cell ratios (30), and to potently induce T-cell mitosis (37).

The high in-vitro activity of BiTE antibodies suggests that they closely mimic a regular T-cell recognition, which only requires a single digit number of TCR/MHC class I complexes for induction of cytotoxicity (38). Numerous BiTE antibodies have been investigated in immunodeficient mouse models using human T cells or peripheral blood mononuclear cell as effector cells and human cancer lines or metastatic tissue for xenograft establishment (29). Of note, human T cells were in all models negative for activation marker at the time of BiTE treatment, and either mixed to cancer lines before subcutaneous inoculation, or later injected intraperitoneally before BiTE treatment of established tumors. Regardless of whether or not xenografts contained T cells BiTE antibodies, low µg/kg doses given by daily i.v. dosing for 5–10 days induced tumor eradication or a significant delay or complete inhibition of tumor outgrowth.

A high potency of BiTE antibodies was also evident in clinical trials with CD19/CD3-bispecific BiTE antibody blinatumomab (MT103) (39). Serum levels of 1–3 ng/ml triggered partial and complete tumor regressions in patients with relapsed/refractory NHL, and led to the clearance of tumor cells from spleen, lymph nodes, liver, bone marrow, and peripheral blood. Owing to its relatively short serum half-life of 2–3 hours, blinatumomab is administered by continuous i.v. infusion over a period of 4–8 weeks using portable mini pumps to establish stable steady-state serum levels. The ongoing dose-escalating phase I study in NHL patients has tested seven dose levels starting at a dose of 0.0005 mg/m^2 per day up to a dose of 0.09 mg/m^2 per day. Efficacy was observed in patients treated with $60 \text{ µg/m}^2/\text{d}$ with an overall high response rate of 82% (18/22) across all tested indications: 11/12 follicular/marginal lymphoma patients responding, 3/5 diffuse large B-cell lymphoma patients reaching a complete response, and 4/5 mantle cell lymphoma patients showing either a partial response or complete response (40). Responses are still ongoing in 11 of 18 patients (61%) with response durations currently up to almost three years. In this ongoing phase 1 trial, the majority of clinical adverse events are flu-like symptoms, for example, pyrexia (all grades: 74.2%; grade 3 or 4: 3.2%), headache (all grades: 41.9%; grade 3 or 4: 3.2%), and fatigue (all grades: 40.3%; grade 3 or 4: 3.2%). The most relevant clinical adverse events (AEs) are fully reversible central nervous system events at the commencement of treatment that can be managed well.

Blinatumomab was active not only against large lymph node tumors of NHL patients but also against minimal residual disease (MRD) of adult patients with B-precursor acute lymphoblastic leukemia (ALL) (41), and against relapsed ALL of three pediatric patients (42). An MRD-positive status in ALL is a strong and independent predictive marker for hematological relapse and has a poor prognosis for both adults and children. ALL patients were treated with a blinatumomab dose of 0.015 mg/m^2 per day in four-week cycles, which had been found in NHL patients to have high activity in peripheral blood and bone marrow, the primary disease sites in ALL. In a completed phase 2 study, blinatumomab induced a molecular complete response rate, that is conversion from MRD positivity to negativity, in 16/20 (80%) of evaluable patients (40). These responses all occurred within the first treatment cycle. The median disease-free survival has not been reached after a median followup of up to 27.5 months (median of 15 months). Most AEs occurred early (in cycle 1) and resolved during ongoing treatment. Grade 3/4 AEs were very rare, and there were no deaths on study. Inflammatory processes dominated the first few days of treatment; all patients experienced grade 1/2 pyrexia, and 43% chills. As in the NHL study, headache (43%) and fatigue (38%) were observed. All were reported as grade 1/2 AEs with the exception of one grade-3 headache. Two patients discontinued infusion prematurely due to reversible AEs, a seizure on day 2 of cycle 1 and a convulsive syncope during cycle 3. These events resolved without sequelae. Blinatumomab's efficacy in adult ALL patients with MRD and in relapsed/refractory disease is now being explored in a phase II and registrational studies, respectively. Clinical studies investigating other B-cell malignancies are ongoing or planned.

The current clinical data show that polyclonal engagement of T cells by continuous systemic administration of a polyclonal T cell–engaging BiTE antibody is feasible and safe, and can lead to very high response rates in hematological malignancies. Initial side effects upon start of infusion are flu like and most likely related to a modest systemic cytokine release at the onset of T-cell activation. Such AEs are typically self-limiting and cease within days under continued treatment.

Two more BiTE antibodies are currently in dose-escalating clinical phase 1 studies. One is the EpCAM/CD3-bispecific BiTE antibody MT110 (3,17) and the other is the CEA/CD3-bispecific BiTE antibody MT111/MEDI-565 (35). Both BiTE antibodies are under investigation for safety and efficacy in patients with metastatic disease from gastrointestinal carcinoma and other solid tumor indications expressing the respective target antigens. Three more BiTE antibodies for treatment of solid tumors or multiple myeloma are in pre-clinical development in collaboration with large biopharmaceutical companies.

While the first clinically tested BiTE antibody appears to be highly active in hematological malignancies, the immunosuppressive microenvironment of solid tumors and the high tumor load of late-stage patients may pose a significant efficacy hurdle to the treatment of metastatic disease by monotherapy with BiTE antibodies specific for solid tumor targets. Immunogenicity has thus far not been an issue for any BiTE antibody. Nevertheless, a new BiTE platform has been engineered based on a human anti-CD3 scFv that is cross-reactive with CD3 on T cells of non-human primates. This now allows the assessment of non-clinical safety of new BiTE antibodies in pharmacologically relevant primate models, as has recently been exemplified for EGFR-specific BiTE antibodies based on antigen binding domains of Erbitux® and Vectibix® (34).

CROSSLINKED MABS

A straightforward approach for manufacturing of bispecific antibodies has been taken by Lum and colleagues (Fig. 18.1D) by chemically cross-linking the commercial anti-CD3ε mAb OKT3 (Orthoclone®) at a 1:1 ratio with other antibodies recognizing established tumor-associated antigens (43). Using registered antibodies like Herceptin (trastuzmab) or Rituxan®) (rituximab) and a conjugation process following "good manufacturing practices" (GMP), GMP-grade bispecific antibodies can be produced for clinical use. The resulting bispecific, tetravalent antibody conjugates are used to "arm" polyclonal activated T cells (ATC). One conjugate of OKT-3 and Herceptin, called Her2Bi, is being tested in an ongoing clinical phase II trial at the Barbara Ann Karmanos Cancer Center. In cell culture experiments, T cells derived from cancer patients that are ex vivo activated and armed with Her2Bi showed high and sustained cytotoxic activity against HER2-expressing cell lines (44). In clinical practice, T cells are isolated from cancer patients and ex vivo loaded with the bispecific antibody conjugate followed by reinfusion of those armed T cells. This procedure is employed to avoid overt systemic cytokine release reactions, which can otherwise be induced by the OKT-3 moiety of the conjugate. A phase I study in 19 metastatic breast cancer patients with the OKT-3/Herceptin conjugate Her2Bi has resulted in one partial response and 10 disease stabilizations (presentation by Lawrence Lum at Sixth Annual PEGS Summit, Boston, MA, May 20–21, 2010).

SOLUBLE T-CELL RECEPTOR FUSION PROTEINS

While all T cell–engaging antibodies described above recognize surface antigens in the same way regular mAbs do, the U.K.-based biotech company Immunocore Ltd has focused on constructing T cell–engaging antibodies that target MHC class I–peptide complexes as normally recognized by specific T-cell clones. To this end, soluble, disulfide-stabilized TCR molecules are recombinantly fused to an anti-CD3 scFv (Fig. 18.2C). This T cell–engaging bispecific format is called "Immune Mobilizing mTCR Against Cancer" or "ImmTAC". Immunocore's lead product IMCgp100 recognizes melanoma cells expressing a gp100-derived peptide antigen presented by MHC molecule human leukocyte antigen (HLA)-A2, which is expressed by approximately 50% of Caucasians. ImmTACs specific for other peptide antigens are under pre-clinical development. They all use soluble TCRs that have been selected to be of very high affinity (45) in order to assure sufficient binding to particular MHC class I–peptide complexes expressed at only very low levels on cancer cells.

In October 2010, clinical phase I testing of IMCgp100 has commenced in melanoma patients in the United Kingdom (presentation by Rebecca Ashfield at Drug Discovery and Development Week by IBC Lifesciences, San Francisco, CA, August 2–4, 2010). In the absence of animal models for assessment of non-clinical safety, the starting dose for the clinical trial was determined to be 5 ng/kg by the "minimum anticipated biological effect level" (MABEL) approach. The maximum dose is anticipated to be 3.6 µg/kg. Doses are administered once weekly by a 4-hr i.v. infusion. In mice, the terminal serum half-life ranged between 2 and 4 hrs, but due to the high target affinity, retention of IMCgp100 in tumor tissue for >24 hr is expected. In a mouse model, a dose of 10 µg IMCgp100 per kg was required to achieve inhibition of tumor outgrowth. A 10-fold higher dose was required for a MAGE A3-specific ImmTAC. The in-vitro activity of IMCgp100 for redirected lysis (LDH release) was in the range of 10^{-10} M (low ng/ml), and for release of interferon-γ in the range of 10^{-11} to 10^{-12} M. In order to reach an EC_{90} for lysis, >150 MHC class I–gp100 peptide complexes were required per target cell.

Apart from HLA restriction and the notorious absence of animal models for non-clinical safety assessment, an obvious limitation of the ImmTAC format is that a particular HLA–peptide complex may be presented by cancer cells only at very low copy numbers. This situation could be aggravated if cancer cells become selected in late-stage disease for loss or reduced expression of MHC class I, β2 microglobulin, or a transporter associated with antigen loading onto MHC, or for an altered proteasome subunit composition that may no longer allow generation of a particular peptide antigen. Therefore, high-affinity binding by the soluble TCR in combination with high drug concentrations is a prerequisite for maximal occupation of target complexes on cancer cells and ensuing lysis by polyclonal T cells. The engagement by ImmTACs of pre-existing polyclonal effector memory T cells by CD3 binding will avoid certain escape mechanisms intercepting with the differentiation of specific T-cell clones. However, escape mechanisms abrogating presentation of peptide antigens by tumor cells are still expected to have a negative impact on the efficacy of this bispecific antibody format.

BISPECIFIC T CELL–ENGAGING ANTIBODIES AND THERAPEUTIC VACCINES: A COMPARISON

The generation of tumor-specific cytotoxic T-cell clones by therapeutic vaccination is a lengthy multi-step process with many stages for possible interference by tumor cells and normal immune regulatory mechanisms. Vaccination can be facilitated by co-administration of APC-boosting adjuvants such as granulocyte-macrophage colony stimulating factor or toll-like receptor agonists, inflammatory cytokines such as IL-2 or interferon-α, or by antibodies blocking the T-cell inhibitory receptor cytotoxic T lymphocyte-associated antigen 4. Proper timely combination of vaccination with diverse chemotherapies and targeted therapies may further improve generation and subsequent performance of specific T-cell clones. Synergistic effects of conventional therapies may arise from the depletion of regulatory T cells, reduction of tumor load, alterations of the tumor microenvironment, and/or improvement of tumor vasculature and penetration by T cells. Although objective responses have been observed in many trials involving cancer vaccines, a majority of patients typically did not experience a lasting clinical benefit. While there definitely is clinical proof-of-concept that vaccines can induce generation of cytotoxic T-cell clones and can cause objective tumor responses, low response rates and short response durations remain an issue. This limited efficacy could be due to the great variety of possible immune escape mechanisms, which are likely to be selected during disease progression and may continuously increase in terms of frequency, diversity, and multiplexity.

T cell–engaging bispecific antibodies are distinct from therapeutic vaccination approaches which produce tumor-specific regular T-cell responses in a number of fundamental properties, which can potentially improve response rates and duration. Bispecific antibodies can mount a polyclonal T-cell response by engagement of pre-existing effector T cells. Obviously, this allows an instantaneous onset of activity with no need for T-cell co-stimulatory stimuli or lengthy T-cell differentiation. Kinetic studies in cell culture experiments with BiTE antibodies have shown that unstimulated polyclonal CD8[+] T cells from peripheral blood have a lag phase of 4–8 h hours before onset of redirect lysis, whereas CD4[+] T cells have a lag phase of up to 20 h[3]. The time lag seems to be required for increasing the levels of granzymes and perforin in resting CD8[+] and CD4[+] T cells as are needed for lysis. In contrast, a pre-activated T-cell line could immediately start redirected lysis upon BiTE addition (30). The lysis reaction induced by a forced interaction with bispecific antibodies appears to be indistinguishable from the process induced when a specific T cell recognizes its matching MHC class I–peptide complex on a target cell. In both cases, a cytolytic synapse is formed, followed by discharge of cytotoxic granules and the action of perforin and granzymes (31,33). It appears that with the exception of naïve T cells, all T-cell subtypes expressing CD3, perforin and granzymes can be engaged by bispecific antibodies, including central memory and γ/δ T cells (36). Whether regulatory T cells (CD4[+], CD25[high], FoxP3[+]) expressing lytic proteins can also be redirected for cancer cell lysis is currently under investigation.

T cells engaged by bispecific antibodies may not be susceptible to frequently encountered immune escape mechanisms. Studies with BiTE antibodies have shown that K562 cells, which are devoid of MHC class I molecules, are lysed by redirected human T cells (31), and so are human target-expressing hamster cells, which do not express human cross-reactive MHC or co-stimulatory molecules (34). Hence, immune escape mechanisms tampering with peptide antigen presentation by tumor cells will not be able to impact T cell–engaging bispecific antibody-binding to surface antigens. Moreover, once a bispecific antibody has induced a cytolytic synapse between a cancer and a cytotoxic T cell, very little may be able to mechanistically halt the ensuing killing reaction. Of note, all escape mechanisms potentially intercepting with this last step of cytotoxic T-cell action must likewise interfere with T-cell immunity in general, including vaccination. The high response rates observed for catumaxomab in ascites of late-stage cancer patients, and of blinatumomab in ALL and NHL patients may indicate that the mode of T cell–engaging antibody action finds little resistance in patients. In a phase II ALL study with blinatumomab, four relapses among 20 evaluable patients were observed, which could be explained in each case. In two patients, ALL cells repopulated the bone marrow from brain and testes, two immunoprivileged sites; and in two patients pre-existing CD19-negative clones grew out after complete elimination of CD19-expressing ALL cells (41).

Two potential issues of T cell–engaging bispecific antibodies need further discussion. One is the consequence of an overt polyclonal T-cell activation, which may not be an issue for vaccination approaches. The other is escape and selection of target-negative clones, which is an issue for any kind of T-cell therapy. The severe consequences of polyclonal T-cell activation are evident from the side effects of anti-CD3 murine IgG2a mAb OKT-3 (46), humanized anti-CD28 agonistic IgG4 mAb TGN1412 (47), and bacterial super antigens (48). By all three agents, a large proportion of peripheral T cells in humans can be instantaneously activated followed by inflammatory cytokines released at high levels, which can result in a toxic shock syndrome with its complex clinical manifestations. T cell–engaging antibodies for cancer therapy therefore need safe guards. In the case of BiTE antibodies, it has been shown that T cells are only activated by BiTE antibodies when target cells are present but not when BiTE antibodies are binding to isolated T cells (32). This suggests that monovalent binding by certain antibodies to CD3 is insufficient for triggering the TCR, but requires some form of cross-linkage. In the case of a strictly target cell-dependent T-cell activation, the number of target cells will determine the extent of T-cell activation and hence the intensity of adverse events.

T cell–engaging antibodies containing an Fcγ domain will not allow control of T-cell activation by target cells. This is because normal cells expressing Fcγ receptors are ubiquitous and, with bound bispecific antibody, will provide a cross-linking matrix for T cells also in the absence of target cells. A low systemic tolerability is therefore expected for this class of antibodies and has indeed been observed in clinic testing (16).

T cells have the intrinsic property of adapting to an initial stimulation. This will result in only a transient release of cytokines. Levels return to baseline within hours or days despite continued stimulation, or will be much reduced upon repeated stimulation. For instance, while

T cells will no longer respond with cytokine release to continued stimulation by BiTE antibody muS110, they proceed with redirected lysis, and do not become anergic (49). Therefore, attention has to be given in the clinical routine to attenuation of a "first dose effect". This may be achieved by anti-inflammatory co-medication and/or regimens using a low entry dose (50). It is currently not clear to what extent an initial cytokine release by T cell–engaging antibodies can even be beneficial for clinical efficacy. It is likely that initially released pro-inflammatory cytokines and chemokines, can, e.g., improve cytotoxic T-cell performance, attract and activate other immune cells, and enforce lymphocyte adherence, transmigration, and infiltration into target tumor tissue.

Escape of target-negative tumor cells under treatment can be a limitation for any T-cell therapy. In the case of T cell–engaging antibodies binding to surface target antigens of cancer cells, these must be carefully selected to be of some biological significance. Most desirable in this respect are targets to which cancer cells are addicted. Frequently, expression of such targets on tumor tissue has a negative prognostic potential for patients' survival. Target-negative tumor cells left after therapy may have a more benign phenotype, which can translate into prolonged survival. Ideally, targets should also be expressed on tumor-initiating or cancer stem cells as has been shown for the bispecific antibody target EpCAM (51).

It is evident that any kind of target for cytotoxic T cell needs to be highly restricted in its surface expression to target cells, and should be largely absent from or inaccessible on normal cells. This is because T cells will indiscriminately eliminate any dividing or non-dividing cell expressing a critical copy number of the target antigen, be it a MHC class I/peptide complex or surface antigen for bispecific antibodies. As a soluble, pharmacological agent, it should however be feasible to adjust bispecific antibody concentrations in patients such that T cells can discriminate between different target expression levels, which can inform their decision to kill, or not to kill. Such a pharmacological adjustment does not seem possible for specific natural T-cell clones, nor for genetically engineered T cells expressing extra TCRs or TCR/antibody fusion proteins. This may be the reason why in several clinical trials treatment of cancer patients with genetically modified T cells caused severe damage of normal tissues and even fatalities (52).

OUTLOOK

T cell–engaging antibodies are a rapidly evolving area of passive immunotherapy showing increasingly promising results in clinical trials. Key challenges for this therapeutic principle are the management of side effects from initial polyclonal T-cell activation, working out dosing regimens for optimal and sustained T-cell activation, and identifying the right target antigens for treating a large variety of malignant diseases. What needs to be further explored is the possibility that T cell–engaging antibodies themselves work as vaccines eliciting specific T-cell immunity. Unless acute treatment with bispecific antibodies is sufficient to ablate all cancer cells in a patient, an ensuing vaccination effect could be a means to improve response rates and especially prolong response duration.

REFERENCES

1. Renner C, Jung W, Sahin U, et al. Cure of xenografted human tumors by bispecific monoclonal antibodies and human T cells. Science 1994; 264: 833–5.
2. Altenschmidt U, Klundt E, Groner B. Adoptive transfer of in-vitro-targeted, activated lymphocytes results in total tumor regression. J Immunol 1997; 159: 5509–15.
3. Brischwein K, Schlereth B, Guller B, et al. MT110: a novel bispecific single-chain antibody construct with high efficacy in eradicating solid tumors. Mol Immunol 2006; 43: 1129–43.
4. Carpenito C, Milone MC, Hassan R, et al. Control of large, established tumor xenografts with genetically engineered human T cells containing CD28 and CD137 domains. Proc Natl Acad Sci USA 2009; 106: 3360–5.
5. Weber J. Ipilimumab: controversies in its development, utility and autoimmune adverse events. Cancer Immunol Immunother 2009; 58: 823–30.

6. Zhang L, Conejo-Garcia JR, Katsaros D, et al. Intratumoral T cells, recurrence, and survival in epithelial ovarian cancer. N Engl J Med 2003; 348: 203–13.

7. Pagès F, Berger A, Camus M, et al. Effector memory T cells, early metastasis, and survival in colorectal cancer. N Engl J Med 2005; 353: 2654–66.

8. Wahlin BE, Sander B, Christensson B, et al. CD8+ T-cell content in diagnostic lymph nodes measured by flow cytometry is a predictor of survival in follicular lymphoma. Clin Cancer Res 2007; 13: 388–97.

9. Rabinovich GA, Gabrilovich D, Sotomayor EM. Immunosuppressive strategies that are mediated by tumor cells. Annu Rev Immunol 2007; 25: 267–96.

10. Staerz UD, Kanagawa O, Bevan MJ. Hybrid antibodies can target sites for attack by T cells. Nature 1985; 314: 628–31.

11. Müller D, Kontermann R. Recombinant bispecific antibodies for cellular cancer therapy. Curr Opin Mol Ther 2007; 9: 319–26.

12. Seimetz D, Lindhofer H, Bokemeyer C. Development and approval of the trifunctional antibody catumaxomab (anti-EpCAM x anti-CD3) as a targeted cancer immunotherapy. Cancer Treat Rev 2010; 36: 458–67.

13. Ruf P, Kluge M, Jäger M, et al. Pharmacokinetics, immunogenicity and bioactivity of the therapeutic antibody catumaxomab intraperitoneally administered to cancer patients. Br J Pharmacol 2010; 69: 617–25.

14. Lindhofer H, Mocikat R, Steipe B, et al. Preferential species-restricted heavy/light hcain pairing in rat/mouse quadromas. Implications for a single-step purification of bispecific antibodies. J Immunol 1995; 155: 219–25.

15. Hirschhaeuser F, Walenta A, Mueller-Klieser W. Efficacy of catumaxomab in tumor spheroid killing is mediated by its trifunctional mode of action. Cancer Immunol Immunother 2010; 59: 1675–84.

16. Sebastian M, Passlick B, Friccius-Quecke H, et al. Treatment of non-small cell lung cancer patients with the trifunctional monoclonal antibody catumaxomab (anti-EpCAMxanti-CD3): a phase 1 study. Cancer Immunol Immunother 2007; 56: 1637–44.

17. Fiedler WM, Ritter B, Seggewiss R, et al. Phase I safety and pharmacology study of the EpCAM/CD3-bispecific BiTE antibody MT110 in patients with metastatic colorectal, gastric, or lung cancer. J Clin Oncol 2010; 28: 15s, abstract no 2573.

18. Kiewe P, Hasmüller S, Klahert S, et al. Phase I trial of the trifunctional anti-HER-2 x anti-CD3 antibody ertumaxomab in metastatic breast cancer. Clin Cancer Res 2008; 12: 3085–91.

19. Buhmann R, Simoes B, Stanglmaier M, et al. Immunotherapy of recurrent B-cell malignancies after allo-SCT with Bi20 (FBTA05), a trifunctional anti-CD3xanti-CD20 antibody with donor lymphocyte infusion. Bone Marrow Transplant 2009; 48: 383–97.

20. Ströhlein MA, Siegel R, Jäger M, et al. Induction of anti-tumor immunity by trifunctional antibodies in patients with peritoneal carcinomatosis. J Exp Clin Cancer Res 2009; 14: 18.

21. Llewelyn M, Cohen J. Superantigens: microbial agents that corrupt immunity. Lancet Infect Dis 2002; 2: 156–62.

22. Robinson MK, Alpaugh RK, Borghaei H. Naptumomab estafenatox: a new immunoconjugate. Expert Opin Biol Ther 2010; 10: 273–9.

23. Forsberg, G, Ohlsson L, Brodin T, et al. Therapy of human non-small-cell lung carcinoma using antibody targeting of a modified superantigen. Br J Cancer 2001; 85: 129–36.

24. Cheng JD, Babb JS, Langer C, et al. Individualized patient dosing in phase I clinical trials: the role of escalation with overdose control in PNU-214936. J Clin Oncol 2004; 22: 602–9.

25. Borghaei H, Alpaugh K, Hedlund G, et al. Phase I dose escalation, pharmacokinetic and pharmacodynamic study of naptumomab estafenatox alone in patients with advanced cancer and with docetaxel in patients with advanced non-small-cell lung cancer. J Clin Oncol 2009; 27: 4116–23.

26. Shaw DM, Connolly NB, Patel PM, et al. A phase II study of a 5T4 oncofetal antigen tumour-targeted superantigen (ABR-214936) therapy in patients with advanced renal cell carcinoma. Br J Cancer 2007; 96: 567–74.

27. Forsberg G, Skartved NJ, Wallen-Ohman M, et al. Naptumomab estafenatox, an engineered antibody-superantigen fusion protein with low toxicity and reduced antigenicity. J Immunother 2010; 33: 492–9.

28. Baeuerle PA, Reinhardt C. Bispecific T cell engaging antibodies for cancer therapy. Cancer Res 2009; 69: 4941–4.

29. Baeuerle PA, Kufer P, Bargou R. BiTE: Teaching antibodies to engage T cells. Curr Opin Mol Ther 2009; 11: 22–30.

30. Hoffmann P, Hofmeister R, Brischwein K, et al. Serial killing of tumor cells by cytotoxic T cells redirected with a CD19-/CD3-bispecific single-chain antibody construct. Int J Cancer 2005; 115: 98–104.

31. Offner S, Hofmeister R, Romaniuk A, et al. Induction of regular cytolytic T cell synapses by bispecific single-chain antibody constructs on MHC class I-negative tumor cells. Mol Immunol 2006; 43: 763–71.

32. Brischwein K, Parr L, Pflanz S, et al. Strictly target cell-dependent activation of T cells by bispecific single-chain antibody constructs of the BiTE class. J Immunother 2007; 30: 798–807.

33. Haas C, Krinner E, Brischwein K, et al. Mode of cytotoxic action of T cell-engaging BiTE antibody MT110. Immunobiology 2009; 214: 441–53.

34. Lutterbuese R, Raum T, Kischel R, et al. T cell-engaging BiTE antibodies specific for EGFR potently eliminate KRAS- and BRAF-mutated colorectal cancer cells. Proc Natl Acad Sci USA 2010; 107: 12605–10.

35. Lutterbuese R, Raum T, Kischel R, et al. Potent control of tumor growth by CEA/CD3-bispecific single-chain antibody constructs that are not competitively inhibited by soluble CEA. J Immunother 2009; 32: 341–52.

36. Kischel R, Hausmann S, Klinger M, et al. Effector memory T cells make a major contribution to redirected lysis by T cell-engaging BiTE antibody MT110. 100th Meeting of the American Association for Cancer Research, 2009;abstract#3252.

37. Brandl C, Haas C, d'Argouges S, et al. The effect of dexamethasone on polyclonal T cell activation and redirected target cell lysis as induced by a CD19/CD3-bispecific single-chain antibody construct. Cancer Immunol Immunother 2007; 56: 1551–63.

38. Purbhoo MA, Irvine DJ, Huppa JB, et al. T cell killing does not require the formation of a stable mature immunological synapse. Nat Immunol 2004; 5: 524–30.

39. Bargou R, Leo E, Zugmaier G, et al. Tumor regression in cancer patients by very low doses of a T cell-engaging antibody. Science 2008; 321: 974–7.

40. Viardot A, Goebeler M, Scheele J, et al. Treatment of patients with NHL with CD19/CD3 bispecific antibody blinatumomab (MT103): Double-step dose increase to continuous infusion of 60 µg/m²/day is tolerable and highly effective. Annual Meeting of the American Society fo Hematology (ASH) 2010;abstract#2880.

41. Bargou R, Zugmaier G, Goekbuget N, et al. Prolonged leukemia free survival following blinatumomab (anti-CD19 BiTE) treatment of patients with minimal residual disease (MRD) of B precursor ALL: updated results of a phase II study. Annual Meeting of the European Hematology Association, Barcelona, 2010;abstract#598.

42. Handgretinger R, Zugmaier G, Henze G, et al. Complete remission after blinatumomab-induced donor T-cell activation in three pediatric patients with post-transplant relapsed acute lymphoblastic leukemia. Leukemia 2010. [Epub ahead of print].

43. Lum LG, Sen M. Activated T-cell and bispecific antibody immunotherapy for high-risk breast cancer. Bench to bedside. Acta Hematol 2010; 105: 130–6.

44. Grabert RC, Cousens LP, Smith JA, et al. Human T cells armed with Her2/neu bispecific antibodies divide, are cytotoxic, and secrete cytokines with repeated stimulation. Clin Cancer Res 2006; 12: 569–76.

45. Liddy N, Molloy PE, Bennett AD, et al. Production of a soluble disulfide-linked TCR in the cytoplasm of Escherichia coli trxB got mutants. Mol Biotechnol 2010; 45: 140–9.

46. [Available from: http://www.drugs.com/sfx/orthoclone-okt3-side-effects.html].

47. Suntharalingam G, Perry MR, Ward S, et al. Cytokine storm in a phase 1 trial of the anti-CD28 monoclonal antibody TGN1412. N Engl J Med 2006; 355: 1018–28.

48. Blackman MA, Woodland DL. In vivo effects of superantigens. Life Sci 1995; 57: 1717–35.

49. Amann M, D'Argouges S, Lorenczewski G, et al. Antitumor activity of an EpCAM/CD3-bispecific BiTE antibody during long-term treatment of mice in the absence of T-cell anergy and sustained cytokine release. J Immunother 2009; 32: 452–64.

50. Amann M, Friedrich M, Lutterbuese P, et al. Cancer Immunol Immunother 2009; 58: 95–109.

51. Munz M, Baeuerle PA, Gires O. The emerging role of EpCAM in cancer and stem cell signaling. Cancer Res 2009; 69: 5627–9.

52. Baeuerle PA, Itin C. Clinical experience with gene therapy and bispecific antibodies for T cell-based therapy of cancer. Curr Pharm Biotechnol 2011; in press.

19 | Antibodies to peptide–HLA complexes have potential application for cancer diagnosis and therapy

Jon A. Weidanz and William H. Hildebrand

EXISTING IMMUNE INTERVENTIONS FOR CANCER

A majority of cancer patients are still treated by non-specific, higher morbidity options (e.g., chemotherapeutic compounds and radiation) or adjuvant therapies; however, targeted therapies provide the clearest path for successful treatment and disease-free progression. Because of their high affinity and extraordinary specificity, immune interventions provide highly targeted anti-tumor effects when directed against target antigens that are exclusively or preferentially expressed in tumors. A powerful class of targeted therapeutics such as monoclonal antibodies (mAbs) can be directed against targets of diverse chemical composition. Therapeutic mAbs exert anti-tumor effects by killing cancer cells or preventing their proliferation. For example, upon binding their respective antigens on the surface of cancer cells, rituximab (anti-CD20) and cetuximab (anti-epidermal growth factor receptor) directly kill cancer cells by activating complement-dependent cytotoxicity (CDC) and antibody-dependent cellular cytotoxicity (ADCC) (1). Rituximab has also been shown to induce apoptosis of cancer cells (2). Trastuzumab (anti-HER2/neu) and bevacizumab (anti-vascular endothelial growth factor) prevent tumor cell proliferation by binding to and inhibiting cell surface receptors that provide signals for tumor cell survival (3,4). Therapeutic mAbs have shown great promise in treating cancers, but most of the cancer patients do not qualify for these treatments due to insufficient biomarker expression (e.g., trastuzumab) or inconclusive data on clinical efficacy (e.g., bevacizumab). In addition, because mAbs can only access antigens on the cell surface, only a handful of validated tumor-specific proteins are suitable targets for therapeutic mAbs. The identification of tumor-specific target antigens is therefore one of the greatest obstacles to the development of new therapeutic mAbs.

While current therapeutic mAbs target cell surface proteins, T cell–based strategies have attempted to target antigens of intracellular origin through the human leukocyte antigen (HLA) system. The HLA system processes proteins from every cellular compartment and presents samples of those proteins on the cell surface as peptides within the context of an HLA class I molecule. HLA class I complexes are constitutively expressed by all nucleated cells, and thus the HLA system marks the surface of every cell in the body with a snapshot of the inner workings of the cell. Disease states such as viral infection or cancer alter the peptide repertoire presented by the HLA system. Specific recognition of disease-associated peptide–HLA class I complexes by the T-cell receptor of effector T cells initiates a series of events that kills the diseased cell, raising the possibility that cancer cells could be eliminated by therapies that invoke an anti-tumor T-cell response.

Indeed, in April 2010, the Food and Drug Administration approved the first therapeutic cancer vaccine, for the treatment of prostate cancer (5). Sipuleucel-T elicits a T-cell response against prostate cancer by immunizing a patient's own antigen-presenting cells against prostatic acid phosphatase, a specific biomarker present in most prostate cancers. Additional therapeutic cancer vaccines are under development, with 10 protocols currently in phase III clinical trials in the United States. In addition, several groups have shown that human melanoma cells express tumor-specific peptide–HLA class I complexes (6–8), suggesting that T-cell-based therapies could be effective for the treatment of other cancers as well. For example, several groups have demonstrated objective cancer regression after antigen-specific T cells were expanded ex vivo and adoptively transferred to melanoma patients (9–11). As it is difficult to identify tumor-specific T cells in cancer patients, a growing trend in experimental and translational immunology has been to generate genetically engineered T cells for transfer into cancer patients. The potential benefit of this approach was demonstrated in a report published by Morgan et al., which described the objective regression of metastatic melanoma lesions in two patients who received genetically engineered T cells (12). Although these limited early successes provide proof of concept for immunotherapies targeting tumor-specific peptide–HLA class I complexes, considerable obstacles must be overcome before T-cell-based therapies can be broadly applied in the clinical setting. For example, limitations associated with the identification of target-specific T-cell receptors (TCR), the transfer of TCR genes into T cells, and the expansion of genetically altered T cells have hindered the technical feasibility of this prospective therapeutic strategy. Furthermore, the tumor environment often lacks the signals necessary for a successful T-cell response (13,14), regulatory mechanisms that prevent reactions against "self" epitopes could impede immune reactions against cancer cells (15,16), and a widespread systemic immune suppression often occurs in late-stage cancer (17,18). Thus, although immune interventions are a promising source of highly targeted cancer treatments, the broad clinical application of mAbs and T-cell-eliciting therapies requires continued effort.

T-CELL RECEPTOR MIMICS: A THREE-PRONGED APPROACH TO IMMUNOTHERAPY

Since only a minor fraction of the proteome is expressed on the cell surface, where antigens are accessible to mAbs, a key obstacle in the development of mAb therapies has been the scarcity of accessible, validated tumor-specific markers. In contrast, by targeting peptide–HLA complexes, T-cell-eliciting therapies have access to targets derived from the entire proteome (19–21). Expanding the pool of potential targets for mAbs to include peptide–HLA complexes would increase the probability of identifying tumor-specific antigens, and we and others have shown that peptide–HLA complexes are suitable targets for mAbs (22–27). This novel approach to immunotherapy exploits the unsurpassed diversity and specificity of antibody-based therapies and harnesses the targeting power of disease-specific peptide–HLA complexes.

The feasibility of this approach has been enhanced by recent advances in the identification of tumor-specific peptide–HLA complexes and in the efficient generation of antibodies to these complexes. Several groups, including our own, have developed antibodies against specific peptide–HLA complexes (22–27). A variety of methods, including bacteriophage display, have been used to generate these antibodies (26,28,29). Our technique uses immunization with synthetic peptide–HLA complexes followed by high-throughput screening to create and identify hybridomas that secrete antibodies, which we call TCR mimics (TCRms) (30,31). Like the TCRs of cytotoxic lymphocytes (CTLs), our TCRms show fine binding specificity for peptide–HLA complexes, and unlike TCRs, our TCRms display a high binding affinity for the cognate peptide–HLA complex. Moreover, while it was previously a challenge to generate sufficient quantities of mAbs for the clinic, recently developed systems for streamlined production and purification now provide TCRm mAbs in ample quantities for research, diagnosis, and treatment.

TCRms offer a three-pronged approach for advancing the development and application of immunotherapy. First, anti-peptide–HLA complex mAbs could be used to directly validate epitope expression in fresh tissue. In recent years, we and others have used anti-peptide–HLA mAbs for direct detection and visualization of specific peptide–HLA class I complexes on the surface of cells (22,23). Second, anti-peptide–HLA mAbs might improve cancer detection and diagnosis. Our data show a significant correlation between specific peptide–HLA expression and tumor staging. For example, tumor-specific peptide–HLA biomarkers were found uniquely expressed on invasive breast carcinoma cells, but not on ductal carcinoma cells in situ, indicating a potential new cancer detection application (Hawkins et al., manuscript submitted). Third, early testing has shown that anti-peptide–HLA mAbs can exert profound effects on tumor growth, raising the possibility that TCRms could markedly expand the repertoire of therapeutic mAbs for cancer treatment (32).

EPITOPE DISCOVERY

A critical barrier to further progress in the treatment of cancer is the paucity of biomarkers for targeted therapies. Therefore, epitope discovery is key to the development of TCRms and other immunological treatment options. Several indirect and direct strategies have been successfully used to discover new peptide–HLA class I complexes. Indirect epitope discovery analyzes peptides from tumor-associated antigens and prioritizes those that show a high-binding affinity for HLA class I molecules, either with predictive computer algorithms or through experimental binding assays. Indirect strategies are limited by the inability to predict both the host proteins from which HLA will sample peptides and the particular peptides that will be presented. The peptides presented by HLA are difficult to predict because many intracellular variables converge to influence the formation of peptides presented by HLA class I molecules, and these variables are modified during tumorigenesis. In addition, numerous studies of cancer immunology show that levels of gene expression do not correspond to HLA peptide presentation (22,33); thus, one must directly characterize HLA peptide cargo in order to identify ligands that distinguish diseased cells.

For direct epitope discovery, HLA molecules are isolated from the surface of tumor cells, and the peptides eluted from the HLA molecules are identified by mass spectrometric analysis. Several factors make direct epitope discovery challenging. First, each individual cell presents a staggering diversity of peptide–HLA class I molecules. Most cells express six different HLA class I molecules (2 HLA-A, 2 HLA-B, and 2 HLA-C), with approximately 50,000 copies of each class I molecule on the cell surface. The 50,000 copies of each class I molecule present approximately 5000 different peptides. Second, the isolation of any single type of class I molecule, and the isolation and handling of the hydrophobic class I peptide cargo are technically challenging. Finally, available cell lines may not express the desired class I molecule. These factors make it difficult to obtain a protein in sufficient quantity and purity for mass spectrometric analysis.

We have developed a robust system that overcomes the difficulties associated with traditional approaches to direct epitope discovery. By transfecting cells with an expression construct encoding a secreted HLA class I molecule (sHLA), we are able to generate HLA molecules that are loaded with peptide just as endogenous HLA molecules, and are then secreted into the media. The cell's own class I molecules remain on the cell surface, and only the transfected sHLA is harvested. In addition, the cell does not have to be detergent-lysed to obtain class I sHLA. Therefore, the sHLA-transfected cell becomes a continuous producer of the desired class I molecule, and purification is more straightforward. This method yields 10-fold more peptide–HLA complexes than traditional membrane purification methods, a quantity and purity sufficient for mass spectrometric analysis (34).

Figure 19.1 illustrates our strategy for identifying peptide epitopes. Peptides are eluted from the purified peptide–sHLA complexes, and the complexity of the peptide pool is reduced by using reverse phase high pressure liquid chromatography to fractionate the peptides. The peptide fractions are then mapped by mass spectrometry. The maps of tumorigenic and non-tumorigenic cell lines are compared to identify peaks that are unique to cancer cells, and ions unique to cancer cells are sequenced. The computed sequence is confirmed by comparing the MS–MS fragmentation spectrum of the eluted peptide with that of a synthetic peptide of the computed sequence. A competitive binding assay is used to further confirm that the identified peptide binds specifically to the HLA class I molecule.

Most studies to date have been performed on the HLA-A*0201 (HLA-A2) isoform, because the HLA-A2 allele is the most common of the class I molecules (expressed by about 50% of individuals in the U.S. population). This process has been utilized to demonstrate that multiple host protein–derived peptides are uniquely presented by class I HLA molecules during viral infection and by cancerous cells. These host-derived epitopes were not predicted by indirect methods, underscoring the value of direct epitope discovery. Using overlapping immunologic, biochemical, and molecular methods, we have since validated these host-derived epitopes as uniquely presented by the class I HLA of infected or tumorigenic cell lines. Finally, because epitope discovery relies on cultured cells, we use TCRm to validate epitopes in primary tissues.

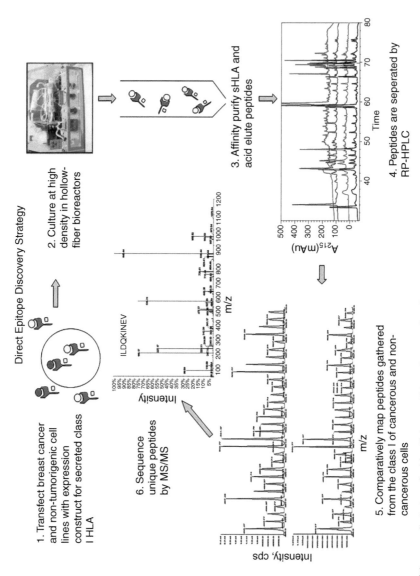

Figure 19.1 View of the overall strategy for identifying peptide epitopes uniquely presented by the HLA A*0201 of breast cancer cells. *Source:* Courtesy of American Chemical Society. From Ref: 34.

EPITOPE VALIDATION BY TCRMS

While mass spectrometry is a powerful tool for epitope discovery, it does not provide information on the immunologic potential of epitopes. We developed TCRm mAbs as a robust and efficient tool for characterizing immune epitopes. This approach was first developed using HIV-infected cells as a model. Using the epitope discovery method described above, we identified a peptide derived from eukaryotic initiation factor 4 gamma (eIF4G) that is presented approximately three folds more abundantly by the HLA-A2 class I of HIV-infected cells than by non-infected cells. We generated 4F7, a TCRm that recognizes the $eIF4G_{720-728}$–HLA complex, to directly characterize the timing, tissue specificity, and comparative level of peptide presentation (23).

Competitive tetramer binding assays confirmed that 4F7 specifically recognized the $eIF4G_{720-728}$–HLA-A2 complex. Since it had previously been reported that eIF4G is overexpressed in malignant cells, we stained a normal human mammary epithelial cell line and a human breast carcinoma cell line (MDA-MB-231) with 4F7. As would be expected based on previous reports, 4F7 stained the carcinoma cell line but not the normal cell line, indicating that cancer cells present the $eIF4G_{720-728}$ peptide in the context of HLA-A2. Next, we used 4F7 to characterize the expression of the $eIF4G_{720-728}$–HLA-A2 complex on HIV-infected (p24+) and mock-infected cells. Flow cytometry showed strong staining of HLA-A2$^+$ HIV-infected cells, weak staining of HLA-A2$^+$ mock-infected or influenza-infected cells, and no staining of HLA-A2$^-$ cells. These results validated the $eIF4G_{720-728}$–HLA-A2 complex as a marker for HIV-infected cells and further confirmed that 4F7 specifically recognizes the $eIF4G_{720-728}$ peptide in the context of the HLA-A2 class I molecule. Finally, we used 4F7 to study the kinetics of $eIF4G_{720-728}$ presentation by primary CD4$^+$ T cells. Within three days post infection, HIV-infected cells showed a two-fold increase in $eIF4G_{720-728}$ presentation compared with mock-infected cells. By the seventh day post infection, infected cells showed four-fold greater $eIF4G_{720-728}$ presentation compared to mock-infected cells. These data indicate that the combination of immunoproteomics and TCRm technology enables the direct identification of new peptide–HLA class I complexes and the validation and characterization of targets that discriminate diseased cells.

While it is well accepted that disease states alter the proteome of the affected cell, it has been difficult to directly study the specificity and timing of changes in HLA peptide presentation following viral infection and malignant transformation. We believe that our approach to epitope discovery and validation provides a valuable new method for the analysis of peptide–HLA complexes on normal, infected, and malignant cells. Unlike other methods for epitope analysis, such as CTL-based approaches, TCRms offer the ability to directly examine and quantify changes in specific peptide–HLA complexes. In addition, TCRms can be used to study peptide–HLA complexes that are present on normal cells, which would not be detectable by CTL-based approaches. TCRms thus offer exciting capabilities for the validation and characterization of novel peptide–HLA class I complexes that are relevant for infections and cancer.

DIAGNOSTIC POTENTIAL OF TCRMS

Because TCRms can recognize tumor-specific peptide–HLA class I complexes with high specificity and affinity, they are ideal candidates for use in cancer diagnostics. Using the epitope discovery method described above, we found that the $YLL_{128-136}$ peptide derived from the p68 RNA helicase protein and the MIF_{19-27} peptide derived from the macrophage migration inhibitory factor protein are presented by the HLA-A2 class I molecule on tumorigenic breast cancer cell lines.

We developed two TCRm, RL6A and RL21A, which specifically recognize the $YLL_{128-136}$–HLA-A2 complex and the MIF_{19-27}–HLA-A2 complex, respectively. For these complexes to serve as diagnostic or therapeutic targets, they must distinguish cancerous cells from benign tissues. Therefore, RL6A and RL21A were used to directly determine the levels of the $YLL_{128-136}$–HLA-A2 complex and MIF_{19-27}–HLA-A2 complex in various primary tissues. Both peptide–HLA-A2 complexes were detected on breast cancer cell lines using our epitope discovery strategy, and immunohistochemical staining of primary tumors confirmed that both complexes were present on neoplastic cells and tumor-associated stroma in breast cancer tissue, but were either absent or expressed at minimally detectable levels on normal adjacent tissue. RL6A staining of various normal, primary tissues indicated that expression of the $YLL_{128-136}$–HLA-A2 epitope was not exclusive to breast tumor cells, but was markedly increased in tumor cells (35). Therefore, by comparing suspected malignancies with normal tissue, RL6A staining of biopsied tissues could provide valuable information regarding malignant cell transformation. Moreover, the YLL peptide has been independently isolated from transformed B cells (36), and our data show strong RL6A staining of neoplastic cells and tumor-associated stroma from metastatic ovarian tissue. These observations suggest that expression of the $YLL_{128-136}$–HLA-A2 target may be broadly upregulated by cancer cells of different histological origins, independently of tumor stage. Future studies will therefore test the possibility that the $YLL_{128-136}$–HLA-A2 complex could serve as a diagnostic indicator for a wide variety of malignant conditions.

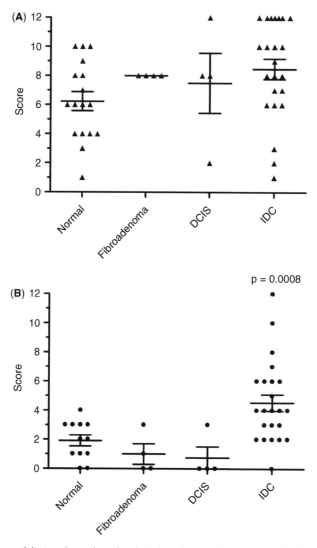

Figure 19.2 RL21A reactivity to primary invasive ductal carcinoma. Cryopreserved, HLA-A*02+ invasive ductal carcinoma (IDC), ductal carcinoma in situ (DCIS), benign fibroadenoma, and matched normal adjacent tissues were stained for (**A**) all HLA-A2 complexes using the BB7.2 antibody and (**B**) the specific HLA-A2/MIF$_{19-27}$ complex using RL21A. (*Continued*)

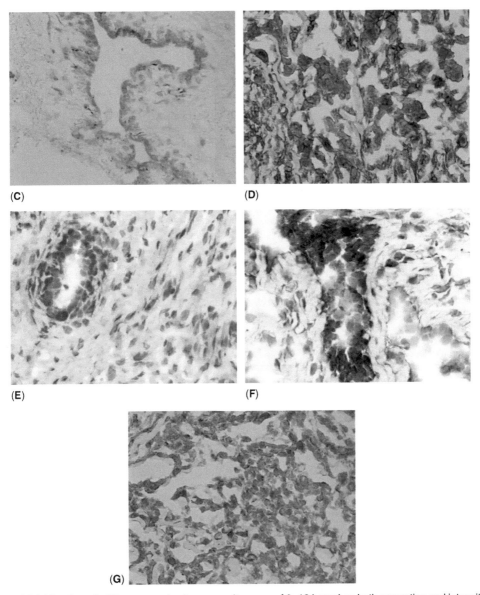

Figure 19.2 (*Continued*)   Tissues received a composite score of 0–12 based on both proportion and intensity of staining. Representative staining of (**C**) normal adjacent tissue and (**D**) IDC tissue by RL21A are shown, with a higher magnified inset. Expression of the MIF1a intact protein is shown using an antigen-specific mAb in panel (**F**) and corresponding control antibody in panel (**E**). Specificity of RL21A staining was confirmed by competition with tetrameric HLA-A2–peptide complexes. Tissue staining was abrogated in the presence of HLA-A2 tetramer containing the MIF_{19-27} peptide (**G**), but not HLA-A2 tetramer containing irrelevant peptides (not shown).

Unlike the $YLL_{128-136}$–HLA-A2 complex, expression of the MIF_{19-27}–HLA-A2 complex is uniquely tumor-specific. Immunohistochemical staining of primary tumors showed that RL21A did not stain fibroadenoma or ductal carcinoma in situ (DCIS), two non-invasive conditions. In contrast, in invasive ductal carcinoma (IDC) tissues, both the tumor tissue and tumor-associated stroma showed strong RL21A staining, while normal adjacent tissues were not stained by RL21A (Fig. 19.2; Table 19.1). Because the MIF protein is expressed by multiple cell

Table 19.1 Key Properties of RL21A TCRm. To assess staining, a total score of 0–12+ based on a target expression score (0–2+=positive staining in ~25% of cells per view field; 3–4+= ~50% of cells; 5–6+=>75% of cells) is added to an intensity score [scale of 0–6+, determined by staining intensity and copy number quantification using the QuantiBRITE™ (BD Biosciences, Franklin Lakes, NJ) bead system]

Property	RL21A result
Isotype	IgG2a (murine)
Protein target	Macrophage migration inhibitory factor 1-alpha
HLA-A*2-Peptide target	FLSELTQQL
Affinity (K_D)	24 nM
In vivo therapeutic efficacy	MDA-MB-231
	BT-20/A2
Secondary effector mechanisms (ADCC/CDC)	MDA-MB-231
	MCF-7
In vitro induction of apoptosis	Annexin V
	Caspase 3
	Poly ADP ribose polymerase
	Jun N-terminal kinase (JNK) phosphorylation
Staining Invasive Grade Breast Tumor Tissue	
All tumor tissue (n=30)	Average 5+ using a 12+ system
Low HER2 tissues: Hercept test score (n=15)	1.5+ using a 12+ system
Staining Normal Human Tissues	
Male donor (20 tissues)	No staining
	(0.0+ on a 12+ system)
Female donor (20 tissues)	(0.0+ on a 12+ system)

types, it is possible that the MIF$_{19-27}$–HLA-A2 complex could be present on a variety of cell types in healthy individuals. However, RL21A showed little to no staining of normal tissues from healthy HLA-A2+ donors, including 18 total white blood cell samples and a panel of 20 cryopreserved tissues each from a male and a female donor (Table 19.1). Therefore, RL21A distinguishes invasive ductal carcinoma from normal and diseased non-invasive breast tissues and from other normal tissues.

To further assess the diagnostic potential of the MIF$_{19-27}$–HLA-A2 complex, the prevalence of RL21A staining was assessed in 30 invasive breast tumors from different donors. We found widespread expression of the MIF$_{19-27}$ –HLA-A2 complex in invasive human breast tumors. Regardless of Her2 status, the average score for RL21A staining of invasive tissues was 4- to 5-fold higher ($P=0.033$) than the score for adjacent normal tissues (Table 19.1). More recently RL21A was shown to stain metastatic ovarian tumors but not normal ovarian tissue, indicating that expression of the MIF$_{19-27}$–HLA-A2 complex is not restricted to cancers of the breast. These findings suggest that our technology can discover prevalently expressed peptide–HLA class I complexes and that TCRms made to these targets might have broad applications for detecting and diagnosing multiple histologically distinct cancers.

The ability to distinguish invasive breast cancer suggests that the MIF$_{19-27}$–HLA-A2 complex could provide an alternative to the three most relevant prognostic and treatment-guiding markers for breast cancer: estrogen receptor (ER), progesterone receptor (PR), and epidermal growth factor receptor (HER-2). Although MIF$_{19-27}$–HLA-A2 has not been directly compared to other breast cancer markers, the MIF$_{19-27}$–HLA-A2 complex showed a degree of overexpression in invasive tissues comparable to HER-2 (~30%). Furthermore, while ER, PR, and HER-2 are often observed in ductal carcinoma in situ, RL21A did not stain this non-invasive tissue type, indicating that RL21A could offer a powerful marker for invasive phenotypes. Future studies will elucidate the full diagnostic value of the MIF$_{19-27}$–HLA-A2 complex.

THERAPEUTIC PROMISE OF TCRMS

In addition to their value for epitope validation and as potential diagnostic tools, TCRms could provide a new class of therapeutics for the treatment of cancer. Breast cancer biomarkers such as HER-2 provide a highly successful precedent for the dual use of peptide–HLA complexes as both prognostic markers and therapeutic targets. Because of their versatility in targeting and their profound anti-tumor effects, TCRms could be used either as direct anti-tumor agents or as targeting agents to enhance the efficacy of other therapeutics.

Direct Anti-Tumor Effects

TCRms exhibit profound anti-tumor activity both in vitro and in vivo. For example, treatment with RL6A or RL21A (Table 19.1) dramatically reduced the tumor burden in two orthotopic breast cancer models (data not shown; Fig. 19.3). In nude mice implanted with the tumorigenic

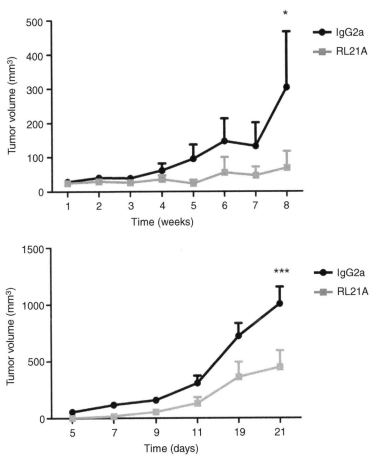

Figure 19.3 RL21A inhibits tumor growth in orthotopic murine models. (*Upper panel*): Athymic nude mice were implanted with MDA-MB-231 tumor cells in the right mammary fat pad in the presence of Matrigel (Sigma-Aldrich, St. Louis, MO). Once-weekly injections of 500 ug of RL6A (n = 10) or control mAb (n = 10) were initiated after tumor volumes exceeded 50 mm^3. Tumor sizes were measured twice weekly using calipers and tumor volumes determined using the standard formula: volume=Lx(b^2)/2 (L=longest diameter; b=shortest diameter, where the mean tumor diameter was measured in two dimensions). Data are plotted as mean tumor volume + SEM. (*Lower panel*): Once-weekly injections with 500 ug of RL6A (n = 10) or control mAb (n = 10) were initiated 48 hours after BT20/A2 tumor cell injection. Tumor sizes were measured twice weekly using calipers, and tumor volumes were determined as described above. *P<0.05; **P<0.001.

MDA-MB-231 cell line, RL6A reduced tumor growth (35), and RL21A treatment inhibited tumor growth by five folds (37). For an orthotopic model using the more aggressive BT-20-A2 cell line, RL21A inhibited tumor growth by more than two folds. Both of these cell lines are phenotypically triple negative (ER⁻, PR⁻, HER-2⁻), suggesting that RL6A and RL21A could be valuable therapeutic tools for breast cancer patients for whom there are currently no targeted therapies. The ability of TCRm treatment to produce significant reduction of tumors in vivo demonstrates that tumor-specific peptide–HLA complexes may offer a prolific source of new targets for successful immune therapies.

Our in vitro and in vivo studies indicate that TCRms directly activate caspases, apoptosis, and cell death by signaling through selective and direct binding to the peptide–HLA class I complex. Inflammatory infiltrate was not obvious in the tumors of xenograft models. Since natural killer cells, monocytes, and macrophages are essential for mAbs to kill tumor cells through ADCC, this suggests that TCRm-mediated killing is at least partly independent of ADCC. In addition, TCRms lacking the Fc fragments were capable of reducing tumor growth, although to a lesser degree than whole TCRms, indicating that TCRm-mediated killing of tumor cells is partially independent of ADCC and complement, but that ADCC and complement-dependent cytotoxicity may contribute to the effects of TCRms. Our in vitro studies indicate that activation of the caspase-dependent intrinsic pathway, disruption of mitochondrial membrane integrity, and Jun N-terminal kinase signaling contribute to TCRm-induced tumor cell apoptosis. The ability of the TCRm to kill tumor cells independently of immune effector cells could provide a significant advantage over the majority of currently approved therapeutic mAbs.

Many current mAb therapies require a functional immune system for tumor cell killing, which is less than ideal for patients who are immunocompromised or in the common scenario, where the tumor is protected from complement-dependent cytotoxicity by high expression of complement regulatory proteins. Like trastuzumab and bevacizumab, TCRms appear to lead to tumor cell apoptosis directly through induction of pro-apoptotic signaling. However, unlike trastuzumab, which shows reduced efficacy when the density of target epitopes on the cell surface is low, TCRms show high efficacy in killing tumor cells despite the relatively low density of target peptide–HLA complexes on the cell surface. This represents an additional advantage of the TCRms, since the expression of tumor-specific proteins is often low. TCRms thus present a promising direction in the development of immune-based cancer therapeutics.

Targeted Drug Delivery

The side effects of non-specific cancer treatments can be minimized by delivering the treatment directly to the tumor. We have found that TCRms coupled directly to poly(lactide-co-glycolide) (PLGA) nanoparticles (<100 nm) containing paxclitaxel can specifically target and poison tumor cells. Furthermore, since differentiated, non-malignant cells produce distinct patterns of peptide–HLA complexes, TCRms directed against cell-type specific peptide–HLA complexes could be used to target specific cell types. For example, highly specific TCRms could potentially be used to deliver drugs to the vascular bed of a specific organ. Indeed, TCRms have been used to target non-malignant cells, and our recent results provide proof of concept for the use of TCRms for brain-specific targeting and overcoming the blood-brain barrier.

The RL6A TCRm recognizes the $YLL_{128-136}$–HLA-A2 complex expressed in brain endothelial cells. The $YLL_{128-136}$ peptide is derived from the p68 RNA helicase protein, which has been shown to have high mRNA expression levels in rat brain microvessels. As an initial model for the blood brain barrier, we used hCMEC–D3 cells, an HLA-A2⁺ cell line derived from human brain endothelium. Flow cytometry analysis showed that hCMEC–D3 cells express the YLL–HLA-A2 complex, and that expression is increased by pretreatment with interferon-γ. Confocal microscopy experiments using both fixed and live cells showed that RL6A bound to the surface of hCMEC–D3 cells and was internalized into vesicles marked by the early endosome marker EEA1. Consistent with these data, primary human brain endothelial cells also bound and internalized the RL6A TCRm, as observed by flow cytometry and microscopy (38).

These results highlight the broad potential of TCRms like RL6A for potential diagnostic or therapeutic applications. It has previously been proposed that the blood-brain barrier could be circumvented by taking advantage of physiological transport mechanisms mediated by endothelial receptor proteins. Although numerous preclinical studies support the promise of this approach, the receptors targeted to date have not been specific to the blood–brain barrier. We predict that specific vascular endothelial cells are marked by unique peptide–HLA complexes, and that the generation of TCRm specific for these markers will allow targeting to select organ vascular beds for diagnostic and therapeutic agents. The internalization of RL6A by brain endothelial cells thus establishes proof of concept, presenting the exciting possibility that TCRms made to peptide–HLA complexes specific to brain endothelium could be used to target diagnostic agents or therapeutics to the blood–brain barrier and brain. Furthermore, the observation that inflammation, proliferation, and other physiological changes influence peptide–HLA expression patterns raises the possibility that tumor neovasculature can be differentiated from normal, resting endothelium. The benefits of targeting tumor vasculature using bevacizumab or other small molecule drugs to block angiogenesis have already been demonstrated in preclinical and clinical settings. Targeting specific peptide–HLA complexes expressed on tumor vascular tissue with TCRms or TCRm-drug conjugates could provide novel strategies for inhibiting angiogenesis. TCRms therefore offer the potential for highly specific targeting of diagnostic and therapeutic agents to the blood–brain barrier, tumor vasculature, and other organ vascular beds.

SUMMARY

Recent developments in soluble HLA production and the generation of TCRms represent significant advances in epitope discovery and validation, and present the potential for powerful new clinical tools. Traditional methods for direct epitope discovery were limited by technical challenges in the purification and identification of peptide–HLA complexes. Using sHLA, we have developed an efficient and reliable method for the discovery of new peptide–HLA complexes that can serve as a novel class of targets for cancer diagnosis and treatment. TCRms can be used to validate these targets, and in the clinical setting, TCRms have the potential to improve cancer diagnosis, directly kill tumor cells, and provide targeted delivery of existing cancer therapies.

Therapeutic mAbs are well-established in clinical practice and have provided a significant advantage over non-specific cancer therapies. However, many patients are not candidates for mAb treatment, and the development of new therapeutic mAbs has been hindered by the paucity of suitable targets. We have shown that peptide–HLA complexes provide a rich source of potential tumor-specific targets, which can be validated with TCRms. Because of their high specificity, TCRms are strong candidates for the diagnosis and targeted treatment of cancer. We have shown that TCRms can distinguish invasive breast tumors from noninvasive and normal breast tissues and from normal tissues. Furthermore, as a new class of mAbs, TCRms exert direct anti-tumor effects, and thus avoid the challenges associated with T-cell-eliciting therapies. TCRms showed a strong anti-tumor activity in orthotopic models of breast cancer, even in the absence of an intact immune response or high target density. Finally, TCRms can be used to target nonmalignant cells, such as tumor neovasculature, and endocytosis of the TCRm–HLA complex by brain endothelium suggests that TCRms could be used to deliver drugs to the blood–brain barrier. In summary, the integration of HLA proteomics and TCRm technology presents the opportunity for a powerful, streamlined approach to cancer therapy.

REFERENCES

1. Nishida M, Usuda S, Okabe M, et al. Characterization of novel murine anti-CD20 monoclonal antibodies and their comparison to 2B8 and c2B8 (rituximab). Int J Oncol 2007; 31: 29–40.
2. Vega MI, Huerta-Yepez S, Martinez-Paniagua M, et al. Rituximab-mediated cell signaling and chemo/immuno-sensitization of drug-resistant B-NHL is independent of its Fc functions. Clin Cancer Res 2009; 15: 6582–94.

3. Lin MZ, Teitell MA, Schiller GJ. The evolution of antibodies into versatile tumor-targeting agents. Clin Cancer Res 2005; 11: 129–38.
4. Dean-Colomb W, Esteva FJ. Her2-positive breast cancer: herceptin and beyond. Eur J Cancer 2008; 44: 2806–12.
5. Carballido E, Fishman M. Sipuleucel-T: prototype for development of anti-tumor vaccines. Curr Oncol Rep 2011. [Epub ahead of print].
6. Celis E, Fikes J, Wentworth P, et al. Identification of potential CTL epitopes of tumor-associated antigen MAGE-1 for five common HLA-A alleles. Mol Immunol 1994; 31: 1423–30.
7. Wolfel T, Hauer M, Klehmann E, et al. Analysis of antigens recognized on human melanoma cells by A2-restricted cytolytic T lymphocytes (CTL). Int J Cancer 1993; 55: 237–44.
8. Kawakami Y, Eliyahu S, Sakaguchi K, et al. Identification of the immunodominant peptides of the MART-1 human melanoma antigen recognized by the majority of HLA-A2-restricted tumor infiltrating lymphocytes. J Exp Med 1994; 180: 347–52.
9. Dudley ME, Wunderlich JR, Yang JC, et al. A phase I study of nonmyeloablative chemotherapy and adoptive transfer of autologous tumor antigen-specific T lymphocytes in patients with metastatic melanoma. J Immunother 2002; 25: 243–51.
10. Rosenberg SA, Dudley ME. Cancer regression in patients with metastatic melanoma after the transfer of autologous antitumor lymphocytes. Proc Natl Acad Sci USA 2004; 101 (Suppl 2): 14639–45.
11. Hughes MS, Yu YY, Dudley ME, et al. Transfer of a TCR gene derived from a patient with a marked antitumor response conveys highly active T-cell effector functions. Hum Gene Ther 2005; 16: 457–72.
12. Morgan RA, Dudley ME, Wunderlich JR, et al. Cancer regression in patients after transfer of genetically engineered lymphocytes. Science 2006; 314: 126–9.
13. Bunt SK, Sinha P, Clements VK, et al. Inflammation induces myeloid-derived suppressor cells that facilitate tumor progression. J Immunol 2006; 176: 284–90.
14. Leen AM, Rooney CM, Foster AE. Improving T cell therapy for cancer. Annu Rev Immunol 2007; 25: 243–65.
15. Powell DJ Jr, de Vries CR, Allen T, et al. Inability to mediate prolonged reduction of regulatory T Cells after transfer of autologous CD25-depleted PBMC and interleukin-2 after lymphodepleting chemotherapy. J Immunother 2007; 30: 438–47.
16. Du C, Wang Y. The immunoregulatory mechanisms of carcinoma for its survival and development. J Exp Clin Cancer Res 2011; 30: 12.
17. Gruber IV, El Yousfi S, Durr-Storzer S, et al. Down-regulation of CD28, TCR-zeta (zeta) and upregulation of FAS in peripheral cytotoxic T-cells of primary breast cancer patients. Anticancer Res 2008; 28: 779–84.
18. Gustafson MP, Lin Y, New KC, et al. Systemic immune suppression in glioblastoma: the interplay between CD14+HLA-DRlo/neg monocytes, tumor factors, and dexamethasone. Neuro Oncol 2010; 12: 631–44.
19. Hayashi E, Matsuzaki Y, Hasegawa G, et al. Identification of a novel cancer-testis antigen CRT2 frequently expressed in various cancers using representational differential analysis. Clin Cancer Res 2007; 13: 6267–74.
20. Xing Q, Pang XW, Peng JR, et al. Identification of new cytotoxic T-lymphocyte epitopes from cancer testis antigen HCA587. Biochem Biophys Res Commun 2008; 372: 331–5.
21. Kessler JH, Melief CJ. Identification of T-cell epitopes for cancer immunotherapy. Leukemia 2007; 21: 1859–74.
22. Weidanz JA, Nguyen T, Woodburn T, et al. Levels of specific peptide-HLA class I complex predicts tumor cell susceptibility to CTL killing. J Immunol 2006; 177: 5088–97.
23. Weidanz JA, Piazza P, Hickman-Miller H, et al. Development and implementation of a direct detection, quantitation and validation system for class I MHC self-peptide epitopes. J Immunol Methods 2007; 318: 47–58.
24. Cohen CJ, Hoffmann N, Farago M, et al. Direct detection and quantitation of a distinct T-cell epitope derived from tumor-specific epithelial cell-associated mucin using human recombinant antibodies endowed with the antigen-specific, major histocompatibility complex-restricted specificity of T cells. Cancer Res 2002; 62: 5835–44.
25. Denkberg G, Cohen CJ, Lev A, et al. Direct visualization of distinct T cell epitopes derived from a melanoma tumor-associated antigen by using human recombinant antibodies with MHC-restricted T cell receptor-like specificity. Proc Natl Acad Sci USA 2002; 99: 9421–6.
26. Andersen PS, Stryhn A, Hansen BE, et al. A recombinant antibody with the antigen-specific, major histocompatibility complex-restricted specificity of T cells. Proc Natl Acad Sci USA 1996; 93: 1820–4.

27. Porgador A, Yewdell JW, Deng Y, et al. Localization, quantitation, and in situ detection of specific peptide-MHC class I complexes using a monoclonal antibody. Immunity 1997; 6: 715–26.

28. Chames P, Hufton SE, Coulie PG, et al. Direct selection of a human antibody fragment directed against the tumor T-cell epitope HLA-A1-MAGE-A1 from a nonimmunized phage-Fab library. Proc Natl Acad Sci USA 2000; 97: 7969–74.

29. Lev A, Denkberg G, Cohen CJ, et al. Isolation and characterization of human recombinant antibodies endowed with the antigen-specific, major histocompatibility complex-restricted specificity of T cells directed toward the widely expressed tumor T-cell epitopes of the telomerase catalytic subunit. Cancer Res 2002; 62: 3184–94.

30. Neethling FA, Ramakrishna V, Keler T, et al. Assessing vaccine potency using TCRmimic antibodies Vaccine 2008; 26: 3092–102.

31. Wittman VP, Woodburn D, Nguyen T, et al. Antibody targeting to a class I MHC-peptide epitope promotes tumor cell death. J Immunol 2006; 177: 4187–95.

32. Verma B, Jain R, Caseltine S, et al. TCR mimic monoclonal antibodies induce apoptosis of tumor cells via immune effector-independent mechanisms. J Immunol 2011; 186: 3265–76.

33. Michaeli Y, Denkberg G, Sinik K, et al. Expression hierarchy of T cell epitopes from melanoma differentiation antigens: unexpected high level presentation of tyrosinase-HLA-A2 Complexes revealed by peptide-specific, MHC-restricted, TCR-like antibodies. J Immunol 2009; 182: 6328–41.

34. Hawkins OE, Vangundy RS, Eckerd AM, et al. Identification of breast cancer peptide epitopes presented by HLA-A*0201. J Proteome Res 2008; 7: 1445–57.

35. Verma B, Hawkins OE, Nethling FA, et al. Direct discovery and validation of a peptide/MHC epitope expressed in primary human breast cancer cells using a TCRm monoclonal antibody with profound antitumor properties. Cancer Immunol Immunother 2010; 59: 563–73.

36. Hunt DF, Henderson RA, Shabanowitz J, et al. Characterization of peptides bound to the class I MHC molecule HLA-A2.1 by mass spectrometry. Science 1992; 255: 1261–3.

37. Hawkins O, Verma B, Lightfoot S, et al. An HLA-presented fragment of macrophage migration inhibitory factor is a therapeutic target for invasive breast cancer. J Immunol 2011; 186: 6607–16.

38. Bhattacharya R, Xu Y, Rahman MA, et al. A novel vascular targeting strategy for brain-derived endothelial cells using a TCR mimic antibody. J Cell Physiol 2010; 225: 664–72.

Index

T - #1081 - 101024 - C296 - 254/175/14 - PB - 9781138112605 - Gloss Lamination